PASS THE SITUATIONAL JUDGEMENT TEST

This book is dedicated to our families, without whose support and patience we would not have been able to write it.

Content Strategist: Pauline Graham
Content Development Specialist: Helen Leng
Project Manager: Srividhya Vidhyashankar
Designer: Christian Bilbow

PASS THE SITUATIONAL JUDGEMENT TEST

A Guide for Medical Students

Cameron B Green BSc(Hons), MBBS
Academic Foundation Year 2 Doctor,
North Central Thames Foundation School,
London, UK

Aaron Braddy BSc(Hons), MBBS
Honorary Clinical Teacher,
University of Sheffield Medical School;
Academic Foundation Year 2 Doctor,
South Yorkshire Foundation School,
Sheffield, UK

Edited by

Professor C Michael Roberts MBChB, MA(MedEd), MD, FRCP, ILTHE, FAcadMEd
Professor of Medical Education for Clinical Practice, Barts and The London
School of Medicine and Dentistry, Queen Mary University of London;
Programme Director, AHSN Programme Director for Education and
Capability UCL Partners; Consultant Respiratory Physician, Whipps Cross
University Hospital, Barts Health NHS Trust, London, UK

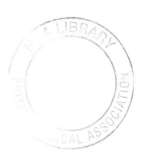

ELSEVIER

Edinburgh   London   New York   Oxford   Philadelphia   St Louis   Sydney   Toronto 2016

ELSEVIER

ISBN   9780702067006

British Library Cataloguing in Publication Data
A catalogue record for this book is available from the British Library

Library of Congress Cataloging in Publication Data
A catalog record for this book is available from the Library of Congress

Last digit is the print number: 9 8 7 6 5 4 3 2 1

Contents

Foreword

The Situational Judgement Test (SJT) was first introduced as part of the selection process for the UK Medical Foundation Programme in 2013. It carries equal weighting with the Educational Performance Measure (EPM) and when combined these provide each applicant with an opportunity to score up to 100 points, which constitutes the overall application score. These points will be used to rank you against each and every other candidate who applies in the same year and may determine your entire medical and possibly your personal future!

For each applicant it is really important to understand that the overall application score will carry with it three critical outcomes. Firstly, for those candidates who score below an agreed level, their performance will be deemed unacceptably poor and will disqualify them from achieving any foundation post in that application round. You do not want to be one of those people. Secondly, for the vast majority who exceed that minimum score, you are now in competition with each and every other candidate to gain entry to your foundation school of choice. A single point can make all the difference between getting your first choice … and another school. For many candidates at this stage their goal is achieved and they see no further, but do not forget there is a key allocation yet to be completed and that is for the specific rotations within your allocated school. Most foundation schools will use the overall application score to allocate preferences for your choice of post, so this remains a final but vital reason for you to achieve the maximum score possible.

Statistics being what they are, approximately half the readers of this book will find themselves in the lower half of the academic rankings within their undergraduate medical school and so at a relative disadvantage in the application process when compared with the 50% in the higher deciles. This is not, however, a disaster because you still have this opportunity to take your future into your own hands at this late stage by outperforming others in the SJT. Don't forget that 50% of the marks are still there to be won! For those in the higher academic deciles, do not feel smug yet. Each year I find myself counselling high achievers who fail to get their first preferences at foundation school because they have simply bombed the SJT, to their total amazement. No matter who you are, your performance in the SJT will have a major impact on your future life, determining in which part of the country you will work and which medical specialties you will experience. The place you work may in turn determine where you spend the rest of your life, and who with. It's high stakes!

So, if you are one of the people who likes to trust to luck, or to fate, then read no further, close the book, turn on the TV or go out for the night. I wish you happiness in your future

FY1 post … wherever that may be! For those who feel that they can influence their own futures and wish to do so, read on.

This book will provide you with a structured and organised approach to your preparation for the assessment and an invaluable framework that will anchor your responses on the day to the competences every successful FY1 doctor needs.

Professor C Michael Roberts

Preface

We wrote this book with one simple aim: to provide medical students with a one-stop guide to succeeding in the Situational Judgement Test. Some of you will have been at medical school for as little as three years (direct dental entrants) or as long as nine years (integrated PhD entrants) and yet half of the score currently allocating your Foundation Programme training post will be based on your performance in a single test lasting just 2 hours and 20 minutes. This book will give you all the relevant preparatory information and guidance, along with practice questions interspersed with our own personal tips and advice, to allow you to achieve your best score.

William Osler (1849–1919, physician) famously quoted 'The best preparation for tomorrow is to do today's work superbly well'. Do not allow yourself to be fooled into thinking this is a test that cannot be prepared for. Although not requiring you to recall the aetiology of diseases, or their management plans, the SJT is no different to any other exam sat at medical school. We have structured this book on the concepts and 'rules' we devised in preparation for our own SJT in December 2013. We both scored in the top 5% of candidates in the 2013–14 academic year, and wholeheartedly attribute this success to this preparatory material. Although we hope you appreciate we cannot guarantee you a similar score, we are confident that by using this book as an aid you will feel as well prepared as we did for your SJT.

We have included guidance set out by the GMC in easy-to-digest segments. Read them and become familiar (if you are not already) with what is expected of you as a doctor. Our 'top tips' chapter is aimed at giving you 'rules' to work to when you are unsure. Of course there will always be situations where you cannot apply every rule, but by having a structure in your mind you will (hopefully) make the correct decision when the options seem all too vague. And finally: practise, practise, practise. This book includes 250 practice questions divided into the five core domains of the SJT. You will find helpful cues throughout the questions to remind you of salient GMC guidance or some of our top tips to assist you. Each question is accompanied by a full and thorough explanation as to the justification behind each answer, as well as the scoring matrix so that you can easily calculate what you will have scored for each question.

We wish you the very best of luck in both the SJT and your final exams!

See you on the wards soon.

Cameron and Aaron

List of abbreviations

A&E	accident and emergency	FFP	fresh frozen plasma
AAU	adult assessment unit/acute assessment unit	FP	Foundation Programme
		FY1	foundation year 1
ACS	acute coronary syndrome	GI	gastrointestinal
ADL	activities of daily living	GMC	General Medical Council
ALS	advanced life support	GP	general practitioner
APTT	activated partial thromboplastin time	HDU	high-dependency unit
		IBS	irritable bowel syndrome
ARCP	annual review of clinical progression	ISFP	Improving Selection to the Foundation Programme
BiPAP	bilevel positive airway pressure	ITU	intensive therapy unit
BMA	British Medical Association	IV	intravenous
BNF	*British National Formulary*	IVDU	intravenous drug user
BNP	brain natriuretic peptide	MAU	medical assessment unit
CCU	coronary/critical care unit	MCA	Mental Capacity Act
CDU	clinical decision unit	MDT	multidisciplinary team
CMT	core medical training	MHA	Mental Health Act
CPAP	continuous positive airway pressure	MMC	Modernising Medical Careers
CPR	cardiopulmonary resuscitation	MRCP	Member of the Royal College of Physicians
CT	computed tomography		
CTPA	computed tomography pulmonary angiogram	MRCS	Member of the Royal College of Surgeons
CXR	chest x-ray	MRI	magnetic resonance imaging
DNACPR	do not attempt CPR	NBM	nil by mouth
DNAR	do not attempt resuscitation	NHS	National Health Service
DOB	date of birth	NOAC	new oral anticoagulants
DSU	day surgery unit	NOK	next of kin
DVLA	Driver and Vehicle Licensing Agency	OGD	oesophagogastroduodenoscopy
		OT	occupational therapist/therapy
DVT	deep vein thrombosis	PALS	patient advice and liaison service
ECG	electrocardiogram	PCR	polymerase chain reaction
EEG	electroencephalogram	PEG	percutaneous endoscopic gastrostomy
EPM	Educational Performance Measure		
ERCP	endoscopic retrograde cholangiopancreatography	PPI	proton-pump inhibitor
		PT	physical therapist/therapy
EUA	examination under anaesthesia	QIP	quality improvement project

SAU	surgical admission unit
SBAR	situation, background, assessment, recommendation
SHO	senior house officer
SJT	Situational Judgement Test
SLE	supervised learning event
TB	tuberculosis
UKFPO	United Kingdom Foundation Programme Office
UTI	urinary tract infection

1. Introduction

The UK Foundation Programme (FP) is a 2-year vocational training programme that bridges the gap between medical school and specialist training, administered by the UK Foundation Programme Office (UKFPO; website: http://www.foundationprogramme.nhs.uk/pages/home). Its main aim is to provide newly qualified doctors with a safe, supportive and well-supervised educational environment to allow them to embellish upon what they learned as an undergraduate, as well as developing and enhancing their clinical and communication skills at the same time as exploring a range of career options.

The FP itself was initially proposed in 2002 by the Chief Medical Officer, Sir Liam Donaldson, in his document *Unfinished Business*. His recommendations were introduced as part of the Modernising Medical Careers (MMC) training programme in 2005.

From 2006, newly qualified doctors were allocated to the FP through a nationalised application system with applicants being awarded scores based on academic quartile rank (40%) and answers to open-ended 'white-space' questions (60%). However, this system was critically reviewed by the Department of Health in the document *A High Quality Workforce: NHS Next Stage Review*. It was deemed that this system had issues regarding its reliability, validity, comparability, longevity, the risk of plagiarism and the amount of National Health Service (NHS) consultant time required to mark the questions.

The Improving Selection to the Foundation Programme (ISFP) project was established in 2009 to design the best method of selecting applicants to the FP. Part of the group's remit in establishing a new method of selection was to undertake a detailed analysis of the clinical and administrative duties performed by foundation year 1 (FY1) doctors. From this analysis were derived the characteristics and attributes required to be a good FY1 doctor; this in turn was to form the basis of examinable content of the new selection process. This analysis was conducted using a detailed review of General Medical Council (GMC) clinical practice guidelines combined with the pre-existing FP content triangulated with interviews of current trainees (Patterson et al, 2010).

The characteristics and attributes discerned in the ISFP report could be broadly defined by nine themes:

1. **Commitment to professionalism** – e.g. honesty, confidentiality, challenging unacceptable behaviour, awareness of own potential misconduct, managing risk, awareness of equality and diversity, managing own professional development
2. **Coping with pressure** – e.g. dealing with pressure, developing resilience and adaptability, managing uncertainty, staying calm in confrontation, developing coping strategies to deal with heavy demands, clear judgement under pressure, showing initiative, offering assistance in an emergency
3. **Effective communication** – e.g. communicating clearly, sensitively and effectively with patients, developing and maintaining effective professional relationships, acting as an effective interface between other clinical teams / specialties, developing active listening, ability to handle difficult patient interactions
4. **Learning and professional development** – e.g. managing self-directed learning, responding constructively to appraisal, teaching peers and students, contributing to the appraisal of colleagues, developing confidence and competence, developing professional attitudes
5. **Organisation and planning** – e.g. demonstrating good time management, prioritising clinical need appropriately, maintaining accurate record keeping, developing a well-organised and resourceful approach to completing tasks
6. **Patient focus** – e.g. taking responsibility for patient care, recognising patients' knowledge, showing respect to all patients, working in partnership with patients
7. **Problem solving and decision making** – e.g. developing clinical judgement and reasoning, task prioritisation, information assimilation
8. **Self-awareness and insight** – e.g. recognising personal and professional limitations, demonstrating willingness to ask for help, developing an intellectual curiosity, learning from own experiences
9. **Working effectively as part of a team** – e.g. respecting colleagues and recognising the important role they play in the multidisciplinary team (MDT), developing effective leadership, adapting to different levels of support.

Situational Judgement Tests (SJTs) have been around for some 140 years and are widely used in the business sector for the selection of employees from large pools of candidates. Research has demonstrated that SJTs are generally well accepted by applicants, who see them as relevant to the job for which they are applying (Lievens & Sackett, 2007; Weekley & Ployhart, 2005). This acceptability by candidates is reinforced by an acknowledgement of fairness as the test is standardised; in the main, all candidates answer the same questions at the same time and the exams themselves are marked in the same way. Finally research has reinforced the validity of the SJT demonstrating that candidates who score highly are likely to be good FY1 doctors, with the test having better predictive value than other potential assessments such as structured interviews (McDaniel et al, 2001).

The SJT, in a similar way to the UK Clinical Aptitude Test that the vast majority of doctors took pre medical school, is designed to sift and rank a large volume of candidates (in 2014, 7974 applications were made for the Foundation Programme) for entry not in this case to undergraduate but to postgraduate training schools. It is used in conjunction with the Educational Performance Measure (EPM) to assist with foundation programme allocations through three mechanisms. The first mechanism is initial entry to any FP training post in the UK. Importantly, if a candidate scores very poorly they will be removed from the application process for that academic year. The second mechanism (and the one most candidates focus on) is allocation to a particular foundation school. Finally, the third mechanism, which is not universally applied, is allocating specific posts within a foundation school once a candidate has gained entry to that school.

The SJT was first introduced as part of the selection process for entry to UK foundation schools in 2013 following a pilot scheme involving 8000 final year students from 15 UK and 2 non-UK medical schools held between October 2010 and April 2011. The SJT uses hypothetical but realistic scenarios faced by FY1 doctors and requires candidates to make judgements about the potential responses posed; therefore the test assesses (a) a candidate's ability to choose the most effective behavioural response in a work-relevant scenario, rather than focusing on clinical knowledge or skills, and (b) the ability to recognise the most important concerns in any situation.

Following the ISFP job analysis, the nine 'attribute themes' were consolidated to five key domains, which form the basis for the Situational Judgement Test; they are:

- Commitment to professionalism
- Coping with pressure

3

- Effective communication
- Patient focus
- Working effectively as part of a team.

Questions for the SJT are developed through a cyclical process. Questions are designed initially in accordance with the FY1 job analysis and then scrutinised by a panel of experts. A scoring key is agreed and the questions piloted. These pilot questions are then included within the next SJT exam but are not counted in the candidates' final scores (in the exam you will sit there will be 10 questions in development – you will not be able to distinguish these questions from the actual questions; however, your score will be derived only from previously approved questions). The exam responses to the pilot questions are psychometrically analysed and quality assured, and if validated and found to be reliable are included in future tests as live questions.

The SJT is a written pencil and paper test that is marked electronically. It consists of 70 questions to be answered over 140 minutes, giving candidates on average 2 minutes to answer each question. The exam is comprised of two question styles: 'ranking questions', in which five responses are arranged in order from the most appropriate to the least, and 'multiple-choice questions', in which three appropriate responses are chosen from a selection of eight. The paper is weighted as two-thirds 'ranking questions' and one-third 'multiple-choice questions'. The justification for using two question styles is that different scenarios lend themselves to being tested in different ways; therefore a greater variety of responses can be elicited by the exam if more than one question style is used.

For the ranking questions, your responses are marked against a model answer as determined by an expert panel. Each individual response is worth a maximum of four points and a minimum of one point. This scoring is determined by how accurately each response is ranked in comparison with the model answer. For example, if you select option C as the most appropriate response, but the model answer has it placed as the second most appropriate response, you will score three points instead of four. If the model answer had placed option C as the third most appropriate answer you will have scored two points, and so on. Therefore, the closer your responses are to the model answer the greater your score will be. This is a fundamental difference, compared with traditional medical school questions, as credit is awarded for near misses. Furthermore, there is no negative scoring in the SJT.

Therefore you **should** attempt to answer **all** questions.

EXAMPLE 'RANKING STYLE' QUESTION

You are the FY1 on hepatobiliary surgery. Your registrar has invited you to assist with an ERCP (endoscopic retrograde cholangiopancreatography) tomorrow. You are keen to impress your new team and so you thank the registrar for this opportunity and agree to meet her in theatre tomorrow morning. The registrar explains that to learn the most from this procedure you should read up on how the ERCP is performed. The following morning you meet the registrar in theatre as agreed. During the time out, it becomes evident that the consent form that was signed in the pre-operative assessment has been mislaid. Your registrar asks you to quickly consent the patient as they have already been told the risks and it's merely a formality as they have previously consented.

Rank in order the following actions in response to this situation (1 = most appropriate; 5 = least appropriate):

A. Remind your registrar that FY1s are not allowed to consent and suggest that they consent the patient.

B. Agree to consent the patient, as it is only signing the form; the registrar has already explained the risks and benefits previously.

C. Explain to the registrar that you are unable to consent as an FY1 but you'd be keen to shadow the registrar to learn.

D. Agree to consent the patient if the registrar will be able to answer any questions the patient may have.

E. Tell the registrar that FY1s do not consent.

In this example question, the correct order of responses is C A E D B. You will answer each question on a grid similar to one below. The most appropriate response is marked in column 1, with each subsequent response continuing across the columns to the least appropriate response, which is marked in column 5.

	Most				Least
	1	2	3	4	5
A	=	■	=	=	=
B	=	=	=	=	■
C	■	=	=	=	=
D	=	=	=	■	=
E	=	=	■	=	=

Remember, for each 'ranking question' the maximum score is 20 and the minimum is 8. The SJT is not negatively scored and even if you rank the responses in the complete opposite order to the model answer you will still score 8 out of 20. Therefore attempt every question even if you are unsure.

The question will then be scored according to the following algorithm.

	Your rank choice				
Ideal order	1st	2nd	3rd	4th	5th
C	4	3	2	1	0
A	3	4	3	2	1
E	2	3	4	3	2
B	1	2	3	4	3
D	0	1	2	3	4

For the multiple-choice questions, again your answers are marked by comparing your response with the model answer determined by an expert panel. You have the potential to achieve a maximum of 12 points per question, with each of the three correct responses worth 4 points. However, an important difference with the multiple-choice questions is that the score for each response is **not** graded and there is **no** reward for near misses (i.e. you will either score 4 points for a correct response or 0 points for an incorrect response). Therefore, you can score a total of 0 points for a question if you select three incorrect responses. Furthermore, you must choose *only* three responses; choosing any more will mean you forfeit all the marks for that question.

EXAMPLE 'MULTIPLE-CHOICE STYLE' QUESTION

Q35. You are working on the adult assessment unit (AAU). You and your consultant see Mrs Bloomsbury. She is a 97-year-old lady who has been admitted because her son is worried that she has been experiencing visual hallucinations. Your consultant diagnoses Charles Bonnet syndrome and explains to Mrs Bloomsbury that treatment is not required and she can be discharged home. You complete the discharge summary and tell the nurse in charge that she can go. Later that day the ward occupational therapist (OT) James tells you that he doesn't think Mrs Bloomsbury can go home because she was very 'wobbly' on her feet. She seemed fine when you saw her earlier in the day.

Choose the most suitable **three** options from the following list:

A. Discuss James's concerns and ask whether Mrs Bloomsbury has any further need for therapy input.

B. Acknowledge James's concerns and ask the GP to monitor blood pressure.

C. Inform your consultant about James's concerns.

D. Ask the on-call senior house officer (SHO) to assess Mrs Bloomsbury.

E. Ask the staff nurse to assess Mrs Bloomsbury and to let you know if she has any concerns.

F. Acknowledge James's concerns but discharge Mrs Bloomsbury as your consultant has already made his decision.

G. Re-assess Mrs Bloomsbury.

H. Ask James to re-assess Mrs Bloomsbury later to see whether she is steadier.

In this example question, the correct response is A C G. You will answer each question on a grid similar to one below. Each correct response is selected as shown. There is no order or ranking of responses in the multiple-choice questions.

	A	B	C	D	E	F	G	H
Q35	▬	=	▬	=	=	=	▬	=
Q36	=	=	=	=	=	=	=	=
Q37	=	=	=	=	=	=	=	=

The question will then be scored according to the following point scheme:

A	B	C	D	E	F	G	H
4	0	4	0	0	0	4	0

The individual score for each question will then be combined to give you a total score, which is standardised against a national distribution curve resulting in a final SJT score of between 0 and 50. This is combined with your EPM score to give you an overall score for your Foundation Programme application.

KEY LEARNING POINTS

- Attempt every question.
- Maximum score in 'ranking' question is 20.
- Minimum score in 'ranking' question is 8.
- Maximum score in 'multiple-choice' question is 12.
- Minimum score in 'multiple-choice' question is 0.

2. Preparing for the SJT

Before committing yourself to day after day of mindless practice questions, and in order to succeed at the SJT, you will require a thorough understanding of the 'non-clinical' elements of healthcare provision in the UK. This is because, unlike many clinical questions asked in medical school examinations where there is a clearly correct answer, and only one correct answer, many of the possible responses in the SJT are 'the best possible answer' or 'the most appropriate response'. To understand why a response may be 'the best possible answer' as opposed to definitively correct, it is important to fully understand the context of medical practice within the UK – that is, its ethics, culture and legal basis including the differences between the Mental Capacity Act 2005 and the Mental Health Act 2007. This is outlined within key guidance from the General Medical Council (GMC) and essential information has been summarised below.

GOOD MEDICAL PRACTICE

Good Medical Practice (GMC, 2013a) provides an overview of the expected duties of a doctor registered with the GMC. It is important that you are familiar with these duties as they not only form the basis of the material assessed in the SJT, but also, more importantly, provide a framework for your behaviour as a doctor throughout your career. You are personally accountable for such behaviour and should therefore be prepared to justify any decision you take if it contradicts these guidelines. These duties are categorised into four sections: knowledge, skills and performance; safety and quality; communication, partnership and teamwork; and maintaining trust. The salient points from each section are summarised below.

1. KNOWLEDGE, SKILLS AND PERFORMANCE

This section focuses on your duty to maintain safe and current clinical practice. It states that you have a duty to act within your competency by maintaining your clinical knowledge, being aware of current guidelines and protocols (including legal aspects of healthcare) and participating in activities that maintain your training and competency. When providing care you should act, when possible, in accordance with best practice, and treat only patients with whom you are familiar and understand their full history. Importantly, you should not prescribe medications, even as a repeat prescription, unless you are familiar with that medication. Wherever possible, you should avoid providing care for somebody with whom you share a close relationship. You should also avoid treating yourself unless absolutely necessary. You must ensure that you have valid consent to carry out all examinations and investigations. Finally, you have a duty to record medical information accurately, clearly and, most importantly, legibly.

2. SAFETY AND QUALITY

This section focuses on your duty to promote patient safety (GMC, 2012) and quality care. As a doctor, you have a duty to improve patient care by participating in regular audits and quality improvement projects (QIPs). You must always act with the patient at the centre of your decision making and promote patient safety, including reporting incidents. You must create an environment whereby your colleagues feel comfortable raising their concerns about patient safety. You have a duty not to put your patients or colleagues at risk because of your own health. Finally, you have a duty to contribute to the safe transfer of patient care between providers by sharing relevant information, competently handing over between shifts and ensuring, to the best of your ability, the competence of the receiving healthcare providers.

3. COMMUNICATION, PARTNERSHIP AND TEAMWORK

This section focuses on your duty to communicate effectively, work in a team, and form and maintain partnerships with patients. The GMC states that you have a duty to communicate effectively with patients, relatives and colleagues. In order to do this, you must be able to speak fluent English. You must listen carefully and provide information that is requested from you. You have a duty to meet the patient's communication needs by use of interpreters or non-verbal communication tools. You must work well in a team and be respectful, non-discriminatory and willing to give advice when required. You must be willing to provide training to doctors and students, and assist when staff members are having difficulties with their performance or health.

4. MAINTAINING TRUST

This section focuses on your duty to form and maintain trust with your patients. You must maintain confidentiality at all times, even after a patient has died. You must be polite, respectful and honest with your patients at all time. You must not use your position of trust to form an emotional or sexual relationship with a patient or somebody they are close to. You must not express your personal beliefs to a patient if that is likely to impair their trust in you or the care that you may provide. You must act with integrity at all times, including if participating in disciplinary matters, or when dealing with finance.

As *Good Medical Practice* is only an overview, the following guidelines have also been summarised to provide more detailed information.

TOMORROW'S DOCTORS

This important document (GMC, 2009a) outlines both the intended outcomes for graduating UK medical students and the standards for undergraduate learning, teaching and assessment.

The overarching outcomes it states are within three domains:

1. The doctor as a scholar and a scientist
2. The doctor as a practitioner
3. The doctor as a professional.

1. THE DOCTOR AS A SCHOLAR AND A SCIENTIST

This domain describes the application of both biomedical and psychological knowledge to explain, investigate, manage and communicate the ill health of patients at both the individual and the societal level. It also explains the knowledge, skills and attitudes needed to conduct medical research.

2. THE DOCTOR AS A PRACTITIONER

This outcome describes the consultation skills required to communicate effectively with patients and other medical colleagues. It focuses on the deliberative processes required to formulate management plans acceptable both to you as the doctor and to the patient. It also covers your ability to manage acutely unwell patients, perform practical procedures and prescribe both effectively and economically.

3. THE DOCTOR AS A PROFESSIONAL

This outcome focuses on your awareness of your role as the doctor and the roles of other healthcare professionals. It describes how you should be an effective member of the wider multidisciplinary team, should reflect, learn from and teach others, protect patients and strive to improve patient care.

CONFIDENTIALITY

As a doctor, you have access to sensitive personal information about patients and you have a legal and ethical duty to keep this information confidential, unless it is in the patient's interest and the patient consents to the disclosure, or disclosure is required by law or is necessary in the public interest (GMC, 2009b).

Your duty of confidentiality relates to all information you hold about your patients, including demographic data, the dates and times of any appointments your patients may have made, and the fact that an individual may be under your care.

1. DISCLOSURE REQUIRED BY LAW

In some circumstances, you are obliged to disclose information to comply with a statutory requirement with or without a patient's consent (e.g. to notify certain communicable diseases). However, only relevant information should be disclosed and about that specific patient only (i.e. not about the patient's relatives). Additionally, personal information should not be disclosed to a third party (e.g. solicitor, police officer) without the patient's expressed consent unless it is required by law or can be justified in the public interest.

2. DISCLOSURE IN THE PUBLIC INTEREST

In some cases it is in the public interest to disclose information revealed during a consultation (e.g. involvement in a violent crime with injury to another). In these cases, consent for disclosure should still be sought but, even if not given or where consent cannot be given (e.g. a patient is unconscious or not contactable), then, if the benefits from disclosure outweigh the risks from doing so, it may be justified to disclose the information even without the patient's consent.

Such circumstances usually arise where there is a risk of death or serious harm to the patient or others. If possible, you should inform the patient of the disclosure before doing so. Examples of such a situation would include one in which disclosure of information may help in the prevention, detection or prosecution of a serious crime. A competent adult's wishes should generally be respected if they refuse to allow disclosure and no one else will suffer.

CONSENT

Good medical care is dependent on a strong patient–doctor relationship. This is founded on openness, trust and good communication between both parties. Doctors must listen to and act upon patients' views on their current and ongoing health and any decisions that are made regarding their care. Ultimately doctors must ensure patients are fully informed to enable them to make decisions about their care and must ultimately respect their decision (GMC, 2013a).

Informed consent is the process through which doctors obtain permission from a patient to perform an investigation or instigate management and it comprises four key factors:

- Competence
- Disclosure
- Voluntariness
- Consent (GMC, 2008).

Competence includes both that of the doctor to explain and perform the investigation or treatment and that of the patient to be able to make an informed decision about what is being proposed.

To obtain consent you need to be suitably trained to perform the procedure or have undergone training to consent for the procedure, have sufficient knowledge of what is being proposed so that you understand the risks and benefits (outcome of no action, side effects, complications and failure of intervention to achieve desired aim) and give this information in a balanced way to the patient so as to avoid bias.

A patient, in order to give informed consent, should be able to understand and retain this information, use or weigh up the information and communicate the information. This may be hampered by nervousness, pain, medication taken, terminology, information overload or lack of competence.

Disclosure of information needs to be adequate to engage patients in healthcare decisions. Patients need a thorough explanation with details of relevant risks, benefits and uncertainties. Do not withhold any information necessary for making decisions, but establish what information a patient wishes to be privy to and tailor this to their needs, wishes, priorities, level of knowledge and understanding about their condition. You should provide patients with resources and opportunities to enable them to gather further information. You should answer questions as fully as possible and escalate unanswerable questions to a senior colleague.

Voluntariness means that the patient's decision must be free from coercion and doctors should be diligent in assessing whether this is present (it can come from family, friends, employers, clinical staff, etc.).

Consent can be presumed, implied, verbal or written (GMC, 2008). Presumed consent is not actively sought; it relates to a procedure that can occur without consent explicitly being given. Presumed consent is withdrawn when a patient (or their legally appointed representative) actively declares an objection to it in advance. An example of presumed consent is organ donation in many countries, whereby organ harvesting will take place in suitable donors unless they have previously 'opted-out' of the scheme. Implied consent relates to the action of an individual that leads others to believe they are giving consent – for example, extending an arm to allow a blood test to be taken. Verbal and written consent relates to a patient giving informed consent by mouth or by signing a consent form. As a general rule of thumb, a high-risk intervention should have written consent (high risk could involve an invasive intervention, one with greater risks or one that has the potential to have significant consequences on a patient's life). It is important to remember that a patient can withdraw consent at any time and you should thoroughly document any discussion surrounding consent, including what was discussed and with whom.

MENTAL CAPACITY ACT (2005)

The Mental Capacity Act (MCA) was introduced in 2005 to legislate treatment of patients aged over 16 years who were believed to lack capacity (Humphreys et al, 2014). This act allows the compulsory and (if necessary) restrained treatment of any **physical condition** without consent, if it is believed to be in the patient's best interest, in individuals meeting the criteria for lack of capacity.

The MCA has five fundamental principles that must be adhered to:

1. A person must be assumed to have capacity unless it is established that they lack capacity.

2. A person is not to be treated as unable to make a decision unless all practicable steps to help them to do so have been taken without success. This may include translators, patient advocates, third-party advisers, communication aides, and different members of the multidisciplinary team.

3. A person is not to be treated as unable to make a decision merely because they make an unwise decision. The autonomy of the patient should still be respected.

4. Any act done, or decision made, under this Act on behalf of a person who lacks capacity must be done, or made, in their best interests.

5. Before the act is done, or the decision is made, regard must be given to whether the purpose for which it is needed can be as effectively achieved in a way that is less restrictive of the person's rights and freedom of action.

If a patient is suspected to lack capacity a formal assessment must take place. This is often governed by local hospital guidance and forms; however, as a minimum it must involve a formal cognitive assessment and assessment of their decision-making process (i.e. comprehension, retention, consideration, and communication). The results of this assessment and the decision taken should be clearly documented in the patient notes. Any subsequent decisions to be made about the patient would require an additional capacity assessment.

MENTAL HEALTH ACT (2007)

The Mental Health Act (MHA) was originally introduced in 1983 and amended in 2007. It is designed to govern **mental disorders**, which are described as any disorder or disability of the mind. Similarly to the MCA, the MHA allows the provision of compulsory and (if necessary) restrained assessment and treatment to any individual aged over 16 years suffering from a mental disorder in order to protect them from harm (Humphreys et al, 2014). An important distinction from the MCA is that the MHA can be used to protect others from harm if it is believed the patient poses a risk to them. Key sections are summarised as follows:

- **Section 5(2)** – this section is for use in inpatients who are already admitted and develop a mental disorder that is presenting as an emergency. It is used when time does not permit a more formal assessment of the patient's mental state. It requires a single doctor and should be used only if all other restrictive measures have been attempted. The maximum duration of this order is 72 hours and it should allow for a Section 2 or 3 to be completed.
- **Section 2** – this section is for use in individuals who require compulsory admission to a psychiatric facility for assessment of a mental disorder. The maximum admission is 28 days duration and it requires two approved mental health professionals to complete.
- **Section 3** – this section is for use in individuals who require compulsory treatment of a mental disorder at a psychiatric facility. The maximum admission is 6 months duration and it requires two approved mental health professionals.
- **Section 136** – this section is for use by police officers who believe themselves to be dealing with a patient with a mental disorder in a public place who they believe requires psychiatric treatment. This act allows the patient to be brought to an approved site of safety until a formal assessment can occur.

COMMON LAW (DOCTRINE OF NECESSITY)

Common law is a fundamental principle in medicine that enables immediate action to be taken to prevent loss of life or limb in an emergency situation, where time for formal MCA / MHA assessment is not available. Common law is based on case/tort law, not statutory law, and thus may have to be argued in a court whereby the judgement passed will decide the law. It can be used for both physical and mental disorders, and to protect the patient or others.

FINANCIAL AND COMMERCIAL RECOMMENDATIONS

The GMC has clear guidance for medical professionals with respect to financial and/or commercial gains. *Good Medical Practice* (GMC, 2013b) states that all doctors should be 'honest in financial and commercial dealings with patients, employers, insurers and other organisations or individuals'. The section 'Financial and commercial arrangements and conflicts of interest' (GMC, 2013c) explores this further and gives the following specific recommendations with respect to 'Gifts, bequests and donations':

1. You must not encourage patients to give, lend or bequeath money or gifts that will directly or indirectly benefit you.
2. You may accept unsolicited gifts from patients or their relatives provided:
    a. this does not affect, or appear to affect, the way you prescribe for, advise, treat, refer, or commission services for patients
    b. you have not used your influence to pressurise or persuade patients or their relatives to offer you gifts.[†]

THE DRIVER AND VEHICLE LICENSING AGENCY (DVLA) AND YOUR DUTIES AS A DOCTOR

The GMC has issued additional guidance in association with its guidance on confidentiality to advise doctors of their duties towards patients and the DVLA (GMC, 2009c). The DVLA is legally responsible for deciding whether individuals are 'medically fit to drive'. This includes private motor vehicles, commercial goods vehicles and passenger-carrying vehicles. Part of its decision will be based on a patient's physical and mental health. It must therefore be informed if a patient has a condition, or is undergoing treatment for a condition, that may affect their ability to drive.

The list of medical conditions and advice regarding their effect on driving are included in DVLA guidance (DVLA, 2013). These are divided into group 1 and group 2 licence holders. Group 1 licence holders include motor cars and motor cycles. Those in group 2 include large goods vehicles and buses.

[†]The acceptance of gifts by general practitioners in all four UK countries is subject to statutory regulation. General Medical Service's contract regulations state that a register should be kept of gifts from patients or their relatives which have a value of £100 or more unless the gift is unconnected with the provision of services. The register of gifts should include the donor's name and nature of the gift. NHS trusts set their own policies on gifts.

Your duty as a doctor is to explain to patients that their medical condition and/or treatment may affect their driving and they are legally obliged to inform the DVLA immediately. If they refuse to do so, or continue to drive against the DVLA's recommendation, you must inform the DVLA's medical advisor immediately. As with all disclosures of patient confidentiality, you should inform patients, both verbally and in writing, that you are required by law to disclose their medical information. This should also be documented thoroughly in a patient's medical record.

It would be impractical for you to attempt to learn every single condition that warrants involving the DVLA. More importantly, you should be aware of this guidance and rest assured that, in the SJT question, it will be made clear that the patient should have reported their medical condition to the DVLA and therefore you can simply proceed as indicated by the guidance above (e.g. inform the patient that you will have to inform the DVLA if they do not).

FITNESS TO PRACTICE

The public is entitled to expect that their doctor is fit to practice – i.e. they follow the principles of *Good Medical Practice*. To be fit to practice, a doctor needs to develop and maintain their professional knowledge and skills, be able to communicate effectively with patients, work in collaboration with their medical and non-medical colleagues, contribute to and comply with systems to protect patient safety – including declaring when their own health or conduct impacts on this – and work without discriminatory prejudice (GMC, 2013d).

When doctors fail to meet the GMC's expectations through poor performance, ill health, misconduct or a criminal conviction, patients are at risk of harm and distress and the medical profession is at risk of being undermined. The GMC accepts that, from time to time, people make mistakes and that doctors are not immune from this. Although these incidents should be investigated to ensure that the mistake does not happen again and so that lessons can be learnt, in most cases the investigation would not reveal an underlying fitness to practice issue. Fitness to practice and your professional registration is questioned, however, when there are serious or persistent failures to follow GMC guidance.

Questions regarding fitness to practice are commonly raised for the following reasons:

1. **Performance risks patient safety** – e.g. a series of incidents that raise concern locally
2. **Deliberate or reckless regard to clinical care** – e.g. unwillingness to practice ethically or lack of insight into self-limitations

17

3. **Doctor's practice is impaired by health** – being ill does not necessarily inhibit your ability to practice, but fitness to practice is questioned if a doctor has a medical condition (including drug and alcohol misuse) and does not heed medical advice or take steps to prevent harm to patients that may subsequently arise
4. **Patient's trust, autonomy or fundamental rights have been violated**
5. **Doctors have behaved dishonestly, fraudulently or in a way such as to mislead others.**

RAISING CONCERNS AND WHISTLEBLOWING

Raising concerns in the workplace, whether these are about one of your colleagues, resources or procedures, or management, is one of the most difficult situations faced by a doctor. To ensure that concerns are raised, *Good Medical Practice* (GMC 2013e) requires doctors to 'promote and encourage a culture that allows all staff to raise concerns openly and safely' and encourages us to take 'prompt action if you think that patient safety, dignity or comfort may be seriously compromised'.

The reasons concerns remain unraised is that we perceive nothing will be done to resolve the problem, we will gain a reputation as a complainer and thus our relationships with colleagues, and potentially our careers, will be negatively impacted. What we must hold at the forefront of our conscience is that we first have a duty to our patients and should act to protect them, before considering conflicting personal or professional loyalties. As long as you are honest and raise a concern based on reasonable belief through the correct protocols, legislation protects you from victimisation. A good tip is that if you notice a pattern of behaviour or repeated events that you feel threaten patient safety you should keep a thorough record of your concerns and the actions you took to resolve them. You must also remember that raising a concern about patient safety is very different from addressing a personal grievance.

When raising a concern, the acuteness of the situation dictates how it is reported. For example, if a patient is imminently at risk of harm then you must act immediately by involving senior staff to prevent the act from happening. If you notice repeated near misses/adverse events, reporting these formally through organisational 'serious untoward events' protocols allows these to be notified via the appropriate governance structure within the organisation (e.g. a hospital or a clinical commissioning group).

You should, as a junior doctor, raise your concern appropriately through the escalation ladder (see Chapter 3, tip 4). If you are, however, not sure whether to or how to raise your concern you should initially try to gain advice from a senior or impartial colleague, the GMC's confidential helpline, your medical defence body or your professional college. If you cannot raise the issue with the person responsible or body locally because you believe them to be part of the problem, or if you have exhausted your escalation ladder and your concern remains, you should involve the GMC as your regulatory body. You should make your concern public only if you have completely exhausted your local escalation ladder and have contacted your regulatory body and believe patients are at risk. Remember that, at all times, when divulging information public you should maintain confidentiality.

What is of upmost importance is that you do raise concerns and that you raise them via the correct channels and to the appropriate person in the correct hierarchical order; this will be the main basis of questions that assess this area in your SJT.

USE OF SOCIAL MEDIA

Social media are websites and applications that enable users to create and share content to participate in social networking. These include blogs, internet forums, content communities and social networking sites.

The rise, ease of access and impact of social media have required our regulatory bodies to set out guidelines for how doctors should act on them and what is expected of us. The GMC makes it quite clear that when communicating through social media the 'standards expected of doctors do not change'; we must still ensure good conduct, maintain patient confidentiality and make sure that any medical information we publish is factual (GMC, 2013f).

The first issue raised by social media is that of **privacy** – the boundaries between our private and professional lives are certainly more blurred with patients, medical colleagues and our employers, having access to information we choose to publish online.

It is important to bear in mind that social media sites do not guarantee **confidentiality** or **anonymity**; therefore what we publish is attributable and traceable back to us. Additionally the poster may hand over ownership of what is published to the owner of the site or application; which may make it difficult to have information removed if an issue should arise. The main message is that you should never post anything that you think has the potential to be damaging. Accordingly, when posting on social media, doctors must not contravene patient confidentiality and must not post inflammatory or defamatory comments about colleagues.

A worrisome feature of social media is the ability of patients to find and make contact with their doctor through it. It is imperative that, should this happen, you 'indicate that you cannot mix social and professional relationships and, where appropriate, direct them to your professional profile' (GMC, 2013 g).

Ultimately, however, social media has the benefits of allowing the medical profession to engage with the public in open discussions, to form networks of national and international colleagues to drive developments in clinical practice and research, and facilitates 'patients access to information about health and services' (GMC, 2013 h). In other words, We can use social media for the benefit of our patients; just be sensible about what you post, and think 'Would I be happy for my patients to read this?'

3. Top tips for mastering the SJT

The Situational Judgement Test has been designed to assess your qualities as a junior doctor, in comparison with a nationwide body of foundation year 1 (FY1) doctors. It is therefore crucial that you are familiar with the content of the test, as well as the appropriate guidance covered in Chapter 2 'Preparing for the SJT'.

However, the following 'top tips' will aid your success in the SJT.

1. PRE-REVISION REVISION

Before you begin practising for the SJT it is important to understand the application process to become a FY1 doctor. You should read and understand the Foundation Programme *Applicant's Handbook* (downloadable at http://www.foundationprogramme.nhs.uk/pages/home) and the 'How to apply' section of the UKFPO website (http://www.foundationprogramme.nhs. uk/pages/home/how-to-apply). This provides the most up-to-date information relevant to your application. It also includes an area specifically on the SJT and two official practice papers.

You are able to complete these practice papers more than once, but the questions do not change. A good technique is to complete the first practice paper early in your preparation for the SJT to give you an accurate idea of the time required to answer each question and the type of questions likely to be included in the SJT. You should complete the second practice paper close to the actual date of the SJT to consolidate the practice you have completed in the interim.

2. UNDERSTAND THE ROLE, EXPECTATIONS AND LIMITATIONS OF A FOUNDATION YEAR 1 DOCTOR

Tomorrow's Doctors (GMC, 2009a) clearly explains the expectations of all graduates from UK medical schools. This includes a list of procedures that you must be competent with, for example urinary catheterisation and electrocardiogram (ECG) interpretation. It is vital for patient safety that you therefore do not attempt to practise outside of these competencies, but there is a balance here in that you **should** attempt to practise what should be within the competence of an FY1 doctor. This is different from what you currently feel comfortable with as a final-year medical student.

For example: 'You are bleeped by the ward sister to place a urinary catheter in a female patient after the nurses have been unsuccessful'. In the question, which might ask 'What would you do?', the correct answer will be to attend the ward and attempt to place the urinary catheter before escalating to your registrar, as this is a skill you **should** be competent with. As a student you would not attempt this and, of course, in reality as a newly qualified FY1 you would probably ask your registrar for assistance as the procedure is almost certainly going to be complicated if the experienced nurses have already failed by this stage. Remember, the SJT is based on **what you should do, not what you would do!**

Your commitment to professionalism and development is also a key factor throughout the SJT. If a question is based on a competency outside of *Tomorrow's Doctors* it is important that you take the opportunity to learn, as long as it is safe, purposeful and poses no harm to the patient. This will often be in the guise of carrying out a procedure with which you are not currently competent under the direct teaching and supervision of your registrar or consultant. Remember: **See one, do one, teach one!** The key here would be that this was done under supervision.

At the other end of this scale of competence there are several specified limitations to your role as an FY1 and you must be familiar with these. They are common themes for SJT questions and include the following:

- Consenting for procedures
- Breaking bad news
- Discharging patients
- Taking referrals from other teams.

If these themes are involved in the question then the answer will always be to involve your senior!

3. PATIENT-CENTRED CARE

The absolute overriding principle of clinical medicine is '*primum non nocere – first do no harm*'. You must always have the safety of the patient at the centre of every question you answer in the SJT. Therefore, whenever the question allows it your first option must always be to assess, review, treat or refer the patient to ensure they are cared for appropriately. Generally, this will also mean your last option should be acting dangerously, avoiding the problem, watching and waiting or not acting at all (unless acting would be dangerous) as these options would compromise the patient's outcome.

Remember: **Patient safety! Patient safety! Patient safety!**

4. ESCALATION LADDER

There will be many situations that you encounter as an FY1 where you will need to ask for advice from your senior, or possibly deal with a complaint that involves external agencies and professional bodies. It is therefore logical that this element of practice became a common theme in the SJT. The key to succeeding with these types of questions is to follow the escalation process below and again focus on the language used.

The patient should always be the centre of your concerns as a doctor. However, you also need to ensure that you are caring for your own health and wellbeing, as indicated in *Good Medical Practice* (GMC, 2013a). When you decide you do need to gain assistance, you must try to stay within **your** team and progress in order of seniority (i.e. bleep your senior house officer (SHO) before contacting your registrar). Therefore, if a question has an option of **your** registrar and the **on-call** registrar then the correct option would be to contact **your** registrar first. If the problem is not patient-based but instead is regarding another issue (such as your mood, or harassment, or if you are concerned about another member of the team) then you should involve your clinical supervisor too. Generally, you should be contacting hospital management or external agencies only if you have escalated appropriately already and feel the problem has still not been dealt with.

The order of priority and escalation is as shown in Figure 3.1.

5. UNDERSTAND THE SUBTEXT OF THE QUESTION

A key domain that is being assessed in the SJT is professionalism. This has many different aspects but an important factor is avoiding confrontation and exploring the ideas, concerns and expectations of others in order to arrive at a consensus. Many questions about issues of professionalism may have options that appear to be the same answer but the difference is in the language used.

It's never a waste of time to consider the language used. For example, in the context of professionalism and potential conflict it is best to attempt to diffuse the situation. Generally, this will involve choosing options with words such as **explore**, **explain**, **discuss** or **suggest**. It is also important to try to avoid conflict. This can be achieved by avoiding options that contain words such as demand, confront, tell, shout, dismiss or ignore. Analysing language is not a guaranteed strategy to selecting the correct response, but often is helpful in excluding a particular response or favouring one over another.

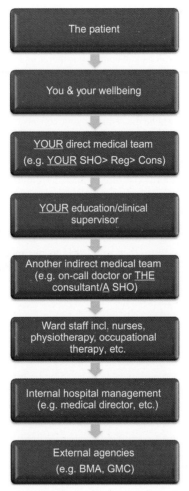

Figure 3.1 Recommended escalation process when seeking advice or raising concerns.

6. DISCLOSING CONFIDENTIAL INFORMATION

The importance of maintaining patient confidentiality and when to disclose information has been covered in Chapter 2 'Preparing for the SJT' and the

GMC's guidance *Confidentiality* (GMC, 2009b). However, the following key examples are commonly examined throughout the SJT and are occasions where disclosing confidential information is required:

- Required by law
  - Communicable diseases (e.g. enteric fever, meningococcal septicaemia)
  - Ordered by a judge
- Protect your patient
  - Safeguarding adult/child
  - Patient with mental health disorder lacking insight
- Protect others
  - DVLA disclosure
  - HIV-positive patient not willing to tell their partner
  - Domestic violence
- Public interest
  - Reporting knife/gun crime
  - Terrorism.

Remember, you should have made every effort to convince your patient to disclose the relevant information themselves unless you believe it poses a risk to the patient, their spouse, their children, or the public. Your conversation and any decision reached should then be clearly documented in the patient's medical notes.

7. PROFESSIONALISM

Professionalism is a very commonly encountered theme in the SJT as it forms a cornerstone of medical practice. There are countless scenarios on which questions can be based but the following simple advice will help you identify the best options for that question.

A large proportion of your time as an FY1 will be spent as the ward doctor responsible for liaising with allied healthcare staff, patients and their relatives. If confronted with concerns or queries it is important to explore these before simply reassuring them – there may be a genuine problem that has arisen. It is also bad practice to ask a member of the allied healthcare staff to speak to the patient and/or their family on your behalf. Remember confidentiality if you do speak with relatives and at all times involve the patient fully in all discussions. Honest and polite answers will always be the best option; failing that you need to be at least honest in your approach to talking with relatives. Completely avoid being untruthful or evasive in your answers.

Handover is another vital skill that involves the entire team and is crucial for patient safety. Questions can be based on handing over in the presence or absence of appropriate staff and also how to hand over correctly so that patient safety is not compromised. It is best practice to hand over in person to the next appropriate member of the team, such as the FY1 taking over the care of that patient. Failing that, you should next attempt to hand over information to a different doctor involved in the patient's care, such as the SHO or registrar. Avoid handing over to a staff member who has no direct responsibility for that patient. Occasionally, it will be impossible to safely hand over in person and so your next best choice would be to make a full entry into each patient's notes before leaving the ward. You should avoid leaving notes on boards.

Finally, it is important to understand the workings of a hospital and your interaction as an FY1. Here are a few common issues included in SJTs.

- You should avoid excessive overtime if possible as this will ultimately affect your wellbeing and patient safety.
- When urgent problems occur, you should act immediately, then reflect and learn later.
- Although it is important to maintain your education and development, this should not be to the detriment of patient safety.
- 'On-call' doctors are a resource to call on generally for emergencies when you can't get hold of your own seniors or for out-of-hour requests.
- Crash calls are for an arresting or non-responsive patient, not simply an unwell patient.

8. CONFRONTATION

Confrontation is sometimes unavoidable in an organisation as large and demanding as a hospital. It is therefore important that you are able to manage these occasions as well as possible.

Generally, the best option is always to discuss your concerns calmly with the individual involved. However, it is counterproductive to do this if the question states you have already tried, or if the issue is clearly inflammatory (e.g. claims of racism or patient neglect). If speaking to the individual is not productive or isn't an option, the next best option would be to speak to **your** clinical supervisor for advice. You should avoid reporting the individual to their supervisor as this often starts a formal process that can be avoided by local discussion and problem solving. It may be appropriate to gain advice from a colleague; however, it is important that you do not 'gossip'. Telling other members of your team, who are not in a position to help you, about an issue is not appropriate. Therefore, if the option does not specifically relate to asking for advice or help it should be avoided. As with many themes in the SJT, the worst options are to do nothing, ignore your concern or problem, attempt to blame or incriminate another member of the team, or report the individual concerned directly to their supervisor or an external organisation.

Finally, if the question is worded such that you are the colleague that somebody else is confiding in for advice, then you should advise that they act as above. It is best not to take on a responsibility outside your competence and get directly involved with resolving the situation.

9. INFORMATION, INFORMATION, INFORMATION

FY1s have an important administrative responsibility within the clinical team and your role will involve completing forms, giving information, receiving information and liaising with members of other teams. It is a key skill to be able to gather, retain and handle this information appropriately, and importantly to know at what point you need to act upon it.

For example if a patient is deteriorating but not imminently at risk then you must escalate your concern to your appropriate team member. However, first gather more information! It is more useful to be able to provide your SHO or registrar with sufficient information for them to be able to make a fully informed plan rather than simply relay a message that you may have been passed by the nurse caring for the patient. If the options allow, it is advisable to assess the patient, take a full history and familiarise yourself with any relevant results before escalating your concern.

10. WHEN IN DOUBT…?

If you become stuck answering a 'ranking question' remember to stay calm and focus on the best and worst options. If you manage to identify these options correctly even if you cannot distinguish the order of the middle three options this will still guarantee you a minimum of 16/20 score for that question.

When answering the 'multiple-choice questions' it can be helpful to try and identify three overriding themes in the question before reading the options. If you successfully identify three problems then choosing the three options that are most likely to solve these will give you the likely correct options. Finally, when there are

> **Practical tip!**
>
> You may find it useful to bring a highlighter to identify the three problems within the question text itself.

two mutually exclusive options available then only one is likely to be the correct answer! Therefore don't put both in your response.

> **Practical tip!**
>
> If you're unsure of your answer, make a note of the question on your exam paper and try to revisit it; consider changing your answer as the evidence would support doing so.

If you are truly unsure with an answer you've put down and think you should change it then you are probably right to do so. Over 70 years of research has shown that in exams most answer changes are from wrong to right (Kruger et al, 2005). However, most people are happier to go with their first answer rather than change, because the fear of regret from changing a right answer to a wrong answer is generally greater than the fear of failing to change a wrong answer to a right answer (i.e. if we are going to err at something, we would rather err by failing to do something). Our advice to you is this: the SJT is a very time-pressured exam; if you're confident with your answer then move on to the next question and forget about the one you've just answered.

4. Domain 1 – commitment to professionalism

Following the Foundation Programme year 1 analysis that was conducted prior to implementing the SJT, it was determined that successful candidates should be honest, trustworthy, reliable and possess a high degree of integrity. They should demonstrate an awareness of confidentiality and ethical issues and be able to challenge unacceptable behaviour appropriately, including any that may threaten patient safety. Finally, they should demonstrate commitment and enthusiasm for their role and be able to take responsibility for their own actions. These attributes can be broadly categorised into three major areas. These will form the basis of the questions involving this domain.

1. Commitment to learning and professional development
2. Confidentiality
3. Challenging inappropriate behaviour

Many medical students feel the pinnacle of their training and development occurs once they receive the golden envelope indicating they have passed their finals. However, an important aspect to your future career is learning and development as a professional.

There will be many different question themes that can address this, including:

- Punctuality and reliability
- Honesty when a mistake has been made and taking responsibility for own actions
- Demonstrating enthusiasm and motivation in your role
- Understanding the responsibility and limitations of an FY1
- Awareness of your own limitations, both professionally and personally (including health)
- Honesty when dealing with patients and colleagues
- Trustworthiness
- Ability to challenge others' knowledge appropriately.

A fundamental pillar of good medical practice is the confidentiality expected by patients, relatives, colleagues and the GMC. This can be a complex issue and is a very popular theme for SJT questions. As discussed in Chapter 2 'Preparing for the SJT', there are defined examples of when confidentiality may be broken and how this should be conducted. In every other example confidentiality must be upheld without error.

Finally, this domain also encompasses the ability of candidates to challenge inappropriate behaviour in a professional and reasonable manner. This behaviour may be in the form of bullying, prejudice (racism, sexism or homophobia), inappropriate relationships, recurring punctuality or reliability concerns, accepting financial gifts from patients, unsafe medical practice, inappropriately speaking to another colleague, or organisational concerns including shift patterns, hours worked, targets enforced, ward structure and foundation school training.

The following practice questions have been developed to provide an opportunity for you to demonstrate how to deal correctly with these topics. Remember, what counts is what you **should** do, not what you **would** do!

Q1. You are the on-call FY1 on the medical assessment unit (MAU) coming to the end of your 12-hour shift. You arrive at the handover to find the replacement FY1 has not yet arrived. It is currently 15 minutes before the end of your shift and the ward clerk informs you that the incoming FY1 has called to inform you that they are not well and will not be able to make it into work. You have managed to see all of the acute admissions and they are stable. You have amended the handover list and were hoping to leave on time today as tomorrow morning you are due to sit your MRCP part 1 exam. This is the only exam slot available that will be in time for your core medical training (CMT) post application.

Rank in order the following actions in response to this situation (1 = most appropriate; 5 = least appropriate):

A. Telephone the on-call registrar to inform them of the issue and ask them to take the FY1 bleep so that you can leave.

B. Call human resources and ask for a replacement FY1 and stay whilst this is arranged.

C. Leave so that you are well rested for your membership exam, informing the ward clerk before you leave.

D. Wait 30 minutes at the handover before leaving a written copy of outstanding jobs with the ward clerk, then leave and prepare for your membership exam.

E. Stay and work the next 12-hour on-call shift.

> Are you prioritising patient safety?

Q2. You are the FY1 on the cardiology ward. A patient is admitted with central crushing chest pain that is suspected to be a heart attack. He undergoes emergency treatment and is transferred to the coronary care unit (CCU). Whilst on the ward you receive a telephone call from the patient's wife asking for an update. She tells you that as she works as a school teacher she is unable to take leave until suitable cover is arranged. You can tell she is clearly anxious. You believe the patient is doing well but have not been to see him yet.

Rank in order the following actions in response to this situation (1 = most appropriate; 5 = least appropriate):

A. Tell the wife that the patient is doing well following his heart attack but you haven't yet seen him on the ward round.

B. Explain to the caller that you will need to speak to the patient first but will call her back once you have received permission to speak with her.

C. Demand that the caller comes to the ward if they wish to know information as you are very busy and do not have time to take calls.

D. Explain to the caller that you are unable to disclose patient information over the phone and would like to arrange a time that is convenient for the patient, the caller and you to meet on the ward to discuss the patient's health.

E. Ask the caller a series of questions to confirm her identity and then proceed with giving her information as requested.

Q3. You are the FY1 on the breast surgery firm. Your team sees Mrs Peters, a 65-year-old lady with breast cancer, on the morning ward round. She is due to have a mastectomy with sentinel lymph node excision and biopsy. Your consultant mentions that she was previously a glamour model and is particularly sensitive about the aesthetic appearance of her breast following the operation. Owing to local policy she was unable to have a concurrent reconstruction. As the consultation with Mrs Peters finishes you overhear the registrar quietly comment to the nurse that 'at her age aesthetics shouldn't matter'. You are uncomfortable with such an insensitive attitude.

Rank in order the following actions in response to this situation (1 = most appropriate; 5 = least appropriate):

A. Immediately tell the consultant what you have heard and express that you are not comfortable with this level of insensitivity.

B. After the ward round has finished demand that the registrar apologises to Mrs Peters.

C. Ignore what the registrar has said as you would just get a name as a troublemaker.

D. Once the ward round has finished ask to speak with the registrar privately, and politely explain that you were uncomfortable with the comment made as you feel it was unprofessional.

E. After the ward round has finished ask to speak with the consultant privately to discuss your feelings and ask for his advice.

Q4. You are the on-call medical FY1 on the acute assessment unit (AAU). Mr Gurung has been admitted to AAU for suspected pneumonia. You have clerked him, arranged appropriate investigations and contacted your registrar to update him on the case. As you are waiting for the registrar to come to AAU, the nurse in charge tells you that he is now very short of breath. You review Mr Gurung, as well as the results of his investigations, and diagnose a pleural effusion, not pneumonia. You know that the correct treatment is a chest drain and you bleep your registrar twice to explain the situation. He does not respond to his bleep and has not yet arrived at AAU. You are very worried so you contact the on-call consultant who tells you to insert the chest drain and next time not to waste his time for such a trivial request.

Rank in order the following actions in response to this situation (1 = most appropriate; 5 = least appropriate):

A. Bleep the on-call registrar again.

B. Research how to place a chest drain and do as the consultant has requested – placing the chest drain with the nurse's assistance.

C. Call the consultant back and explain that as an FY1 this is not a skill with which you are confident and would like him to come in as you feel the patient cannot wait further.

D. Call the on-call anaesthetic registrar, apologetically explaining the situation and request they attend to assist with the chest drain. Observe the procedure and enter this as a reflection in your e-portfolio.

E. Ask the nurse to monitor the patient more closely until the registrar attends AAU and continue with your remaining job list.

Q5. You have been working on your medical firm for 3 weeks. Over the past 3 weeks you have been late to work four times as you are still getting used to the local bus routes. The matron in charge of your ward has noticed this and tells you that it is not acceptable and if you do not improve she will have no option but to report you to human resources. You feel it is unacceptable for a nurse to make such comments and explain that it is none of her business. She is upset by your comments and leaves the ward to attend a meeting.

Rank in order the following actions in response to this situation (1 = most appropriate; 5 = least appropriate):

A. Download the local bus timetable and plan to catch the earlier bus to ensure you are on time from now on.

B. Ignore the nurse's comments as she has no right to chastise a doctor.

C. Apologise to the nurse for your comments and explain that you will make a conscious effort to be on time from now on.

D. Report the nurse to human resources as you are not happy that she has been monitoring your punctuality.

E. Adhere to your current morning routine as being late four times in 3 weeks is acceptable.

Q6. You are due to start working on the liver transplant unit as the medical FY1. On your first day a patient is admitted with liver cirrhosis due to chronic alcohol use. It is decided that, as the patient is not abstinent from alcohol, he will be treated medically, not surgically, and is passed to your team. You are upset by this decision as your father passed away from alcoholic liver cirrhosis 3 months ago and this case reminds you of this. You have been finding it very difficult to cope with day-to-day life since your father passed away and you have little motivation for work.

Rank in order the following actions in response to this situation (1 = most appropriate; 5 = least appropriate):

A. Continue your duties and work as an FY1 as your responsibility as a doctor should come before your own concerns.

B. Arrange an appointment with your general practitioner (GP) to discuss how you are coping with your father passing away.

C. Refuse to treat this patient as it is too difficult for you.

D. Arrange an appointment with your educational supervisor to discuss whether this is the best placement for you at this time.

E. Arrange an appointment with your consultant to discuss your current concerns and difficulties.

> Perhaps you should speak to somebody?

Q7. You are the on-call FY1 for care of the elderly. You have been called to see Mr Patel, an 83-year-old patient with a known history of insulin-controlled type 2 diabetes. He has been admitted with a hypoglycaemic emergency and treated successfully in accident and emergency (A&E). You have been bleeped to prescribe his regular insulin now that he is eating and drinking again. You prescribe his insulin and inform the nurse to bleep you if there are any problems; 2 hours later the nurse bleeps you as Mr Patel has become unresponsive. You review Mr Patel and to your horror realise that you have prescribed 10 times too much insulin. You treat Mr Patel for hypoglycaemia and he recovers without complication.

Rank in order the following actions in response to this situation (1 = most appropriate; 5 = least appropriate):

A. Re-write your prescription on a new drug chart, telling the nurse you do not know why Mr Patel became hypoglycaemic again.

B. Accuse the nurse of drawing up too much insulin and tell her that it is best she doesn't mention this to anyone as she may get into serious trouble, but don't worry as you corrected the chart in case.

C. Re-write your prescription and apologise to the patient, explaining what has happened. Inform the nurse you have corrected your error, and there is a new prescription to use.

D. Enter a reflection into your e-portfolio but do not tell the nurse you have made a mistake.

E. Re-write your prescription on the same drug chart, inform the nurse of the error and ask her not to tell anyone as you are still new.

Q8. You have been allocated renal medicine as your medical rotation for FY1. You really want to become a cardiologist and are very unhappy about this decision. Your CV is already well developed for a post in cardiology and you feel a rotation in FY1 would be the final addition. You have asked for a transfer but this is not possible.

Rank in order the following actions in response to this situation (1 = most appropriate; 5 = least appropriate):

A. Tell your consultant you are not happy in renal medicine and demand they authorise a transfer to the cardiac unit. In the mean time, do your job to the best of your ability.

B. Arrange an appointment with your educational supervisor and see what advice they can offer.

C. Discuss your career aspiration with your consultant and ask that, if any renal patients are admitted with cardiac disease, you are able to have the opportunity to look into their cardiac care.

D. Resign from your renal placement if the hospital is unable to transfer you to cardiac care.

E. Do not mention this to your consultant but show little interest or motivation during your renal placement to prevent any future placements with this team.

Q9. You have nominated yourself as the doctors' mess representative for your hospital. You are planning the first event at a local bar as a simple welcome party. During the night Nick, a fellow FY1, tells you that he thinks he may be gay and doesn't know what to do. His parents are very strict and keep asking him about when he is going to get married. You tell Nick that you are happy to help but think it would be best to meet after work so that people at the mess event do not see him upset. During your coffee break the next morning Rachel, another FY1, asks what you and Nick were discussing last night as she loves a bit of gossip.

Rank in order the following actions in response to this situation (1 = most appropriate; 5 = least appropriate):

A. Gossip with Rachel about Nick as it's all going to come out eventually.

B. Tell Rachel you were talking about work and it is nothing exciting.

C. Explain to Rachel that you do not think gossiping is professional and that she wouldn't like it if it were the other way round.

D. Make an excuse to leave the room and call Nick to see whether he wants Rachel to know.

E. Demand Rachel shows more sensitivity in the future and tell her that you will submit a formal grievance if you find out she is gossiping.

Q10. You are in general practice as an FY1 for your second rotation. You have now been working at the practice for 3 weeks and your GP supervisor has explained that it is normal practice to have a 4-week induction period. You have still not been able to spend any time with patients as you are often used to carry out filing in reception. One morning in particular you were asked to work on reception as the normal receptionist was unwell. You feel that the practice is not supporting your learning and you are unsure whether you can last an additional 3 months.

Rank in order the following actions in response to this situation (1 = most appropriate; 5 = least appropriate):

A. Resign from your post with the foundation school and submit a formal complaint to UKFPO for placing you at this surgery.

B. Contact your clinical supervisor at the foundation school to discuss your concerns about this practice.

C. Confront your GP supervisor and ask that he allow you to run clinics under his supervision as you have educational requirements whilst at the practice.

D. Complete the final week of your induction and if you still do not have any patient contact ask to discuss this with your GP supervisor.

E. Stop attending the practice as it is clearly going to be of limited benefit to your training.

Q11. You are seeing a known epileptic patient in A&E who has been admitted with a seizure. After stabilising the patient, you discuss his medication with him and he admits to avoiding his anti-epileptic medication. He explains that he finds it difficult to remember to take it each morning and generally doesn't like to take pills as they make him feel pathetic. You explain the risks of not adhering to his treatment plan and ask him about driving. He admits to you that he still drives as his work depends on it. You explain the DVLA requirements to him but he refuses to disclose his diagnosis.

Rank in order the following actions in response to this situation (1 = most appropriate; 5 = least appropriate):

A. Explore the patient's concerns regarding his epilepsy and try to persuade him to disclose his diagnosis to the DVLA.

B. Explain to the patient that if he does not agree to disclose his diagnosis to the DVLA, you are required by law to do so.

C. Agree not to inform the DVLA on this occasion but ask that if the patient has another seizure he liaises with his GP immediately.

D. Tell the patient he is putting other people's lives at risk, and that you will be disclosing his diagnosis to the DVLA.

E. Agree not to inform the DVLA on this occasion but include this development in the discharge summary that is sent to the patient's GP.

> Is this an occasion when you should breach patient confidentiality?

Q12. You are the surgical FY1 on hepatobiliary. You are bleeped to review a patient in the AAU who is believed to have gallstones. You are very busy on your ward and tell the nurse that it will be at least an hour before you will be able to come to AAU. The nurse explains that the patient is very unwell and she doesn't think the patient can wait. You attend AAU and complete the admission clerking based on the A&E doctor's findings. You hand over your instructions to the nurse and return to the ward. The nurse is worried that you have not fully assessed the patient and informs your registrar, who then asks you what happened.

Rank in order the following actions in response to this situation (1 = most appropriate; 5 = least appropriate):

A. Deny the accusation and tell the registrar you assessed the patient fully and found similar findings to the A&E doctor.

B. Admit that you felt overworked and took the shortcut as the A&E doctor is likely to be correct owing to their experience.

C. Review the patient immediately and correctly document your findings. Admit that you made a mistake and apologise to the patient, nurse and registrar.

D. Admit that you have made an error and ask the registrar not to tell anybody further as you can promise you will never do that again.

E. Tell the registrar that you examined the patient fully and have no idea why the nurse would accuse you of falsifying clinical findings. Proceed to AAU and demand the nurse retracts her allegation.

Q13. You have just started your final FY1 rotation in urology. You have always been very interested in urology and you hope to apply for core surgical training after your foundation programme. You recently recall reading an article in *BMJ Best Practice* regarding the investigation and treatment of haematuria. On the ward round this morning your team saw Mr Philips, a 68-year-old man with a history of painless haematuria. You recall from the article that the recommended investigation is cystoscopy but your consultant asks you to arrange an alternative scan. You feel that Mr Philips should be sent for cystoscopy.

Rank in order the following actions in response to this situation (1 = most appropriate; 5 = least appropriate):

A. Wait until the ward round has finished and re-read the *BMJ Best Practice* article to check your impression.

B. Explain to the consultant that you are interested in urology and would he be able to explain the rationale behind his choice of scan, as you are keen to learn more.

C. Once the ward round has finished, tell the consultant what you recently read and discuss the benefits of both scans, focusing on which scan is best for Mr Philips.

D. Ignore what your consultant has told you as he is clearly not aware of current best practice and arrange cystoscopy in accordance to the guideline.

E. Whilst still with Mr Philips, ask the consultant why he has chosen a suboptimal scan choice, bearing in mind the *BMJ Best Practice* guidance.

Q14. You have received your rota for the next 3 months and notice that you have been scheduled to work the weekend of your sister's wedding. You are very upset with the rota as you submitted your request for time off at the start of FY1. You arrange to meet with the manager of human resources but she refuses to change your shift as the rotas have already been finalised. When you try to explain the importance of the request the manager tells you that she is 'tired of doctors thinking they can change everything to suit themselves and they never think of people who have to run around to arrange these things'.

Rank in order the following actions in response to this situation (1 = most appropriate; 5 = least appropriate):

A. Speak with other FY1s and arrange to swap your shift. Inform the HR manager that you have swapped your shift and apologise for any inconvenience caused.

B. Wait until your scheduled weekend and call in sick for work, allowing you to attend your sister's wedding.

C. Discuss your concerns with your clinical supervisor, and ask that they support your request for time off.

D. Submit a formal grievance in response to what the manager said and demand that you are given the time off.

E. Explore the concerns the HR manager has and ask that if you arrange appropriate cover will she approve the shift change.

Q15. You are working as an FY1 in A&E when Mr Jones is admitted with vomiting. You know Mr Jones from your previous rotation in oncology and are aware that he has a terminal diagnosis of renal cell carcinoma. You recall Mr Jones's case as he has a very demanding family that were often very rude to you. Your registrar asks you to assess Mr Jones and treat him as necessary. It is decided that Mr Jones needs to be admitted for observation and he is moved to a medical ward. Before this can happen, Mr Jones's daughter arrives at A&E and is demanding to see the doctor who saw her father. When you arrive she asks you why her father has been admitted for an 'upset stomach', as her father is a fit and healthy man and will recover perfectly well at home.

Rank in order the following actions in response to this situation (1 = most appropriate; 5 = least appropriate):

A. Ask the daughter to wait in the relatives' room and call the specialist palliative nurse to join you. Explain to the daughter that the father has a terminal diagnosis and is very unwell.

B. Tell the daughter that you are not allowed to disclose a patient's medical details, even if she is family.

C. Ask the daughter to wait in the relatives' room and ask Mr Jones if he would like you to explain his situation to his daughter.

D. Explain to the daughter that Mr Jones requires observation owing to his vomiting and he has agreed to be admitted.

E. Ask the senior nurse to tell the daughter you are too busy to speak with her at this point and admit Mr Jones as planned.

Q16. You are an FY1 in general surgery. Your consultant has asked you to assist in theatre today and you are sitting in the coffee room between procedures. You are very keen to impress the team as you are hoping to apply to core surgical training after the Foundation Programme. You are talking with your surgical registrar when the consultant anaesthetist from your theatre joins you. The next patient is of Asian ethnicity and when you discuss the surgical case with your registrar, the anaesthetist tells you he is 'sick of these damn immigrants always coming to our country to get free healthcare, and there is nothing we can do about it … They don't even deserve treatment anyway.' You and the registrar are clearly uncomfortable but the registrar doesn't say anything.

Rank in order the following actions in response to this situation (1 = most appropriate; 5 = least appropriate):

A. Agree with the consultant anaesthetist. You don't want to get a name as a troublemaker and these types of doctor are the old generation.

B. Stay quiet with the registrar hoping that the consultant anaesthetist realises you are both uncomfortable with his views.

C. Politely explain to the consultant that you do not think his views are appropriate and he definitely should not be discussing them in a work environment.

D. Submit a formal grievance to human resources as the consultant anaesthetist should be reprimanded for his comments.

E. Speak to your educational supervisor for advice as you are not comfortable with the situation.

> Is this comment in accordance with the professional standards expected by the GMC?

Q17. You have just started your final shift on care of the elderly. You have really enjoyed your training and one patient in particular, Mrs Wong, has made a real impact on you. She has been an inpatient for 7 weeks owing to a complex medical history and several failed attempts to discharge her. She is aware that today is your last day as her FY1 and she has arranged for her neighbour to bring in a gift for you. You are very flattered and explain that you will open it later after the ward round. When you open the gift, you see that it is a very expensive-looking antique watch, at least £3000–£4000 in value.

Rank in order the following actions in response to this situation (1 = most appropriate; 5 = least appropriate):

A. Accept the gift as you have been working hard to provide Mrs Wong with good care and she would be offended if you tried to return it.

B. Speak to your consultant to explain the situation and ask for their advice.

C. Return the gift to Mrs Wong and explain that, whilst you are very appreciative, a gift of this nature is not necessary as it was your pleasure to treat her.

D. Politely return the gift explaining to Mrs Wong the GMC's guidance on accepting gifts.

E. Thank Mrs Wong and accept the gift but declare it to the hospital's gift register.

Q18. You are an FY1 currently on the acute admissions unit. Your colleague, James, has finished clerking a young, attractive, female patient. She has presented with a simple urinary tract infection (UTI) and has been discharged with a course of antibiotics. On the way out of the department, you see her giving her telephone number to James. You speak to James about the situation and he tells you that he will throw the number away as he knows it's unprofessional. Three weeks later you bump into James in town. He is with the patient who gave him her number. James tells you to ignore it as she was barely a patient anyway and she seems to really like him. You are not comfortable with the situation and tell James you think he is making a mistake.

Rank in order the following actions in response to this situation (1 = most appropriate; 5 = least appropriate):

A. Arrange an appointment with your educational supervisor to get their advice.

B. Ignore what you saw as it was outside of hospital premises and unlikely to cause a problem.

C. Tell James that if he doesn't stop seeing the patient that you will have no option but to report him to the hospital.

D. Inform the GMC of what James has been doing as you know it will act in accordance with the guidelines.

E. Ask your registrar for advice.

Q19. You are an FY1 in general practice. You have been working in this practice for 2 months and you feel things are going well. You are being allowed to run six clinics a week with the supervision and guidance of your GP tutor. This morning, your GP tutor is on a training course and you have been scheduled to be supervised by an older GP partner. He is very polite and seems to be liked by his patients, but twice this morning you have noticed that his management plans were not in accordance with current guidelines and you feel his choice of medication is woefully inadequate. You know that had your GP tutor been supervising this clinic the most recent treatment would have been followed.

Rank in order the following actions in response to this situation (1 = most appropriate; 5 = least appropriate):

A. Ignore what you are thinking as the GP partner is very experienced and probably knows more than the recent guidelines anyway.

B. Wait for your GP tutor to return and raise your concerns with him.

C. Respectfully raise your concerns with the GP partner and openly discuss the guidelines together.

D. Tell the GP partner that you think his management is woefully out of date and that he should make a better effort to stay abreast of recent changes.

E. Inform the GMC that you have serious concerns about the GP partner.

Q20. You are in your final rotation as an FY1 and you receive an email informing you of your upcoming e-portfolio review with your academic supervisor. You have been aware of the requirements of the e-portfolio throughout FY1 but have often ignored them. You are concerned that in the email there is a reminder that FY1s who have not completed the recommendations could face being delayed in their progression to FY2. You check your e-portfolio and see that you have approximately 24 objectives to meet. Your review is planned for 2 weeks' time.

Rank in order the following actions in response to this situation (1 = most appropriate; 5 = least appropriate):

A. Email your academic supervisor immediately, explaining exactly what you have left to do and asking whether you may delay your review to allow you time to complete the requirements.

B. Ignore the email as you haven't heard of anybody not completing FY1.

C. Speak to your registrar and explain the situation. Ask if they can help you meet the requirements in time for your review. Apologise sincerely and hope they are compassionate.

D. Speak to other FY1s and see whether they are also in a similar position. If they are, ask whether you can work together to maximise your effectiveness.

E. Work hard in the next 2 weeks to complete your requirements but do not inform anybody as it will make you look unprofessional.

Q21. You are the medical FY1 on call in accident and emergency. Mrs Patel, a 35-year-old patient, attends A&E alone. She has told the triage nurse that she has fallen and bumped her head. When you examine Mrs Patel you feel that her history is not consistent with her injuries. You are worried that she is suffering from domestic violence. She explains that she has two young children at home that she has left with her husband's sister. She is in a hurry to be discharged because she tells you that she needs to get back to her children before her husband returns from his social club. You sensitively raise your worries with Mrs Patel, who breaks down into tears explaining that her husband has been hitting her. She begs you not to tell the police because 'it will just make him more angry'. You are concerned for the safety of Mrs Patel and her young children.

Rank in order the following actions in response to this situation (1 = most appropriate; 5 = least appropriate):

A. Agree not to disclose any information but give Mrs Patel an advice leaflet for local women's domestic violence centres.

B. Try to ascertain more information about whether the husband has ever been violent towards his children as this will indicate further risk.

C. Explain to Mrs Patel that you are worried about the safety of her and her children and have to inform social services.

D. Explain to Mrs Patel that you are worried about her and her children and try to reach an agreement to disclose this information.

E. Ask Mrs Patel to wait in the cubicle and call the police so that they can arrest Mr Patel.

> Is this an occasion when you should breach patient confidentiality?

Q22. You are the FY1 on paediatric gastrointestinal surgery. You have assisted with several procedures but unfortunately every procedure lead by Professor Woodson has ended with a poor outcome. You note that he has a very obstructive attitude towards raising concerns and you are worried that his actions are responsible for the poor outcomes. You raise your concerns with your consultant, who dismisses you immediately. You are very unhappy with this outcome so discuss your worries with your clinical supervisor. He advises that, as you are concerned, you have very little option but to discuss this with a member of the hospital management team. You speak with the medical director, who immediately advises you to liaise with your clinical supervisor. Feeling that you are not progressing with your concern and Professor Woodson is still operating, you contact the GMC. They inform you that they will begin an investigation but Professor Woodson will not be prevented from operating as this is a hospital decision and they have not reached any conclusion yet.

Rank in order the following actions in response to this situation (1 = most appropriate; 5 = least appropriate):

A. Contact your deanery and ask to transfer posts.

B. Inform the medical director that you have had no option but to raise your concerns with the GMC.

C. Accept that you have done all you can and hope further patients are not affected by the current situation.

D. Raise your concerns in the public domain as the medical director has not acted.

E. Contact your medical defence organisation for advice.

Q23. You are on call and are bleeped by one of the ward nurses, June, who explains that Mrs Coff has not passed urine for several hours and is complaining of severe lower abdominal pain. June and her colleague, Mary, have attempted to catheterise her but have been unsuccessful as Mrs Coff is very agitated and overweight. They have asked you to perform the female catheterisation. You explain to June that you have one patient to see first but will come as soon as you can. You have not had many opportunities to catheterise female patients but did pass the OSCE station in your medical school exams.

Rank in order the following actions in response to this situation (1 = most appropriate; 5 = least appropriate):

A. Contact the urology SHO and explain the situation asking if they would mind trying as the patient must be difficult.

B. Bleep your registrar and explain that you are not confident with urinary catheterisation on female patients so would they be able to attend to assist.

C. Complete your current task as planned and attend Mrs Coff. Attempt to catheterise her with the assistance of the ward nurses.

D. Call June on the ward and explain that you are not happy with being asked to catheterise Mrs Coff as the ward nurses should be able to perform this skill.

E. Complete a reflective entry to your e-portfolio about urinary catheterisation in difficult female patients.

Q24. You are working on care of the elderly as an FY1 and you feel that your registrar is lazy and often not available for advice when you need it. You have tried to raise your concerns with him about this but he tells you that it is because you are such a competent FY1 that he feels he can trust you on the ward, allowing him to work on his e-portfolio for consultancy. You explain that although this is very flattering you would prefer him to be available for advice more freely. He agrees to attend the ward more often but after 3 weeks you do not see an improvement. Your registrar then informs you that he requires 360-degree feedback from all members of the team, including you, as part of his registrar assessment.

Rank in order the following actions in response to this situation (1 = most appropriate; 5 = least appropriate):

A. Tell the registrar that you are unwilling to complete the feedback as you do not feel he took your concerns seriously.

B. Agree to complete the anonymous feedback and truthfully score the registrar.

C. Explain to the registrar that you are willing to complete the feedback but will have to honestly answer the teamwork and leadership elements and that these will not be positive.

D. Agree to complete the feedback and score the registrar well in all domains as you wouldn't want to affect his future position.

E. Discuss your concerns with your registrar and agree to complete the feedback once he demonstrates that he is able to support the team more appropriately.

Q25. You are an FY1 on a cardiology firm in a tertiary referral centre. You are in your final week of this rotation and have spent the previous 4 months working very hard and often past your scheduled hours. You have a day off in lieu scheduled for Friday and you have planned a long weekend to relax before starting your next rotation. You receive a call from the rota coordinator explaining that owing to staff illness you are required to work on call on Friday. She apologises and explains that you can take an additional day off in your next rotation. You explain that you already have confirmed plans but she reminds you that only annual leave days are protected and not days off in lieu.

Rank in order the following actions in response to this situation (1 = most appropriate; 5 = least appropriate):

A. Tell the rota coordinator this is unacceptable and that you will not be in work as you have already paid for a short break.

B. Complete a retrospective hours monitoring exercise and submit your findings to the deanery so that future FY1s may be protected.

C. Speak with your consultant and explain the situation.

D. Call in sick on Friday with diarrhoea and vomiting reminding the rota coordinator that you must remain away from work for at least 48 hours as per hospital policy.

E. Cancel your short trip and work as requested.

Q26. You are on call in the acute admission unit clerking new patients into the hospital. You have been working for 9 out of your 13 hours and have seen several patients that your registrar has been impressed with. He explains that, as you are nearing the end of your FY1 training, it would be a good exercise to hold the registrar pager for an hour to develop your prioritising skills. You agree without thinking too much of it and carry on seeing new patients. Twenty minutes into the new arrangement you realise that the patient you are seeing is deteriorating despite your intervention and you have a GP waiting to refer a second patient via switchboard. As you are trying to respond to this referral, the pager goes off with a cardiac arrest call on the 7th floor.

Rank in order the following actions in response to this situation (1 = most appropriate; 5 = least appropriate):

A. Call the medical registrar as you make your way to the cardiac arrest. Explain the situation and ask for him to relieve you of the pager immediately and to swap with you at the cardiac arrest so you may attend the unwell patient in the admission unit.

B. Ask the GP to call back in 5 minutes giving you time to re-assess the unwell patient in the admission unit. Ignore the cardiac arrest as the rest of the cardiac arrest team will attend that.

C. Briefly ask the senior nurse on the admission unit to repeat observations on the deteriorating patient and start intravenous (IV) fluids. You will review the patient after attending the cardiac arrest.

D. Attend the cardiac arrest immediately, assess your need to stay once the rest of the cardiac arrest team arrive, and if possible return to the deteriorating patient in the admission unit. Once the situation has settled, call the registrar and discuss your actions.

> Are you prioritising patient safety?

E. Turn the registrar pager off for the remainder of the hour.

Q27. You are an FY1 in a district general hospital. You are on your second rotation and are enjoying your new role. Your FY1 colleague Carol is talking to you about her current rotation and seems apathetic about it. You ask her what is wrong and she explains that her registrar took her to one side last week and told her that she thought Carol was a terrible FY1 and didn't understand how she had passed medical school. Carol was very upset by this comment but the registrar simply told her to improve her act or she'd have no option but to report Carol to her educational supervisor. Up until now Carol had received glowing feedback from her previous team. Carol is unsure of what to do and tells you that she will probably just forget about the comment made.

Rank in order the following actions in response to this situation (1 = most appropriate; 5 = least appropriate):

A. Advise Carol not to ignore the comment made as it was clearly inappropriate and should be investigated. She should speak to the registrar directly and explain that she was upset by the comment.

B. Tell Carol that you will help and approach the registrar yourself asking why she criticised Carol without cause.

C. Agree with Carol that it is probably best to ignore the comment as everybody else Carol has worked with has been so impressed.

D. Arrange a meeting with Carol's clinical supervisor to explain what has happened.

E. Advise Carol to arrange a meeting with her clinical supervisor to explain what has happened and to ask for advice.

Q28. You are on call in the medical assessment unit overnight. It is the start of your shift and your co-worker James has failed to attend. You ask your registrar and the ward matron whether anybody has heard from him and they tell you that he hasn't called in sick. This is the third time you and James have been scheduled to work together and both previous times James has not attended his on-call shift. The shift is very busy and even though the whole team plough through the workload you do not finish until 2 hours after the end of your shift. When you eventually get home the next morning you are looking through Facebook when you notice pictures of James at a party last night. You are concerned that a pattern is developing with his attendance for on call shifts.

Rank in order the following actions in response to this situation (1 = most appropriate; 5 = least appropriate):

A. Explain to James that you are not impressed by his actions last night and he needs to improve his attitude towards working.

B. Inform James's clinical supervisor that he did not attend his on-call shift but was at a party instead.

C. Discuss your concerns with the on-call coordinator as this is not the first time this has happened.

D. Speak to James next time you see him and advise him that if he is going to miss work he shouldn't incriminate himself on Facebook afterwards.

E. Speak to your registrar and explain what has happened. Ask what they think the best course of action is.

Q29. You are the FY1 on call covering the wards for medicine. You are called to see Mrs Kildin, a 36-year-old woman who has been admitted for pyelonephritis. When you arrive on the ward the nurses explain that they are very worried because it appears Mrs Kildin has received double the maximum daily dose of the antibiotic gentamicin owing to a prescription error. You are aware that gentamicin can cause renal damage and ototoxicity. You review Mrs Kildin, who appears well and isn't displaying any signs of side effects. You can see that the error occurred following gentamicin being prescribed on the A&E prescription chart as well as the inpatient prescription chart when Mrs Kildin was admitted to the ward. You order a gentamicin assay level and kidney function test to see whether any damage has occurred.

Rank in order the following actions in response to this situation (1 = most appropriate; 5 = least appropriate):

A. Ignore what has happened to Mrs Kildin as she is not displaying any signs of any adverse effects.

B. Wait for the results of your blood tests and if the gentamicin assay and kidney function are normal then there is no need to tell Mrs Kildin what has happened.

C. Explain what has happened to Mrs Kildin and apologise for the error occurring.

D. Inform your consultant of the incident and explain that you have assessed the patient and ordered bloods to assess any damage.

E. Complete a serious incident report so that this type of error can be investigated by the hospital trust and possibly be prevented in the future.

Q30. You are the FY1 on a general medical ward. It is 4.45 pm on Friday afternoon and your FY1 anaesthetic colleague comes to the ward to explain that your ward is going to be receiving an ITU patient who is now suitable for ward-based care. The anaesthetic FY1 is not with the patient, who is still on ITU. She begins to give the patient handover and explains that the patient will need to be seen over the weekend by the on-call team and have daily blood tests. You explain that you are not happy accepting this referral without the patient present and because you are only an FY1. You explain very clearly that you have not accepted this referral and the anaesthetic FY1 should bleep your registrar and handover, and also arrange weekend review with the on-call team. When you come into work on Monday you find that the patient is on your ward, but that they haven't had any blood tests or been reviewed over the weekend. In the patient's notes you see that the anaesthetic FY1 has documented your name and bleep as the doctor who accepted her handover.

Rank in order the following actions in response to this situation (1 = most appropriate; 5 = least appropriate):

A. Confront the anaesthetic FY1 and explain that you are very unhappy with what has happened as the patient was put at serious risk.

B. Complete a serious incident report.

C. Inform the ward manager/senior nurse that an inappropriate transfer has taken place.

D. Immediately assess the patient to ensure they are not unwell. Take some urgent blood tests and inform your registrar of what has happened.

E. Complete a reflective entry in your e-portfolio.

Q31. You are the FY1 on hepatobiliary surgery. Your registrar has invited you to assist with an ERCP tomorrow. You are keen to impress your new team and so you thank the registrar for this opportunity and agree to meet them in theatre tomorrow morning. The registrar explains that to learn the most from this procedure you should read up on how the ERCP is performed. The following morning you meet the registrar in theatre as agreed. During the time out, it becomes evident that the consent form signed in the pre-operative assessment has been mislaid. Your registrar asks you to quickly consent the patient as they have already been told the risks and it's merely a formality as they have previously given consent for the procedure.

Rank in order the following actions in response to this situation (1 = most appropriate; 5 = least appropriate):

A. Remind your registrar that FY1s are not allowed to consent and suggest that they consent the patient.

B. Agree to consent the patient as it is only signing the form; the registrar has already previously explained the risks and benefits.

C. Explain to the registrar that you are unable to consent as an FY1 but you'd be keen to shadow the registrar to learn.

D. Agree to consent the patient if the registrar will be able to answer any questions the patient may have.

> What are the limitations for an FY1?

E. Tell the registrar that FY1s do not consent.

Q32. You are the on-call medical FY1 covering the wards on the weekend. You receive a bleep from a member of the discharge team asking that you assess Mr Hurst's suitability to be discharged. They explain that there were 14 patients in A&E overnight and several have breached the government 4-hour target. You are told that Mr Hurst was seen by his consultant on Friday and his observations have been stable over the weekend. The discharge coordinator explains that he is due two more doses of IV antibiotics but the patient is happy to attend the ambulatory care centre tomorrow as an outpatient for these to be administered. The discharge coordinator reminds you that the hospital is fined every time a patient breaches a government target.

Rank in order the following actions in response to this situation (1 = most appropriate; 5 = least appropriate):

A. Call your supervising registrar on call and explain what has happened. Ask whether they are able or willing to assess Mr Hurst.

B. Agree to assess Mr Hurst. If he is stable and happy to come back into the hospital tomorrow he can be discharged this evening.

C. Call Mr Hurst's consultant and ask whether they are happy with the suggested plan.

D. Explain to the discharge coordinator that if the consultant has not documented their discharge plan in the notes you are unwilling to review this patient.

E. Tell the discharge coordinator that you are the on-call doctor and discharges are not your priority.

Q33. You are due to be working on call this weekend. This will be the third on-call weekend that you have worked and they are always very busy. There is minimal medical cover and you often feel overwhelmed and have to stay late to complete your tasks. Your SHO and registrar colleagues also feel the same and if anybody misses an on-call shift they are often given a hard time when they return to work. You have developed diarrhoea and vomiting overnight but it has now stopped. Apart from feeling tired you are feeling better and think it must have been a passing viral illness. You do not want to let your team down but because you didn't get much sleep overnight you'd rather take today and tomorrow off to recover. You are aware that the hospital guidance is not to return to work until you have been diarrhoeafree for 48 hours.

Rank in order the following actions in response to this situation (1 = most appropriate; 5 = least appropriate):

A. Call James, another FY1, and ask if he can cover you this weekend in return for one of his future weekend shifts.

B. Attend your on-call shift as you do not think you'll be infectious any longer and you do not want to affect the on-call team.

C. Attend your on-call shift but go home immediately if you have any further episodes of diarrhoea.

D. Inform your educational supervisor that the on calls are understaffed and you are put under too much pressure.

E. Call in sick as you are aware the trust has a 48-hour policy with diarrhoea and/or vomiting.

Q34. You have started working in infectious diseases. Mr Mullin, who you have been seeing for several weeks for pyrexia of unknown origin, is diagnosed with human immunodeficiency virus (HIV). He explains that he was an intravenous drug user (IVDU) when he was younger but hasn't ever had an HIV test. As you are discussing what treatment options there are he mentions that he has recently started seeing a new partner. You explain that the partner is at high risk of contracting HIV if they are having unprotected sex. Mr Mullin explains that they haven't been but were planning to stop using barrier contraceptives shortly. You explain that, due to the nature of HIV,

Mr Mullin is required to disclose this information to his partner so that they can make an informed decision about having unprotected sexual intercourse. Mr Mullin explains that he does not want to tell his partner as he thinks they will leave him.

Rank in order the following actions in response to this situation (1 = most appropriate; 5 = least appropriate):

A. Explain to Mr Mullin that if he doesn't disclose this information you will have to as you have a duty to protect his partner from harm.

B. Tell Mr Mullin that you think his behaviour is appalling.

C. Sensitively stress that it is important that if Mr Mullin is planning on having unprotected sexual intercourse with his partner he must disclose his HIV status beforehand.

D. Agree not to disclose any information about Mr Mullin but call his partner offering an impromptu sexual health screen.

E. Respect Mr Mullin's wishes as you have a duty to maintain patient–doctor confidentiality.

Q35. You have just finished your final on-call night shift following a week on call. Once you get home you realise that you have left the patient handover sheet in the hospital coffee shop. You are aware that the hospital has a very strict policy about this and an FY1 colleague was disciplined for a similar error 2 months ago.

Choose the most suitable **three** options from the following list:

A. Ignore the handover sheet as it was probably thrown away.

B. Drive back to hospital to ensure the list has been removed.

C. Call the on-call FY1 and ask them if they are able to collect the handover sheet.

D. Enter a reflection in your e-portfolio about this incident.

E. Wait until the morning and visit the coffee shop to see whether it was collected.

F. Inform your consultant of your mistake.

G. Ensure that you inform the patients the following day and apologise for leaving their personal details in the coffee shop.

H. Call your mum to discuss what she thinks you should do.

Q36. You are an FY1 on haemoncology. James Peters has been admitted for an elective bone marrow transfer. You are asked by your registrar to complete the admission clerking and you notice that James is neutropenic and has a fever. You give him immediate intravenous penicillin as per the trust policy for neutropenic sepsis. Twenty minutes later you receive a bleep from the nurse looking after James explaining that she has given the antibiotics but now James isn't looking too well. She isn't sure what is going wrong but she asks whether it could have anything to do with his allergy. You don't recall asking James if he had an allergy during your clerking as you were distracted by his blood results.

Choose the most suitable **three** options from the following list:

A. Inform your registrar of what has happened.

B. Explain to James that you didn't realise he had an allergy and apologise for not asking beforehand.

C. Tell the nurse that she shouldn't be bothering you unless she has a full set of observations available.

D. Destroy James's drug chart. Re-write it with the allergy clearly stated and a non-allergic antibiotic prescribed.

E. Ask the nurse to give some fluids and you will assess James soon but will need to finish the task you are currently doing.

F. Immediately return to the ward and assess James.

G. Ask the nurse to call the cardiac arrest team so that you have help when you arrive.

H. Update James's drug chart and medical notes with his allergy status.

> Are you prioritising patient safety?
>
> What should you do if you make an error?

Q37. You have been called to AAU as the on-call surgical FY1. A patient has been admitted with suspected acute pancreatitis following an alcoholic binge. The patient is still intoxicated and is refusing to be cared for by a Nigerian nurse. The patient is shouting profanities and threatening to assault the nurse if he attempts to treat him. The patient is in bed but is disturbing other patients.

Choose the most suitable **three** options from the following list:

A. Tell the patient that he is disturbing other patients and is being offensive towards the staff. Explain that this will not be tolerated and if he continues to be disruptive he may not be treated.

B. Call security.

C. Call the police.

D. Prescribe a sedative so that you and the nurse can carry on with your duties.

E. Ensure that the other patients are not upset.

F. Tell the nurse to ignore the patient and ask whether there is another nurse to care for the patient until he is discharged.

G. Explore the patient's concerns and reasoning behind his comments and try to calm him down by explaining that everyone is trying to help him.

H. Tell the patient to leave the hospital immediately.

Q38. You are starting your second rotation as an FY1 when you have your meeting with your new clinical supervisor Dr Gregson. He suggests to you that it may be a good idea for you to start a journal club as the department currently doesn't have one. You are not keen to take on the extra responsibility but agree as you want to make a good impression. It is agreed that the club will be organised for every second Wednesday lunchtime. Two weeks later Dr Gregson asks you how the first journal club meeting went as he is looking forward to attending the next meeting. You realise that despite agreeing to organise the meeting you have forgotten to do so.

Choose the most suitable **three** options from the following list:

A. Tell Dr Gregson that the meeting went well and that you are looking forward to seeing him at the next meeting.

B. Explain to Dr Gregson that you forgot to arrange the previous journal club and that you are sorry.

C. Tell Dr Gregson you were unable to organise the meeting as the education department did not have any classrooms available.

D. Deny any memory of this arrangement.

E. Explain that you will begin preparation to organise the next meeting immediately.

F. Tell Dr Gregson that you are sorry for not arranging the meeting but did not want to take on this responsibility in the first place.

G. Contact the education department to book a classroom for the meeting.

H. Email all members of the department advertising the journal club.

Q39. You are an FY1 on the urology ward. Your shift pattern seems unfair compared with your colleagues in general surgery as your shift starts at 6.30 am and finishes at 7.30 pm every day. You have been working for 3 weeks and are feeling very tired and low in mood. You are worried that you are not coping with the pressures of your shift and notice that you are arriving late more frequently. Your SHO has also noted this and quietly speaks to you enquiring whether there is a problem. You break down in tears as you feel exhausted and that you are weak for not being able to cope.

Choose the most suitable **three** options from the following list:

A. Take annual leave and rest from your long working hours.

B. Contact the British Medical Association (BMA) about unfair working hours.

C. Arrange an appointment with your GP to discuss your mental wellbeing.

D. Arrange a meeting with your educational supervisor to discuss your shift pattern.

E. Discuss your concerns with your FY1 colleague, explain that you do not feel that you are coping and ask for their advice.

F. Call in sick tomorrow as you are too tired to continue working.

G. Resign from your foundation training post.

H. Discuss starting an 'hours monitoring exercise' with your Medical Personnel department.

Q40. You are the FY1 on a care of the elderly ward. This placement was not in your top 10 choices and you are struggling to enjoy the role as you feel you are not getting to see any "real medicine". Your registrar asks if you would like to get involved in the ward quality improvement project (QIP), which is focusing on nutritional assessment in patients admitted to the ward. You are aware that junior doctors are encouraged to participate in audits and QIPs, but you are not enjoying this placement and would prefer to wait until your acute medical placement before starting additional projects. Your registrar asks that you get back to her by the end of the week.

Choose the most suitable **three** options from the following list:

A. Decline the offer to get involved with the QIP.

B. Agree to help with the QIP but tell the registrar that if there is somebody more enthusiastic on the ward you are happy to withdraw.

C. Agree to help with the QIP and research how these are performed so that you can show initiative when sharing your ideas.

D. Explain to the registrar that you are not enjoying care of the elderly and you are doing this placement only because you have to.

E. Discuss your concerns about your placement with your educational supervisor as you feel you are not seeing the appropriate amount of medicine.

F. Submit a request to the deanery to change placements.

G. Use this placement to fully understand how the Mental Capacity Act works and how social services are linked with healthcare provision.

H. Do not reply to the registrar's email and hope she doesn't ask you again.

Q41. You are working as the surgical FY1 on a trauma and orthopaedic rotation. Your registrar calls you from theatre and asks you to review Mr Pantous. He is due to have a right knee arthroscopy as he has been complaining of his knee 'giving way'. He came into the day assessment unit this morning and is due to be taken to theatre this afternoon. Your registrar explains that she was due to assess Mr Pantous herself but has been held up in A&E with a trauma call. Mr Pantous has already had his anaesthetic assessment but needs to have a brief review and his right knee site-marked.

Choose the most suitable **three** options from the following list:

A. Agree to assess Mr Pantous and site-mark his leg.

B. Agree to assess Mr Patnous but leave his leg unmarked. The registrar can do this in the anaesthetic room before his procedure.

C. Explain that you are happy to assess Mr Pantous to ensure he is still medically fit but FY1s are not allowed to site-mark.

D. Offer to carry out any jobs that need to be done in A&E so that the registrar can assess Mr Pantous before his afternoon procedure.

E. Call your SHO and ask whether they would be willing to assess Mr Pantous, including site-marking his leg.

F. Tell the registrar that you do not want to assess Mr Pantous because you can't site-mark so do not see the point.

G. Read about arthroscopy to enhance your understanding.

H. Ask the registrar whether you can assist with the arthroscopy as you are keen to learn more about trauma and orthopaedics.

> What are the limitations of an FY1?

Q42. You have started working at a district general hospital as an FY1. When you accepted the post you hadn't been to this hospital before. You have been working for 2 weeks now and have realised that the transport links are poor and you have been late to work several times as the buses are infrequent. You often miss the 7.50 am bus, meaning that you have to get the 8.20 am bus instead, which results in your arriving to work no earlier than 9.15 am. Your registrar has taken you to one side to express his disappointment with your punctuality.

Choose the most suitable **three** options from the following list:

A. Investigate closer accommodation so that you do not need to rely on public transport to get to work.

B. Set your alarm earlier so that you are able to make the 7.50 am bus.

C. Explain the bus-timetabling situation to your registrar and ask whether you can work 15 minutes later each day to make up the time.

D. Tell the registrar that he is being unduly strict; 15 minutes doesn't really make much of a difference to the day.

E. Ignore your registrar because it isn't your fault that transport links are poor in this area.

F. Explain that you will improve your punctuality but accept that you'll probably be late occasionally.

G. Apologise to the registrar and explain that you will improve your punctuality.

H. Ask your SHO whether you can arrange a car-pooling agreement.

Q43. You are on call and are called to see Mr Atiz, a 78-year-old man with chronic colitis and rectal bleeding. The day team has asked you to review his blood results and implement any necessary management. You review his blood results and find that he has become severely anaemic. However, when you assess Mr Atiz he seems well. You briefly examine him but as he is so well-looking you do not feel that a rectal exam is required. You arrange a routine blood transfusion for tomorrow until he can be fully investigated. Later in the day, your cardiac arrest bleeper goes off and you arrive to find that Mr Atiz has gone into cardiac arrest. The on call medical registrar is already in attendance.

Choose the most suitable **three** options from the following list:

A. Discuss your mistake with Martin your FY1 colleague.

B. Discuss your mistake with your educational supervisor.

C. Tell the medical registrar that this is most likely due to his low haemoglobin and explain that you didn't perform a rectal exam.

D. Do not admit your mistake as there are several reasons a patient may go into cardiac arrest.

E. Do not assist with the cardiac arrest as it may complicate any future investigation into Mr Atiz's care.

F. Offer to carry out chest compressions but do not admit you may have missed a rectal bleed.

G. Complete a reflection in your e-portfolio about this case so that you can learn from your mistake.

H. Suggest that they check Mr Atiz's haemoglobin but do not give a reason.

Q44. You have been working on the endocrine ward for 2 months. You work closely with Jane, the second FY1 allocated to endocrinology. You have been getting on well and have been out for several drinks. This morning you notice Jane is behaving very strangely. She keeps making mistakes and seems very agitated. You ask Jane what is wrong and she admits that she took cocaine early this morning whilst she was out with friends. She asks you to keep this information to yourself as she will be fine after lunch.

Choose the most suitable **three** options from the following list:

A. Agree not to tell anybody and keep an eye on Jane.

B. Ignore what Jane has told you and carry on with your tasks.

C. Tell Jane that she must go home immediately as she is not fit to work.

D. Ask your registrar for advice.

E. Report Jane to the police as this is a criminal offence.

F. Inform occupational health about Jane.

G. Inform the GMC that Jane worked under the influence of illicit drugs.

H. Explain that you are not comfortable with this information and tell Jane that she should seek help towards illicit drug use.

Q45. You are sitting in the doctors' mess with Jeff, your FY1 colleague. You overhear a conversation that two other doctors are having. They have read an article in the local newspaper about immigration. You can hear that they are expressing a very negative view towards migrants and at points this becomes evidently bigoted. You and Jeff feel very uncomfortable hearing this conversation as you do not think this is an appropriate discussion in a work environment. Jeff tells you to ignore the other doctors but you are upset with what they have said.

Choose the most suitable **three** options from the following list:

A. Demand that the two doctors leave the mess immediately.

B. Discuss your concerns with your clinical supervisor.

C. Inform human resources (HR) what you have heard and ask them to send an email reminding everyone of the trust's policy.

D. Shout across the mess that the two doctors are ignorant and should keep such bigoted views to themselves.

E. Inform the doctors that their views are bigoted and a breach of GMC and trust policy.

F. Leave the mess with Jeff as saying something will cause a scene.

G. Politely ask which wards the two doctors work on and inform their consultants of what has happened.

H. Quietly speak to the doctors explaining that you do not think such a conversation is appropriate in a work environment.

Q46. You are the FY1 on call in the acute admission unit. You have been very busy throughout the day when a patient's relative approaches you and asks whether you could spare a moment to discuss Mr Bonty in bed 13. You ask what relation they are to Mr Bonty and they explain that they have been close friends for many years and live next door to each other.

Choose the most suitable **three** options from the following list:

A. Explain why Mr Bonty has been admitted and ask his friend to send your regards to the patient.

B. Document your discussion with Mr Bonty's friend in his medical notes.

C. Arrange for the staff nurse to speak with Mr Bonty and his friend as she is likely to know the case better.

D. Politely explain that as the on-call doctor you do not know Mr Bonty well and it would be better for them to speak to his regular doctor.

E. Read Mr Bonty's medical notes so that you are familiar with his case.

F. Tell the friend that you do not have the time to discuss patients as the on-call doctor.

G. Explain that you are happy to meet with Mr Bonty and his friend but do not have time at the moment. You will try to come back to the ward later once you are less busy.

H. Ask the close friend to wait while you confirm whether Mr Bonty is happy for you to speak to them about his medical condition.

> Should you disclose confidential information without discussing this with the patient?

Q47. You are the FY1 in dermatology. You have been working with a small team and have become very close. Your SHO asks you whether you are able to attend a team meeting on their behalf. It is a chance to discuss the exciting research that the team has been involved in. You agree to attend the meeting and prepare a short talk to give. You are aware that there will be several large groups of dermatologists from around the country present. On the day of the talk you are called by your education centre staff to remind you of a compulsory training session you must attend this afternoon.

Choose the most suitable **three** options from the following list:

A. Call your SHO immediately and inform them of the clash in schedule.

B. Call in sick to the training session so that you can attend the team meeting.

C. Arrange for your training session to be rescheduled so that you can attend the dermatology meeting.

D. Attend the morning session of the dermatology meeting and the compulsory training afternoon.

E. Tell your SHO that you attended the talk but there were no points for the team raised.

F. Ignore the training session as attending the dermatology talk will gain you more points on your SHO application.

G. Forward the prepared talk to your SHO.

H. Do not attend your training session as you are now committed to the dermatology meeting.

Q48. You are starting your first rotation as an FY1. You have been given a document explaining that a requirement for you to pass your FY1 year is a 75% attendance at the compulsory FY1 teaching sessions on Tuesday lunchtimes. Five weeks into your rotation you are sent an email as you have not attended any of the compulsory teaching sessions. The email explains that if you do not meet a minimum 75% attendance you will be required to meet with your educational supervisor and also complete an e-learning module to compensate for the reduced attendance.

Choose the most suitable **three** options from the following list:

A. Email the education department requesting a list of what you have missed and complete the associated e-learning modules.

B. Reply to the email explaining that you are too busy on your ward to attend FY1 teaching.

C. Ignore the email from the education department.

D. Reply to the email explaining that you didn't realise the teaching was compulsory.

E. Email your educational supervisor explaining that you didn't realise your error and get advice on moving forward.

F. Discuss this issue with your FY1 colleague for advice.

G. Arrange a meeting with your clinical supervisor to ensure that you are released from ward duties to attend teaching from now on.

H. Ensure that you attend all future compulsory teaching sessions.

Q49. You and Samantha have been friends throughout medical school and have both secured jobs at your first-choice hospital. Although you have been close friends with Samantha you have never worked with her; however, she has always achieved high grades in her exams. You are both working on the vascular surgery ward and notice that the nurses keep asking you to amend prescriptions. You eventually realise that all these prescriptions are written by Samantha.

Choose the most suitable **three** options from the following list:

A. Inform Samantha's clinical supervisor that she is making repeated mistakes with her prescriptions.

B. Tell Samantha to pay attention when prescribing.

C. Speak to Samantha privately. Explain that nurses are struggling with her prescriptions and she should consult the *British National Formulary* (BNF) more often.

D. Tell the other FY1s that Samantha is a dangerous prescriber and they should monitor her prescriptions as well.

E. Tell the nurses that they are being unduly cautious and Samantha's prescriptions are fine.

F. Seek advice from your registrar about how to approach Samantha.

G. Ignore what you have realised; you are both FY1s and are learning.

H. Explain to the ward sister that if the nurses are concerned they should raise their concerns through the appropriate channels.

Q50. You are the FY1 working on medical care of the elderly. You are approached by Jasmine, the general surgery house officer. She explains that one of her patients, 89-year-old Ms Carey, has recovered from her elective colectomy and is now surgically fit for discharge. However, owing to her ongoing reduced mobility as an inpatient, she now requires assessment by physiotherapy (PT) and occupational therapy (OT) before she can be discharged home. This is the only reason she has not been discharged. Jasmine therefore feels that this would be better dealt with by medical care of the elderly.

Choose the most suitable **three** options from the following list:

A. Tell Jasmine that you are sick of surgical patients being palmed off onto medicine. She can call PT/OT for an assessment.

B. Show Jasmine how to refer to PT/OT so that Ms Carey in future may not need to be referred to a medical doctor.

C. Tell Jasmine she should arrange for Ms Carey to be transferred to the trust's rehabilitation hospital for assessment.

D. Agree that this would be better dealt with by your team and accept Jasmine's referral.

E. Review Ms Carey on the surgical ward and decide whether she is suitable for medical care of the elderly.

F. Explain to Jasmine that she will need to refer to your registrar before you can accept care of Ms Carey.

G. Discuss the referral with the registrar and, if they accept Ms Carey, arrange for her to be transferred to your ward.

H. Arrange for Ms Carey to be transferred to your ward and brief the registrar on what you have agreed when they return to the ward.

ANSWERS

A1. This question initially focuses on your commitment to developing your career as a doctor. Currently it is beneficial to have sat at least part 1 of your postgraduate exams (e.g. MRCP/MRCS) before applying for further training posts following your Foundation Programme. In this question you have your exam tomorrow morning. It is clearly important that patient safety is always your priority, but it is also vital you are well-rested. This requires you to find replacement cover but without compromising patient safety by simply leaving (**answer B**). Failing this, the next best option would be the on-call registrar (**answer A**). This would still preserve patient safety as the FY1 tasks would be completed, and the problem is kept within your team – remember the 'escalation ladder'. Leaving notes is generally frowned upon; however, in this question it is the next best option (**answer D**). If a replacement does eventually turn up they will be able to action outstanding jobs. This question also assesses your ability to recognise your limitations as an individual. Working 24 hours straight does not lead to a safe working environment. Therefore, although far from ideal, failing all attempts to find replacement cover and having left all outstanding jobs in a written handover, it is best to leave (**answer C**). The worst option is to work the additional 12 hours (**answer E**).

Ideal order	Your rank choice				
	1st	2nd	3rd	4th	5th
B	4	3	2	1	0
A	3	4	3	2	1
D	2	3	4	3	2
C	1	2	3	4	3
E	0	1	2	3	4

A2. This question focuses on confidentiality. In this question the key is recognising that, although the caller has identified herself as the patient's 'wife', that doesn't automatically grant her access to his medical information. Before disclosing any patient information it is required that you gain the patient's consent. However, it is equally important to be polite and professional to relatives at all times. These are both best achieved by **answer D**. The next best option is **answer B**. This maintains the patient's confidentiality whilst also giving the relative an understandable reason for not disclosing information. She is likely to be appeased by your calling back with an update. **Answer C** is the next best option because, although it is unnecessarily rude, it still maintains confidentiality – which should be your priority here above all else! The final two options are both flawed. However, **answer E** is the better of the two. If the caller is able to answer a series of questions about the patient the chances are she is indeed his wife, and therefore probably next of kin. **Answer A** is the worst option as it is not necessarily true and could cause all manner of problems if the patient has deteriorated or, even worse, passed away since you last saw him.

Ideal order	Your rank choice				
	1st	2nd	3rd	4th	5th
D	4	3	2	1	0
B	3	4	3	2	1
C	2	3	4	3	2
E	1	2	3	4	3
A	0	1	2	3	4

A3. This question focuses on challenging inappropriate behaviour. It is important in healthcare not to feel bullied or pressured into agreeing with a senior's beliefs. However, there is an accepted approach to challenging such behaviour. The favoured option, if practical, is to openly discuss your feelings with the individual concerned in private and come to an agreement that avoids formal proceedings (**answer D**). Unfortunately, this isn't always practical, or you may feel uncomfortable with a potentially confrontational situation. You should always aim to gain advice from your team in order of seniority. Normally, this would be your SHO or registrar. However, as the registrar is in question, your only option is your consultant. In any case, this is also best done in private (**answer E**). If you feel the situation cannot wait until a private opportunity becomes available then still follow the chain of seniority (**answer A**). A direct but often flawed approach is to attempt to challenge the behaviour immediately (**answer B**). This is inflammatory and unlikely to work with an individual so willing to air a controversial opinion. However, the worst option is to ignore the comment to protect your reputation (**answer C**) as you have a duty to the patients and other staff members to develop a professional environment free from bias.

Ideal order	Your rank choice				
	1st	2nd	3rd	4th	5th
D	4	3	2	1	0
E	3	4	3	2	1
A	2	3	4	3	2
B	1	2	3	4	3
C	0	1	2	3	4

A4. This question is focusing on procedural limitations of an FY1. *Tomorrow's Doctors* (GMC, 2009a) clearly defines the practical skills that all FY1s must have on completion of their undergraduate training. Performing a chest drain is not on this list and is an invasive procedure not to be attempted unless one is fully trained. Generally, the approach to developing your practical skills, which is clearly important, is 'see one, do one, teach one'. In reality this translates to: see many, do many more with direct supervision, do some more with less supervision, finally do some unsupervised, and possibly teach one later on! In this question, the best option (although daunting) is **answer C**. The consultant may be unhappy but you have been honest, professional, patient-centred and kept within your limitations. **Answer D** should be your next plan of action. This patient requires urgent treatment and, although not the anaesthetists' responsibility, they are often available and willing to help inexperienced junior staff members with critically ill patients. Failing these two options, your next course of action should be to do nothing (**answer E**) – remember 'first do no harm'. You will do more harm than good if you attempt an invasive procedure without the correct training. Bleeping the registrar (**answer A**) is unlikely to change the situation as he is already not responding. However, the absolute worst and most dangerous option would be to attempt this procedure (**answer B**).

Ideal order	Your rank choice				
	1st	2nd	3rd	4th	5th
C	4	3	2	1	0
D	3	4	3	2	1
E	2	3	4	3	2
A	1	2	3	4	3
B	0	1	2	3	4

A5. This question assesses your ability to maintain professional relationships as well as time keeping – a crucial skill all junior doctors must possess. In this scenario the ward matron has every right to comment on your lateness as it directly affects patient safety as well as all members of the team, including the nursing staff. The matron has acted correctly by asking you to improve your punctuality and has simply reminded you of the protocol if you do not. Taking this into consideration, the best option would therefore be **answer C** as this would (hopefully) prevent any further action being taken whilst maintaining professional relationships with the nursing staff. Following this, the next best option would be **answer A** as this would at least attempt to correct the underlying cause for complaint. The next option, whilst far from ideal, would be to ignore the nurse's comments so as to minimise any further antagonism (**answer B**). The final two options are both poor choices. It is unacceptable to be late this frequently and making no attempt to change is impertinent (**answer E**). However, as the nurse has not done anything wrong reporting her to human resources is clearly unacceptable. Therefore, your final choice should be **answer D**.

Ideal order	Your rank choice				
	1st	2nd	3rd	4th	5th
C	4	3	2	1	0
A	3	4	3	2	1
B	2	3	4	3	2
E	1	2	3	4	3
D	0	1	2	3	4

A6. This question demonstrates your ability to recognise the mental pressures that medicine often puts on individuals, and how to correctly deal with them. It is clear that in this scenario your mood is low following the death of your father and you may not be dealing with this correctly. This will affect your work and may also affect the care you are able to provide to your patients. Therefore, the best option would be to involve your own GP as you may benefit from their help (**answer B**). Following this, you should then involve your direct supervisor (**answer E**), who may be able to authorise compassionate leave, or alter your role in the team. You may also feel it is beneficial to discuss your concerns with your educational supervisor (**answer D**) as even with additional support you may require a departmental change. Many doctors will simply ignore their own health concerns and continue working in times of stress (**answer A**). This is bad practice as it puts you and your patients at risk. However, this option is better than refusing to treat a patient (**answer C**) as this will directly put the patient at risk and is unacceptable. Your priority is always to the patient first.

Ideal order	Your rank choice				
	1st	2nd	3rd	4th	5th
B	4	3	2	1	0
E	3	4	3	2	1
D	2	3	4	3	2
A	1	2	3	4	3
C	0	1	2	3	4

A7. This question focuses on your willingness to admit that you have made an error, and your honesty when rectifying the problem. In this question it is clear that you have made an error that has adversely affected a patient. Your first action should always be to assess/treat the patient and ensure they are not at risk of any further harm. In this scenario this would mean correcting the prescription immediately. However, it is also important that you are open and honest as a doctor. You must admit that you have made an error and apologise to the patient. It is always good practice to inform the nurse when you alter a prescription so that you minimise the risk of an additional error. Therefore, the best option is **answer C**. The next best option is then **answer E** as it also maintains patient safety. However, you should always be open and reflective in your practice to learn from your errors and so asking the nurse to 'cover-up' your mistake is not ideal. **Answer A** would be the next best choice. Although you are withholding information from the nurse and patient, you are still protecting them from further harm. **Answer D** is a poor answer as it does not immediately protect the patient; nor does it encourage an open and honest working environment. **Answer B** is the worst option as it is a false allegation.

Ideal order	Your rank choice				
	1st	2nd	3rd	4th	5th
C	4	3	2	1	0
E	3	4	3	2	1
A	2	3	4	3	2
D	1	2	3	4	3
B	0	1	2	3	4

A8. This question focuses on your commitment to learning and your ability to raise your concerns professionally. It is important that you follow your aspirations and develop your career as a doctor. Your application to become an FY1 is only the first of many future application cycles. In this question you have already attempted to swap and this has not been possible. You should try to find a way to continue your career development whilst maintaining your responsibility to your role as an FY1. Therefore, **answer C** is the best option as it professionally informs the consultant of your career aspirations, whilst maximising your chances of furthering your curriculum vitae (CV). Failing this, the next best option is to gain advice from your educational supervisor as they are responsible for assisting your development throughout the Foundation Programme (**answer B**). The next choice is **answer A** as it maintains patient safety, although acting in a confrontational manner towards your consultant is never going to end well. **Answer E**, whilst ignorant and unprofessional, is the next choice as resigning from your post will affect both patient outcome and your career (**answer D**).

Ideal order	Your rank choice				
	1st	2nd	3rd	4th	5th
C	4	3	2	1	0
B	3	4	3	2	1
A	2	3	4	3	2
E	1	2	3	4	3
D	0	1	2	3	4

A9. This question focuses on your trustworthiness and honesty with your colleagues. It is important to remember that as a doctor you are expected to be professional throughout your career and also your personal life. Considering this, it would be expected that you would maintain confidentiality with your colleagues too. It is also important that you challenge inappropriate behaviour correctly. Therefore the best option would be **answer C**. However, occasionally it may be useful to gain advice from your peers. This is different from gossiping if your intent is sincere. However, if you are planning on disclosing any information it is usually best to gain permission first. Therefore, **answer D** would be your next best choice. **Answer B** is then the next most suitable option. Although it may not be completely honest with Rachel, it will maintain confidentiality with Nick and hopefully discourage Rachel from pursuing her questioning. The final two answers both have their problems. However, as your concern should be with protecting Nick's confidentiality, **answer E** is the next option. The worst option is **answer A** as gossiping is unprofessional.

Ideal order	Your rank choice				
	1st	2nd	3rd	4th	5th
C	4	3	2	1	0
D	3	4	3	2	1
B	2	3	4	3	2
E	1	2	3	4	3
A	0	1	2	3	4

A10. This question is focusing on your commitment to your professional development and your ability to challenge the behaviour of your senior appropriately. In this question, you are clearly not going to be able to meet your learning objectives and Foundation Programme requirements if the remainder of your placement continues in this vein. However, it can

63

sometimes be difficult to judge a placement in the early weeks. Therefore, the best option in this scenario would be to get advice from your clinical supervisor (**answer B**). It is also a good idea to openly and politely discuss your concerns with your GP supervisor. You may find that they are planning clinical contact following your induction as they have indicated. Therefore, your next best option would be **answer D**. **Answer C**, whilst confrontational, is the better option next as you do have educational requirements that the practice should meet. The final two options are both unprofessional. However, resigning from your post as an FY1 is detrimental to your career, and as you are not seeing patients at the surgery you are not compromising their safety. Therefore, the next choice should be **answer E** as **answer A** is the worst option.

	Your rank choice				
Ideal order	1st	2nd	3rd	4th	5th
B	4	3	2	1	0
D	3	4	3	2	1
C	2	3	4	3	2
E	1	2	3	4	3
A	0	1	2	3	4

A11. This question is assessing two aspects of professional practice. Firstly, does the candidate understand their legal duties with regards to driving, and secondly, does the candidate understand confidentiality? The GMC gives clear guidance in terms of driving and your role as a doctor. *Confidentiality: reporting concerns about patients to the DVLA or the DVA* (GMC, 2009c) explains that in this case your duty as a doctor is to explain to the patient that epilepsy may affect their driving and they are legally obliged to inform the DVLA immediately. If the patient refuses to do so (as in this case) you must inform the DVLA's medical advisor immediately. As with all challenging consultations, exploring the patient's concerns may provide insight into the problem and lead to a resolution that is agreeable to both patient and doctor. Therefore, the most appropriate course of action would be **answer A**. However, if this is not possible, your only option would be to inform the patient that you will be disclosing this information to the DVLA as it is your legal duty to do so (**answer B**). **Answer D**, although clearly not winning any prizes in communication skills, is an accurate statement and would be the next most appropriate action. **Answer E** is an indirect approach and relies on the GP reading your discharge summary and acting upon this information. This answer is a poor choice because it is your duty to inform the DVLA as you have been made aware of the problem. However, it is more appropriate than **answer C**, which is clearly the least appropriate choice as it would put the patient and the public at risk, and you are failing in your duty as a doctor.

Ideal order	Your rank choice				
	1st	2nd	3rd	4th	5th
A	4	3	2	1	0
B	3	4	3	2	1
D	2	3	4	3	2
E	1	2	3	4	3
C	0	1	2	3	4

A12. This question is focusing on your honesty and integrity. It is not uncommon to feel overworked as an FY1 but in this scenario it is evident that you have made a mistake and this should be dealt with. However, you cannot ignore patient safety, which should be at the forefront of every question you answer. Therefore **answer C** is the most appropriate action to take. This will ensure the patient does not come to harm and that you have acknowledged your mistake. **Answer B** would be the next best option as this shows you are open and honest with regard to your error. **Answer D** should be your next choice as this also shows that you are willing to admit to your mistakes. However, asking the registrar not to disclose this information is far from ideal as it creates an environment of covering up mistakes. **Answer A** and **answer E** are both clearly poor choices as you would be lying and you would find yourself referred to the GMC fitness to practice panel fairly promptly if this were the case. However, as answer E would fictitiously accuse a colleague, this is clearly the least appropriate choice.

Ideal order	Your rank choice				
	1st	2nd	3rd	4th	5th
C	4	3	2	1	0
B	3	4	3	2	1
D	2	3	4	3	2
A	1	2	3	4	3
E	0	1	2	3	4

A13. This question is assessing your ability to challenge a decision made by a senior member of the team both appropriately and respectfully. It is good practice to learn to ask 'why?' so that you can develop your own decision-making skills and to allow the team an opportunity to debate the correct choice for the patient. It is also not unreasonable to recognise that you may think an 'incorrect' decision is being made owing to your lack of experience and knowledge. Therefore, asking in an open and polite manner is a key skill for doctors to possess. In this scenario, **answer C** is the most appropriate choice as it keeps the patient at the centre of your task whilst providing the consultant with the opportunity to explain or even change their decision. **Answer B** would be the next most appropriate choice as this demonstrates your enthusiasm whilst providing the consultant with the same opportunity as answer C. **Answer E** should be your next choice as it still focuses on what is best for Mr Phillips, although this approach would not be well received. **Answer A** is not a sensible solution to this problem. You are told that the best scan is cystoscopy so re-reading the article is on a par with not acting, which is rarely the correct choice. **Answer D** is the least appropriate answer. The care of a patient falls under the named consultant and so they are responsible for the outcome. Unless a situation is actually dangerous you are obliged to follow the requests of your consultant.

Ideal order	Your rank choice				
	1st	2nd	3rd	4th	5th
C	4	3	2	1	0
B	3	4	3	2	1
E	2	3	4	3	2
A	1	2	3	4	3
D	0	1	2	3	4

A14. This question is based on your commitment to professional development. If focuses on dealing with confrontation appropriately and balancing your responsibilities as a doctor and your personal responsibilities away from work. As with all scenarios, the best way to diffuse any situation is to attempt to understand the individual involved. In this case, exploring the concerns of the coordinator may provide an explanation as to why they appear inflexible and by suggesting a compromise you may find this appeases all parties involved. Therefore **answer E** is the most appropriate first choice. **Answer A** is the next logical approach. The hospital still maintains its cover (therefore protecting patient safety) whilst allowing you to attend the wedding. You may, however, face a perturbed rota coordinator on your return. In this situation, escalating your concerns to your clinical supervisor (**answer C**) is the next most appropriate measure to take. You have clearly attempted to solve the problem and could benefit from senior advice. **Answer D** is not an incorrect answer, but it should be low on your list as it will not solve the problem and can therefore be deemed as not acting – an answer generally unpopular with the SJT. Finally, **answer B** is clearly the least appropriate answer as you will put patient safety at risk and leave your team understaffed and overworked.

Ideal order	Your rank choice				
	1st	2nd	3rd	4th	5th
E	4	3	2	1	0
A	3	4	3	2	1
C	2	3	4	3	2
D	1	2	3	4	3
B	0	1	2	3	4

A15. This question is assessing your knowledge on patient confidentiality and also how you will deal with a sensitive situation. The GMC *Confidentiality* guideline (GMC, 2009b) gives clear advice on how to approach this topic. You must gain permission from a patient to disclose medical information to anybody not directly involved in their medical care. Do not assume that the family is privileged to this information. In this scenario you would need to ask for the patient's permission before speaking to his daughter. However, it is also important to understand that family members are often very worried and so you should be polite and caring (**answer C**). The next most appropriate choice would be **answer B** as this maintains the patient's confidentiality; however, it is likely to upset the daughter further. **Answer D** is then a fair third choice. The daughter is already aware that her father has an upset stomach and so you have not disclosed any new information and he is likely to require observations. Therefore, you have not given inaccurate information. However, this is avoiding the problem and should not score highly on your priorities. The final two choices are both poor. **Answer E**, which is the next most appropriate choice, does maintain the patient's confidentiality but is dismissive, and abdicating to a nurse is never a good idea. **Answer A** is clearly the least appropriate choice as it breaks the patient's confidentiality.

Ideal order	Your rank choice				
	1st	2nd	3rd	4th	5th
C	4	3	2	1	0
B	3	4	3	2	1
D	2	3	4	3	2
E	1	2	3	4	3
A	0	1	2	3	4

A16. This question is assessing your willingness to challenge inappropriate behaviour in the workplace, in this case racism. It can be difficult to challenge the behaviour of senior colleagues but you have the right to work in an environment free from prejudice. In this scenario, the anaesthetist is acting totally unprofessionally and in contravention of good medical practice guidance. **Answer C** is the most appropriate action to take. It challenges the behaviour whilst remaining professional. These situations will always be difficult but should result in formal grievance. Therefore it would be wise to have the support of your supervisor so that the formal procedure can be followed correctly. Therefore, **answer E** and **answer D** are the next most appropriate choices respectively. It can seem easier to stay quiet and not challenge your senior, especially as you may be concerned about 'getting a name' for yourself. However, this is incorrect and will be deemed as not acting – a quality that is not desirable for foundation training. However, this is clearly better than agreeing with the consultant and so **answer B** would be deemed more appropriate than **answer A**, which is clearly the least appropriate answer.

Ideal order	Your rank choice				
	1st	2nd	3rd	4th	5th
C	4	3	2	1	0
E	3	4	3	2	1
D	2	3	4	3	2
B	1	2	3	4	3
A	0	1	2	3	4

A17. This question is focusing on your ability to remain professional in the receipt of gifts. This is not an uncommon problem. Many patients like to show their gratitude for the care they have received and it can be perceived as rude to reject a gift. However, the GMC has clear guidance on the acceptance of personal gifts. In this scenario, the main problem is the value of the gift. A 'thank you' card and box of chocolates that can be shared amongst the ward team is generally acceptable. However, expensive individual gifts are not to be accepted as they may complicate the patient–doctor relationship that you have developed. It is important to remain humble and polite so as to avoid upsetting the patient. Therefore, **answer C** is the most appropriate course of action. **Answer D** is then the next most appropriate choice; however, mentioning GMC guidance may make you appear inhuman. Seeking advice would be sensible at this point to ensure that you are following the trust's policy correctly (**answer B**). In certain situations, accepting gifts can be acceptable if they are declared on the gifts register. In this scenario, that would be better than simply accepting an expensive gift and therefore **answer E** is slightly more appropriate than **answer A,** which is the least appropriate choice.

Ideal order	Your rank choice				
	1st	2nd	3rd	4th	5th
C	4	3	2	1	0
D	3	4	3	2	1
B	2	3	4	3	2
E	1	2	3	4	3
A	0	1	2	3	4

A18. This question is assessing your ability to challenge inappropriate behaviour, in this case James's romantic relationship with a patient. The GMC's *Good Medical Practice* (GMC, 2013a) has clear guidelines on not using your position as a doctor to develop emotional or physical relationships with patients. In this scenario, James is in clear breach of this guidance and you have attempted to intervene but to no avail. Therefore, your only option is to escalate your concerns. The most appropriate course of action would be to gain advice from your senior beforehand (**answer E**). A sensible decision following this would be to discuss your concerns with your education supervisor if your registrar isn't able to help (**answer A**). You would then need to confront James directly about his actions (**answer C**) as, so far, he has dismissed your concerns. It is unlikely this would work but you should always attempt to solve problems between you and the individual involved before formally lodging a grievance. Unfortunately, in this scenario you would now have no option but to report James formally to the GMC for breach of duty (**answer D**). Although making a formal complaint will always be difficult, you have a duty as a doctor to report behaviour that you feel is unsafe or inappropriate. The GMC will be fair and show due diligence in these instances taking all matters into consideration. The least appropriate choice would be to do nothing (**answer B**) as you have seen behaviour with which you are clearly uncomfortable.

Ideal order	Your rank choice				
	1st	2nd	3rd	4th	5th
E	4	3	2	1	0
A	3	4	3	2	1
C	2	3	4	3	2
D	1	2	3	4	3
B	0	1	2	3	4

A19. This question is centred on a common issue amongst medical practitioners: staying abreast of current guidelines and treatment regimens. Although this is certainly a challenge, the GMC does expect this from doctors. In this scenario you are in a difficult position. You are uncomfortable with the practice you are seeing but clearly this GP's patients are very fond of him and, as a new doctor, you do not want to seem obnoxious. However, you cannot ignore what you have seen and you will need to challenge the behaviour of the older GP appropriately and respectfully. Your first choice should be to raise your concerns openly with the GP himself and to discuss what you have seen (**answer C**). This will provide a learning opportunity for you both, as well as maintaining your professional relationship. Failing that approach, as you haven't seen anything that is dangerous you can wait until your GP trainer returns in the afternoon and seek their advice (**answer B**). In this scenario, **answer D** would be the next most appropriate choice. It would address your concerns but is unduly rude and could clearly be approached in a more sensitive manner. However, ignoring what you are concerned about (**answer A**) and informing the GMC (**answer E**) are undoubtedly inappropriate. Involving the GMC is the most inappropriate choice as this is a matter that could be easily corrected through the practice.

Ideal order	Your rank choice				
	1st	2nd	3rd	4th	5th
C	4	3	2	1	0
B	3	4	3	2	1
D	2	3	4	3	2
A	1	2	3	4	3
E	0	1	2	3	4

A20. This question is focusing on your commitment to learning and professional development. Starting foundation training is only the beginning of a lifelong agreement with education. Throughout your career you will have revalidation exercises and portfolio assessments. Therefore it is important to meet your academic deadlines. In this scenario it is clear that this has not occurred and so it is best to be completely honest with your supervisor and ask for their advice (**answer A**). You will need the assistance of your senior colleagues to complete your assessments before meeting with your supervisor and so **answer C** would be the next most appropriate choice. **Answer D** is the next appropriate choice as you may be able to arrange group sessions with senior colleagues to go through some of the less individualised assessments, such as core procedures. The final two options are both very risky. **Answer E**, which is the next most appropriate choice, may work if you are able to complete your work but is indefensible if you aren't. Acknowledging your mistakes and asking for assistance is a key quality that you must develop in foundation training. Ignoring a problem (**answer B**) does not make it go away and will ultimately cause you more worry and anguish in the near future.

Ideal order	Your rank choice				
	1st	2nd	3rd	4th	5th
A	4	3	2	1	0
C	3	4	3	2	1
D	2	3	4	3	2
E	1	2	3	4	3
B	0	1	2	3	4

A21. This question is focusing on your knowledge and understanding of the GMC (2009b) guidance on confidentiality. It states that there are certain occasions where disclosing confidential information is required. In this scenario, as you are concerned for the safety of Mrs Patel's children, you are required to disclose this information either to social services or even to the police if you feel they are in imminent danger. However, in most cases where you plan to disclose confidential information, you should initially attempt to negotiate with the patient to come to an agreement and gain their consent (**answer D**). If this is not practical you are required to go against the wishes of the patient and disclose the information nonetheless. You should still inform the patient that you are going to disclose their confidential information (**answer C**). Calling the police without informing Mrs Patel (**answer E**) may seem like a poor choice but in this scenario it would be the next most appropriate answer. From what you have been told, you are worried about the safety of Mrs Patel and her children. Therefore, you cannot morally allow her to leave and return to a possibly dangerous environment. Gaining further history (**answer B**) is irrelevant at this stage as you are already concerned enough to act. Finally, the worst option would be to do nothing and allow Mrs Patel to leave (**answer A**).

Ideal order	Your rank choice				
	1st	2nd	3rd	4th	5th
D	4	3	2	1	0
C	3	4	3	2	1
E	2	3	4	3	2
B	1	2	3	4	3
A	0	1	2	3	4

A22. This question is focusing on challenging malpractice behaviour and your understanding of the GMC whistleblowing policy. In this scenario you are worried that an individual surgeon is causing poor outcomes. You attempt to raise your concerns but are met by an 'organisational wall'. However, having correctly followed the escalation protocol you will have very little option but to raise your concerns publicly as you genuinely feel that patients are at risk as long as Prof Woodson continues to operate. Therefore, it would be sensible to contact your defence organisation for advice (**answer E**). You would then have to raise your concerns publicly in an attempt to protect patient outcomes as advised in the *GMC Policy on Whistleblowing* (GMC, n.d.) (**answer D**). Although it will seem like a very difficult decision, you have acted correctly and out of genuine concern for patient safety – the Francis Inquiry report (Mid Staffordshire NHS Foundation Trust, 2013) is a poignant memory of what happens when this doesn't happen. At this point, it would be polite to inform the medical director (**answer B**) so that they can prepare for the media outcry that is likely to occur. Contacting your deanery to transfer posts (**answer A**) would not be unreasonable as you will likely feel that you have made your current position untenable. The least appropriate action would be simply not to act as this could put patients at risk (**answer C**).

	Your rank choice				
Ideal order	1st	2nd	3rd	4th	5th
E	4	3	2	1	0
D	3	4	3	2	1
B	2	3	4	3	2
A	1	2	3	4	3
C	0	1	2	3	4

A23. This question is assessing the candidate's understanding of FY1 expected core competencies. Urinary catheterisation is a skill that all FY1 doctors should be competent with and therefore your first point of call should be to attend Mrs Coff and attempt the catheterisation (**answer C**). You should then consider asking your registrar for assistance (**answer B**) as this would keep the problem within your team in accordance with correct escalation protocol. At this stage, requesting assistance from a urology SHO would be sensible as they are likely to be more confident with difficult catheterisation (**answer A**). Making a reflective e-portfolio entry about difficult situations and how you overcome them (**answer E**) is an important aspect of continued professional development, but in this scenario should rank low on your list of priorities. Clearly, **answer D** is the least appropriate choice as you should be willing and able to catheterise any patient and the nurses have correctly informed you.

Ideal order	Your rank choice				
	1st	2nd	3rd	4th	5th
C	4	3	2	1	0
B	3	4	3	2	1
A	2	3	4	3	2
E	1	2	3	4	3
D	0	1	2	3	4

A24. This question is focusing on your ability to be open and honest with your colleagues (including your senior colleagues). In this scenario, you have made it clear to the registrar that you feel undersupported and would appreciate more input from him. Despite raising your concerns, the registrar has not changed his behaviour. He is now asking for feedback on his performance and it is important that this is genuine feedback so that the individual involved can develop. Therefore, the most appropriate choice would be **answer C** as this is the most honest approach to take with the registrar and more importantly will give the registrar constructive feedback for him to improve upon. The next most appropriate option would be **answer B** as this will also provide constructive feedback, but is not as open as you could be. In this scenario, **answer E** would be the next most appropriate choice; however, as you had previously asked for more support this is unlikely to make a big difference, but at least you are being honest in your approach. The final two choices are both poor as it would be inappropriate to score the registrar well when you have concerns, but it is also important that you are required to partake in feedback to enable your colleagues to develop. However, in this scenario lying would be far worse and so **answer A** would be your next choice, with **answer D** as the least appropriate answer.

Ideal order	Your rank choice				
	1st	2nd	3rd	4th	5th
C	4	3	2	1	0
B	3	4	3	2	1
E	2	3	4	3	2
A	1	2	3	4	3
D	0	1	2	3	4

A25. This question is focusing on your understanding of commitment to professionalism, in particular punctuality and reliability. This situation is not too uncommon and, although it may seem unfair, it is wise not to arrange leave unless authorised from your rota coordinator. Ultimately the hospital must have its on-call positions filled each day to maintain patient safety. However, it would be wise to discuss this with your consultant first as they may be able to offer assistance and suggest a solution (**answer C**). This may not be productive, in which case the next most appropriate answer is to attend the on call (**answer E**). As it is clear in this scenario that you have been working above and beyond your scheduled hours, it would be a good idea to complete a retrospective hours monitoring exercise (**answer B**). This may provide two benefits. Firstly, the deanery may allocate additional doctors to this firm in the future and secondly you may receive a retrospective back-payment. If you genuinely did plan on not attending the shift, informing the rota coordinator (**answer A**) would allow her to try to find somebody else to cover, thus maintaining patient safety. However, this would likely result in an unauthorised absence and formal disciplinary hearing. The least appropriate option would be to call in sick on the day (**answer D**) as this would compromise patient safety by impairing the on-call service.

Ideal order	Your rank choice				
	1st	2nd	3rd	4th	5th
C	4	3	2	1	0
E	3	4	3	2	1
B	2	3	4	3	2
A	1	2	3	4	3
D	0	1	2	3	4

A26. This question is assessing the candidate's ability to recognise their own professional limitations. In this scenario it is that you are in over your head and need support. However, you also have two very unwell patients who you need to see before thinking about relieving yourself of the added burden of carrying the registrar bleeper. As with all questions, patient safety must be your priority. Therefore the most appropriate action would be **answer D** as this prioritises the cardiac arrest correctly. Following this, the next most appropriate choice is **answer C**. This attempts to maintain patient safety as best as you can in a difficult situation. **Answer A** is the next most appropriate choice. It attempts to maintain patient safety whilst also trying to gain extra support. However, it is ranked lower than the first two answers because it suggests you are not considering the severity of the cardiac arrest. The final two options are both irresponsible. It is indefensible to ignore a cardiac arrest call with the assumption that the remainder of the team will arrive (**answer B**). What if every other member of the team had that thought? However, the least appropriate answer would be to turn off the bleeper as this would pose the most risk to the most patients (**answer E**).

Ideal order	Your rank choice				
	1st	**2nd**	**3rd**	**4th**	**5th**
D	4	3	2	1	0
C	3	4	3	2	1
A	2	3	4	3	2
B	1	2	3	4	3
E	0	1	2	3	4

A27. This question is focusing on challenging inappropriate behaviour correctly. By all accounts the registrar's opinion is likely to be unfounded according to previous feedback and, even if this opinion was correct, the registrar should have discussed her concerns with Carol and, more importantly, given her constructive methods to improve her performance. In these scenarios it is important not to become involved personally but instead to support and guide the individual concerned to take appropriate action. Therefore, the most appropriate action would be for Carol to seek support from her clinical supervisor (**answer E**). Approaching the registrar directly is a fair second choice as it may resolve this grievance (**answer A**). However, this makes the situation worse as the registrar has already spoken out of turn and so this should be advised only after Carol discusses the matter with her clinical supervisor first. Ignoring the comment in this scenario would be the next most appropriate advice to give to Carol (**answer C**). Although it is generally not advisable 'not to act' in the SJT, on occasions such as this ignoring the comment may be a better approach once directly approaching the individual concerns has failed. The key in this question is remembering not to become involved yourself. Therefore the final two choices, which involve becoming directly involved, are the least appropriate choices. However, discussing your concerns with Carol's clinical supervisor (**answer D**) is slightly better than challenging the registrar yourself (**answer B**) – which is the least appropriate answer as it would probably inflame the situation further.

Ideal order	Your rank choice				
	1st	**2nd**	**3rd**	**4th**	**5th**
E	4	3	2	1	0
A	3	4	3	2	1
C	2	3	4	3	2
D	1	2	3	4	3
B	0	1	2	3	4

A28. This situation is focused on reliability but also assesses your ability to act in the correct manner seeing that you are not the individual directly involved. As you are concerned with James's attendance, the most appropriate course of action would to discuss this with your registrar as they will advise you on what to do next (**answer E**). Your next choice should be to discuss your concerns with the rota coordinator so that they are aware of the problems with the on-call rota (**answer C**). This may enable them to make changes and/or provide additional cover in the future. You may find it helpful to approach James to discuss what he has been doing. In this scenario, explaining that you are unhappy with his behaviour would be more appropriate than giving him advice on use of social media (although clearly this would be of benefit to him). Therefore **answer A** and **answer D** are your next two choices respectively. Informing James's clinical supervisor directly is the least appropriate choice (**answer B**). This would be seen as formally complaining about James and, at this stage, trying to resolve conflicts locally is always a better solution.

	Your rank choice				
Ideal order	1st	2nd	3rd	4th	5th
E	4	3	2	1	0
C	3	4	3	2	1
A	2	3	4	3	2
D	1	2	3	4	3
B	0	1	2	3	4

A29. This question is focusing on your ability to be open and honest when dealing with mistakes. Regardless of any adverse events, Mrs Kildin was mistreated by the hospital and should be informed. This should be done openly without any attempt to hide or alter the facts. Therefore the most appropriate action is **answer C**. The next appropriate course of action would be to inform your consultant (**answer D**). This has two purposes; firstly, it will allow the consultant to recommend additional medical management and secondly it escalates the incident correctly within Mrs Kildin's team. When an incident occurs that endangers a patient you must submit a serious incident form (**answer E**). This allows the trust to investigate how the incident happened and attempt to change practice so that future incidents do not occur. Although these forms are important, they do not rank highly in your list of priorities and should come after your clinical tasks. It is inappropriate not to disclose information to patients once an incident has occurred. However, in this scenario waiting for the bloods results would at least reassure you that no harm had come of this incident (**answer B**). However, clearly the least appropriate action would be to ignore the error entirely based purely on a patient's lack of physical signs (**answer A**).

Ideal order	Your rank choice				
	1st	2nd	3rd	4th	5th
C	4	3	2	1	0
D	3	4	3	2	1
E	2	3	4	3	2
B	1	2	3	4	3
A	0	1	2	3	4

A30. This question is assessing your ability to prioritise tasks, escalate appropriately and respond when a clinical incident has occurred. The most appropriate choice is to assess the patient and ensure they have not come to any harm over this incident (**answer D**). Remember, patient safety always comes above any other option. Following this the remainder of the question is focusing on correctly dealing with incident escalation. You should next confront the FY1 involved in this scenario to discuss what happened and to explain that you will be completing an incident report (**answer A**). This will provide an opportunity for both sides of the incident to be discussed, allowing you both to learn from what has happened. Informing the ward manager/senior nurse is a sensible choice at this point as they are responsible for patient transfer and also will be involved in investigating any incident form that is submitted for their ward (**answer C**). At this point you can now submit your incident form (**answer B**). It is important to try to learn from these situations and so reflecting on what has happened should not be ignored (**answer E**). In this scenario, it is the least appropriate action simply because the other four options take a higher priority. There is nothing 'inappropriate' about answer E.

Ideal order	Your rank choice				
	1st	2nd	3rd	4th	5th
D	4	3	2	1	0
A	3	4	3	2	1
C	2	3	4	3	2
B	1	2	3	4	3
E	0	1	2	3	4

A31. This question is focusing on your understanding of your limitations as an FY1. Put simply, you are not allowed to consent for procedures. The GMC describes informed consent as 'the process through which doctors obtain permission from a patient to perform an investigation or instigate management'. In order to do this, doctors must themselves be competent in the investigation and disclose relevant information to the patients, allowing them to voluntarily make an informed choice regarding consent. As an FY1, you will not be able to meet these requirements. However, you do need to learn – remember a key requirement in the SJT is your ability to demonstrate commitment to lifelong learning. Therefore, the most appropriate first choice would be **answer C**. Your next choice would be **answer A** as this still states the salient point but is more receptive than **answer E**, which would be option 3. Consenting the patient yourself is wrong under any circumstances. However, in this scenario recognising that you would not be competent to answer all of the possible questions the patient may have is an attempt at improving the outcome (**answer D**). The least appropriate answer would be **answer B**. Although consent has once been taken, it becomes invalid if the form used to document this consent is absent. There would be no proof of what risks were explained and that the patient agreed to them. Consent must always be gained in accordance with the GMC guidance – even if it is just 're-signing' the physical form.

Ideal order	Your rank choice				
	1st	2nd	3rd	4th	5th
C	4	3	2	1	0
A	3	4	3	2	1
E	2	3	4	3	2
D	1	2	3	4	3
B	0	1	2	3	4

A32. This question is focusing on your understanding of your limitations as an FY1. Although you will often come under pressure to discharge patients, you must remain firm in that FY1s do not have the authority to discharge patients from hospital. Of course, in practical terms the FY1 will complete the discharge paperwork, but a senior doctor has made the decision that the patient is suitable for discharge. In this scenario, there is no documentation that the team caring for Mr Hurst is in agreement with discharge. However, another senior doctor on call may be willing to make this decision. More likely than not, they also will not be willing to make this decision over a weekend as they do not know the patient fully. Therefore **answer A** is the most appropriate choice. The next most appropriate action would be to explain to the discharge team that this is not a decision you are able (or willing) to make. **Answer D** does this in the best manner. **Answer E**, whilst unnecessarily confrontational, would be your next most appropriate choice in this scenario. Calling Mr Hurst's consultant is not appropriate as they are not on call and should not be disturbed over the weekend because of hospital pressures (**answer C**). The least appropriate option is to assess and discharge Mr Hurst as FY1s do not discharge patients (**answer B**).

Ideal order	Your rank choice				
	1st	2nd	3rd	4th	5th
A	4	3	2	1	0
D	3	4	3	2	1
E	2	3	4	3	2
C	1	2	3	4	3
B	0	1	2	3	4

A33. This question is assessing your ability to recognise your own personal limitations. Illness cannot be predicted and you should not feel pressure to work if you are not fit to practice. This will put both yourself and your patients at risk. Generally, hospitals will insist that staff members do not attend the hospital for 48 hours after diarrhoea and vomiting have stopped. This is to limit the risk of spread of infection. In this scenario, the most appropriate option is **answer A**. This will ensure you do not feel obliged to work when you are ill whilst attempting to minimise the impact this has on the on-call team. Of course, if you are unable to arrange cover because you are too unwell or it is too short notice you should simply call in sick (**answer E**). In this scenario, discussing your concerns with your education supervisor is the next most appropriate choice as this may lead to a change in the level of staffing, thereby reducing the pressure put on staff members for legitimately missing work (**answer D**). Attending your shift is inappropriate as you will put colleagues and patients at risk of contracting a diarrhoeal illness. However, **answer C** demonstrates some willingness to monitor your wellbeing and is marginally better than simply working your on-call shift when you may not be fit. Therefore, the least appropriate choice is **answer B**.

Ideal order	Your rank choice				
	1st	2nd	3rd	4th	5th
A	4	3	2	1	0
E	3	4	3	2	1
D	2	3	4	3	2
C	1	2	3	4	3
B	0	1	2	3	4

A34. This question is focusing on confidentiality and is indeed a challenging situation. Remember, there are four occasions when you are required to disclose confidential information. In this scenario, the protection of others (i.e. the partner) from contracting a serious and life-altering condition requires you to act. If at all practical or possible, it is advisable to try to persuade the individual concerned to disclose their information themself (**answer C**). Failing this, you must inform the individual that you are going to disclose their information before doing so (**answer A**). This should be done in writing as well as verbally. The important factor in this scenario is realising that you have a duty to protect the partner. Without barrier protection they are at very high risk of contracting HIV. In this scenario, **answer D** would be the next most appropriate choice. Although it is strongly inadvisable to mislead patients in any way, at least you have made an attempt to protect Mr Mullin's partner from harm. Offering your personal opinion as a doctor is not appropriate as doctors must always be non-judgemental (**answer B**). Respecting Mr Mullin's wishes is clearly the least appropriate choice as it would leave his partner at high risk (**answer E**).

Ideal order	Your rank choice				
	1st	2nd	3rd	4th	5th
C	4	3	2	1	0
A	3	4	3	2	1
D	2	3	4	3	2
B	1	2	3	4	3
E	0	1	2	3	4

A35. This question is focusing on confidentiality. Patient lists contain personal information as well as medical information. In this scenario it is very likely that somebody not involved in the care of your patients will have seen the information on the list. Therefore this is a breach of confidentiality. In this instance, the correct course of action would be to attempt to minimise the breach in confidentiality by removing the list from the canteen (**answer C**). If you do make a mistake it is important to be open and apologise to those involved (**answer G**). It is also important to inform your supervisor/consultant if you make an error so that they are fully informed (**answer F**). This will allow them to identify any training needs but also to be prepared for any formal grievances.

Reflecting on your errors is vitally important to learn from them and to prevent them from recurring. In this scenario, this would have been an appropriate choice **if** you were selecting a fourth option. However, in this case **answer D** is good practice but not a critical action here. Ignoring the matter is not the appropriate approach and this would result in confidential information being exposed. Therefore **answer A** and **answer E** are not correct. Driving back to the hospital would limit the damage of an exposed list but is not practical. You need to develop a balance between work and rest and returning to work is not sensible. The on-call/out-of-hours team is there specifically to continue caring once you have left. Therefore **answer B** is not a suitable choice. **Answer H** is not relevant here. Calling a friend or relative is not necessary. The breach has occurred and you simply need to correct your mistake.

A	B	C	D	E	F	G	H
0	0	4	0	0	4	4	0

A36. The basis to this question revolves around dealing with mistakes. However, you cannot ignore the patient safety element as the nurse is alluding to what could very easily be an allergic reaction and even anaphylaxis. Therefore immediately returning to the ward to assess James must be one of your choices (**answer F**). The remainder of your choices should then focus on dealing with your error appropriately. In this scenario that would be explaining to James what happened and apologising for your error (**answer B**), and updating his medical notes and drug chart in an attempt to prevent this error happening again (**answer H**).

In this scenario the nurse has followed the correct course of action by bleeping you as James has deteriorated. Therefore it would be incorrect to chastise the nurse (**answer C**). Nor would it be appropriate to postpone assessing James as he is likely to have had a reaction to penicillin and could be very unwell (**answer E**). However, it is equally inappropriate to call the cardiac arrest team (**answer G**) as the nurse does not give you any information to indicate that James is peri-arrest. Informing your registrar (**answer A**) is a sensible decision in the overall management of unwell patients but it would not be in the top three priorities in this scenario. Finally, destroying medical notes or drug charts is always incorrect. If an error has been made the document, in this case the drug chart, should be clearly marked as erroneous and filed in the patient's notes. Therefore **answer D** is incorrect.

A	B	C	D	E	F	G	H
0	4	0	0	0	4	0	4

A37. This question is focusing on your ability to challenge inappropriate behaviour correctly, in this case racism. The patient should be told that he is acting inappropriately and this behaviour is not tolerated (**answer A**). However, the best method for calming down agitated or disruptive patients is to talk to them. Exploring the patient's concerns may provide an insight into why he is being disruptive (**answer G**). This may provide a solution to his behaviour. It is important to ensure that other patients have not been disrupted or upset as they will have probably heard the commotion (**answer E**). Remember patient care trumps almost all other choices.

In this scenario the patient is being verbally abusive but is not acting aggressively or attempting to intimidate anybody. Therefore it would not be appropriate to involve the police (**answer C**) or security (**answer B**) at this stage. Of course if the situation escalated then security may be required. Asking the patient to leave the hospital (**answer H**) without explaining that his behaviour is disruptive would needlessly put the patient's health at risk. He may quieten down after his warning, allowing him to receive treatment. Sedating an agitated or intoxicated patient is unethical and dangerous if your only desired outcome is peace and quiet (**answer D**). Sedation should be used only by trained staff members in circumstances where patients are at risk to themselves or others. Asking a member of staff to simply ignore a patient's comments is not appropriate as it is likely to lead to the nurse feeling poorly supported (**answer F**). The patient's behaviour is inappropriate and should be treated as such.

A	B	C	D	E	F	G	H
4	0	0	0	4	0	4	0

A38. This question is assessing your ability to show commitment to your educational and professional development, dealing with mistakes, and being honest as a doctor. Being asked to take on an additional responsibility by consultants is not uncommon. They are often trying to develop your skills as a member of the team and these opportunities should be taken to enable you to develop your career. In this scenario, you have made an honest mistake and it has slipped your mind. You should admit this immediately to the consultant (**answer B**). It is almost certain that the consultant will accept your apology and simply expect the club to start on the next Wednesday. You can further allay any potential disappointment by explaining that you will start planning the first meeting immediately (**answer E**) by booking a classroom for the meeting to take place (**answer G**).

Emailing members of the department (**answer H**) would be a good idea to advertise your journal club. However, it would not be a priority at this stage as you haven't arranged the meeting yet or set an agenda. Therefore it would be better to do that once you can provide some information. The worst approach to this type of situation is attempting to lie or conceal that you may have made a mistake. Honesty and integrity are vital to a career in medicine and a breach in this may result in your referral to a GMC fitness to practice hearing. This may seem trivial but even 'insignificant lies' cast doubt into your colleagues' minds. Therefore **answer A, answer C** and **answer D** are not correct. Shying away from simple responsibilities (**answer F**) is not advisable as you should be attempting to develop your career by seeking out these types of roles.

A	B	C	D	E	F	G	H
0	4	0	0	4	0	4	0

A39. This question is focusing on your ability to recognise your limitations as an FY1, including your own health and wellbeing. In this scenario you are clearly working a high number of hours and this will take its toll on your mental wellbeing. Fatigue is complicated and it is still not fully understood but you are already showing signs of it as your punctuality is deteriorating. You should arrange a meeting with your educational supervisor to discuss your concerns (**answer D**) as they may be able to suggest coping strategies or speak with the rota coordinator. It would also be wise to meet with your own GP (**answer C**). They will be able to assess your mental wellbeing from a non-biased viewpoint and would be able to treat you if necessary. Finally, HR departments routinely conduct hours-monitoring exercises to ensure their trainees are not being put under excessive pressure. You should contact the HR department raising your concerns and asking for your ward to be examined (**answer H**). This may lead to an altered rota and a more appropriate working balance.

In this scenario, calling in sick (**answer F**) and taking annual leave (**answer A**) are not appropriate. If your working hours are too long your aim should be to raise this correctly and allow due process to occur, which will hopefully result in an improved rota. Calling in sick and taking annual leave are only temporary solutions and will not help you in the long run. Contacting the BMA (**answer B**) before allowing your own HR department a chance to act is not necessary and would be deemed unprofessional. Resigning from your foundation training post (**answer G**) is rarely going to be the correct answer. You have trained for many years to become a doctor and long hours are only one of the challenges you'll have to overcome in your career. However, remember to escalate concerns using the appropriate channel before making any rash decisions. Finally, discussing your concerns with your peer (**answer E**) is unlikely to lead to any change and, although this may seem an easy option, it will not tackle your concerns.

A	B	C	D	E	F	G	H
0	0	4	4	0	0	0	4

A40. This question is focusing on your commitment to learning and professional development. All foundation doctors are expected to be involved in quality improvement projects. An important skill to develop is the ability to find learning opportunities in every patient. Less 'acute'/long-stay wards give you the opportunity to learn about the 'non-clinical' elements of healthcare including social services and mental capacity. This should be embraced as you need this knowledge to discharge patients safely later on in your career (**answer G**). You are also being offered the opportunity to easily complete one of the many requirements of your foundation training and you should agree (**answer C**). These two options show that you are motivated and committed to developing as a broad foundation doctor. However, as you have concerns you should raise them (**answer E**). You should not shy away from a problem that you are having and your educational supervisor may be able to suggest helpful advice.

Showing a lack of interest in your work is not advisable as you should always be committed to learning and developing your career (**answer A, answer B, answer D** and **answer H**). Finally, requesting to change your placement (**answer F**) before discussing your concerns with your educational supervisor is too extreme as you haven't given due process a chance.

A	B	C	D	E	F	G	H
0	0	4	0	4	0	4	0

A41. This question is focusing on your understanding of the limitations of an FY1. Obtaining consent and/or site-marking are not to be carried out by FY1s. This is partly to minimise any risk of error occurring but also because you have not been trained in doing so. Remember, in order for you to take consent you must be able to explain the detailed risks and benefits of the procedure. You must also be able to answer any questions that patients may have so that they are fully informed. As an FY1 you will not be in a position to do this. In this scenario the correct action is to remind the registrar of your limitations (**answer C**). However, as the registrar is clearly busy it would be wise to offer to help them with any tasks they have, thus freeing them up to site-mark (**answer D**). Alternatively, you can call your SHO, who is able to site-mark this patient (**answer E**).

Agreeing to site-mark Mr Pantous's leg is incorrect as FY1s do not site-mark (**answer A**). Equally, **answer B** is not appropriate as the purpose of marking a site before the patient reaches the anaesthetic room is to prevent errors occurring. Reading up on the procedure due to take place (**answer G**) and asking to assist (**answer H**) are a good idea whilst on your surgical rotation. They show that you are enthusiastic and willing to learn new skills. However, they are not relevant to this scenario. Finally, telling your registrar that you do not see the point in assessing a patient is confrontational and unnecessarily rude (**answer F**).

A	B	C	D	E	F	G	H
0	0	4	4	4	0	0	0

A42. This question is focusing on your appreciation of the importance of punctuality. You applied for and accepted this post. Therefore it is your responsibility to ensure you are able to meet your contractual obligations of this post, one of which will be your working hours. In this scenario, you have been noted to be repeatedly late and so you must take appropriate action to alter this pattern. You should apologise to your registrar (**answer G**) and make a plan to improve. In this case the simplest method will be setting your alarm earlier (**answer B**). However, a more long-term solution may be moving closer to the hospital so that your commute is more manageable (**answer A**).

Asking to alter your working hours (**answer C**), responding obnoxiously to your registrar (**answer D**) and ignoring your registrar (**answer E**) are not acceptable choices. You have contractual obligations to which you must adhere and it is your responsibility to ensure you are able to do so. The hospital, and the staff that work there, are not obliged to make any exceptions for your choice of accommodation. **Answer F** is an empty response as you are not actually altering your behaviour, which is not an appropriate solution. Finally, although arranging a car-pooling scheme with your SHO (**answer H**) may solve the problem when you are both working, it would not assist your punctuality when either of you are on call or on annual leave. Therefore this is not a sustainable solution to improving your punctuality.

A	B	C	D	E	F	G	H
4	4	0	0	0	0	4	0

A43. This question is assessing your ability to deal with your mistakes. You cannot say for definite that Mr Atiz has gone into cardiac arrest from his anaemia. However, you should tell the registrar as much information as you know openly so that they can act as they see fit (**answer C**). You should also reflect on what happened (**answer G**). This is an important step in acknowledging and learning from your errors. You may find that Mr Atiz actually developed hyperkalaemia secondary to incorrect fluid administration by the nurses, but that still would not excuse your mistake earlier in the day. Take the opportunity to learn and think about what you would do differently in the future. Finally, it is important to discuss with your education supervisor any mistake that may have contributed to a patient having a poor prognosis (**answer B**). They will be able to advise you on any additional action that is likely to occur.

Refusing to admit your error openly (**answer D, answer F** and **answer H**) or assist with a patient in cardiac arrest (**answer E**) is inappropriate. Your only duty at this point is to assist with returning Mr Atiz to a pre-cardiac arrest state if at all possible. Any future development or reprisal should not be your focus. Finally, discussing this with your colleague is not inappropriate as you are likely to feel guilt and need to dissect what has happened (**answer A**). However, it should not be among your top three priorities as Martin is unlikely to be able to offer you any meaningful advice, whereas your educational supervisor will.

A	B	C	D	E	F	G	H
0	4	4	0	0	0	4	0

A44. This question is focusing on your ability to challenge inappropriate behaviour correctly. The GMC has very clear fitness to practice guidelines and drug taking is not acceptable. In this scenario your concerns about Jane are more than a suspicion as she has admitted to taking cocaine. The most important action you must take is telling Jane to go home (**answer C**) as she is not fit to work. You should also advise Jane to seek help with her illicit drug use as you are not the appropriate person for her to approach (**answer H**). In these difficult situations you should gain advice yourself so that you can ensure you have dealt with the situation to the best of your ability. Speaking to your registrar is an appropriate starting point (**answer D**). You may keep names confidential if you like as the registrar doesn't need to know intimate details to give you the correct advice.

Ignoring (**answer B**) or colluding with Jane (**answer A**) is inappropriate as Jane is not fit to practice medicine. She is under the influence of an illicit substance and her judgement is impaired. However, it is also inappropriate to inform the police (**answer E**), occupational health (**answer F**) or the GMC (**answer G**) as it is not your position to do so. Your grievance should be raised through your consultant, thus allowing the hospital to carry out due process. Remember to escalate your concerns by following the escalation ladder.

A	B	C	D	E	F	G	H
0	0	4	4	0	0	0	4

A45. This question is focusing on challenging inappropriate behaviour correctly, in this case bigoted views. As a healthcare professional you are expected to be non-judgemental and it is not acceptable behaviour to share your personal views in your working environment if they may cause offence to other employees or, with respect to healthcare provision, your patients. You should challenge another doctor if you hear bigoted views. This should be done professionally (**answer H**) and in a matter-of-fact way (**answer E**). However, it is also important that this type of behaviour is escalated to ensure that it does not recur. As with any grievance, you should discuss your concerns with your own clinical supervisor (**answer B**) before attempting to speak to the 'offenders'.

It is easy to become agitated when you overhear offensive or bigoted discussions taking place. However, it is important not to become drawn into an argument or confrontation when challenging this type of behaviour. Therefore **answers A** and **D** are not appropriate choices. They would lead to a conflict and is not the professional manner in which you should be acting. However, nor can you leave the mess without challenging this behaviour (**answer F**). It is important not to allow this type of conduct to occur in a professional environment. Informing human resources (**answer C**) or their consultants (**answer G**) is not the correct process. Even if HR sends an email this is unlikely to make a difference. The individuals concerned will be likely to ignore such an email and contacting their consultants will be seen as a formal complaint without having escalated through the appropriate channels.

A	B	C	D	E	F	G	H
0	4	0	0	4	0	0	4

A46. This question is focusing on confidentiality and is a common occurrence. The important factor in this question is recalling that you should not disclose any confidential information, even to next of kin, without the patient's agreement (**answer H**). Not all patients will be comfortable discussing their health with their spouses, siblings, parents or children. It is good practice to familiarise yourself with a patient's medical notes if you are asked to discuss their case with a relative/friend, especially as an on-call doctor (**answer E**). This will enable you to give accurate information when required to do so. Finally, any discussion you have should be clearly documented in the patient's medical notes (**answer B**). Even if your only discussion is that the patient does not want you to discuss their medical information with this relative/friend, it should be documented.

In this scenario, you are the on-call doctor and will be very busy. It may seem tempting either to refuse to speak with the relative (**answer D** and **answer F**) or to ask the staff nurse looking after Mr Bonty to speak with the relative (**answer C**). However, your role as the on-call doctor does involve speaking with relatives if required to do so. If you were very busy and being called away to another ward it would be perfectly reasonable to explain that you are too busy at this time but will try to come back later (**answer G**). However, in this scenario you did not have any other tasks to complete and so should deal with the relative now. Disclosing Mr Bonty's medical information without his permission is a breach of confidentiality and therefore inappropriate (**answer A**).

A	B	C	D	E	F	G	H
0	4	0	0	4	0	0	4

A47. This question is focusing on your ability to display honesty and integrity whilst dealing with your commitment to learning and professional development. In this scenario you have been given the opportunity to develop your CV by attending a regional event. However, your compulsory training does take priority. The key factor in this question is recognising that you need to be honest with your SHO and escalate this problem early (**answer A**). Contacting your educational department to explain what has happened and attempting to reschedule your training is sensible (**answer C**). This may be easily done allowing you still to attend the regional talk, showing commitment to your professional development. Finally, you should email the talk that you have prepared to your SHO so that another member of the team can attend in your place and will still be able to deliver the talk on behalf of the team (**answer G**).

It is highly unprofessional to simply be absent, at either the training session or the conference/regional meeting. Therefore **answer B**, **answer F** and **answer H** are inappropriate choices. As eluded to above, it is not appropriate to lie or to act dishonestly as a doctor and therefore telling your SHO that you attended is not advisable (**answer E**). If your talk was scheduled for the morning session of the regional meeting then a compromise could be viable (**answer D**). However, as this is not clear in the scenario it is not a suitable answer as you may miss your talk.

A	B	C	D	E	F	G	H
4	0	4	0	0	0	4	0

A48. This question is dealing with your commitment to learning. Although you have completed medical school, beginning as a foundation doctor is the start of a lifetime of learning ahead of you. It is common practice for you to have a trust-specific teaching programme throughout your foundation training. Attendance at this teaching is compulsory excluding on-call and annual leave. In this scenario, you have not been attending this teaching and therefore need to make a conscious effort to improve this. It may seem too simple but you must attend future teaching sessions (**answer H**). Discussing your difficulties with your clinical supervisor before your attendance is too poor to correct is advisable (**answer G**). Finally, requesting a list of missed sessions so that you can complete the associated e-module is a sensible approach to make up what you have missed (**answer A**).

Replying to the email with an inflammatory response (**answer B**) or ignoring the email entirely (**answer C**) is not a professional attitude. The educational department is there to assist you with your learning and you should work with them to maximise your time as a foundation doctor. Explaining that you did not realise the teaching was compulsory (**answer D**) may be true but that does not attempt to correct the mistake or make changes to the future and is therefore not helpful. At this point you do not need to email your educational supervisor (**answer E**). You still have plenty of time to attend the remainder of your training and meet the 75% minimum. Finally, it is unlikely that your FY1 colleague will be able to offer you any additional advice other than attending the teaching from now on (**answer F**).

A	B	C	D	E	F	G	H
4	0	0	0	0	0	4	4

A49. This question is focusing on your ability to challenge unacceptable behaviour, in this case Samantha's potentially unsafe prescribing. This type of scenario will always be challenging as you are both FY1s. However, you need to prioritise patient safety, which may be at risk. It would be wise to discuss what you have discovered with your registrar as they will be able to advise you appropriately (**answer F**). However, as this scenario is not confrontational or inflamed an appropriate choice would also be to speak with Samantha privately and inform her of what has been occurring (**answer C**). Finally, as the nurses repeatedly ask you to amend the prescription charts it would be necessary to advise the nurses to escalate their concerns (**answer H**). It is not practical for you to correct every prescription over which they have a concern.

This is not something that you can ignore as patients are potentially at risk (**answer E** and **answer G**). Nor is it appropriate to approach Samantha bluntly (**answer B**) – that shows poor communication skills. Discussing this issue with other FY1s is gossiping and is not appropriate (**answer D**). Finally, raising this issue with Samantha's clinical supervisor without first speaking with her is not the correct escalation process (**answer A**). Unless Samantha's prescriptions were overtly dangerous she deserves the opportunity to improve her practice now that she has been informed of her error.

A	B	C	D	E	F	G	H
0	0	4	0	0	4	0	4

A50. This question is focusing on your understanding of your own limitations as a foundation doctor. You cannot accept referrals from other teams and these should always be directed towards your registrar. They will be able to discuss the cases more appropriately and make an informed plan. Therefore, Jasmine should be directed towards your registrar (**answer F**). You should follow up with your own discussion about Ms Carey (**answer G**) as you will want to start the transfer process to assist the registrar. However, it would also be useful to show Jasmine how to make an OT/PT referral so that in future cases her team may not need to refer to a medical doctor (**answer B**).

Accepting the referral is incorrect – this is not something that FY1s should be doing (**answer D**), nor is it advisable to review this patient (**answer E**). There is no suggestion of a threat to patient safety and therefore any review should be carried out by the accepting clinician (i.e. the registrar). Agreeing to transfer a surgical patient to a medical ward will be seen as a referral acceptance and is also incorrect (**answer H**). OT/PT need to assess this patient before any plans for rehabilitation can be made. Therefore advising Jasmine to transfer Ms Carey to a rehab hospital is not appropriate (**answer C**). Finally, criticising Jasmine is unprofessional (**answer A**). You should always attempt to help your colleagues even if it is simply by showing them how to make a referral – everybody has to learn at some point.

A	B	C	D	E	F	G	H
0	4	0	0	0	4	4	0

5. Domain 2 – coping with pressure

Being a doctor is an extremely stressful role, none more so than in the foundation years. Research has shown that junior doctors in particular struggle with having to take on professional responsibility, dealing with terminal illness and death, breaking bad news, the hours and intensity of work, professional relationships with patients, relatives and the wider multidisciplinary team (MDT) and the potentiality of mistakes by themselves or others (Paice et al, 2002).

In recent times, steps have been taken to reduce working hours of junior doctors and to improve their educational and clinical supervision to abate this stress; however, issues still persist. Therefore the ability of applicants to cope with stress in the work environment whilst still being able to make the correct clinical decision is an important domain to be tested within the SJT (Patterson et al, 2013).

In the SJT, questions will focus on the following topics:

- Your decision-making ability whilst under pressure
- How you deal with confrontation from both patients and relatives
- How you cope with stressful interactions with fellow healthcare professionals
- How you adapt and develop coping mechanisms (i.e. your resilience)
- How you seek support from your seniors
- How you manage clinical uncertainty or ambiguity
- How you respond when you identify that a mistake has been made.

Research has looked into the transitional period from medical school to FY1 doctor and managing the anxiety that is born out of a self-perception of incompetence is a key experience of junior doctors. Hence, FY1 doctors must be able to develop coping strategies and confidence with their own ability.

Remember: patients in hospital are likely to be anxious and worried themselves. These feelings are transferred onto their relatives and other healthcare professionals involved in their care.

Questions relating to this domain will, therefore, in the main, focus on difficult interactions that you may encounter in the workplace.

The following practice questions have been developed to provide an opportunity for you to demonstrate how to deal with these topics correctly. Remember, what counts is what you **should** do, not what you **would** do!

Q51. You are the FY1 on call over the weekend and you are covering six medical wards. Ten minutes ago you were bleeped by a nurse on Acorn Ward to assess a patient they felt had acutely deteriorated. Following your assessment of the patient you deem them to be in sepsis and so begin their medical work-up. Whilst taking the patient's blood your pager goes off again. As you are mid-procedure you don't have a chance to look at the pager and make a note of the number trying to contact you. Unfortunately your pager goes off again, before you have a chance to make a note of the first number. You have given the patient an initial fluid challenge to which they have responded positively, so you take the opportunity to answer your bleep whilst recording your assessment and initial management of the patient in the medical notes. The phone is picked up by a nurse on Birch Ward who has bleeped you twice; she is angry as you have taken 15 minutes to respond to her initial bleep and she has a patient she would like you to assess urgently.

Rank in order the following actions in response to this situation (1 = most appropriate; 5 = least appropriate):

A. Immediately leave Acorn Ward to attend the other unwell patient.

B. Explain to the nurse that you are currently assessing another unwell patient, but obtain further information to allow you to triage your attention to clinical need.

C. Ask the nurse to contact the senior house officer on call if she is acutely concerned with the patient as you are busy with another unwell patient.

D. Refuse to speak to the nurse and insist that she apologises for being rude before taking the referral.

E. Ask the nurse to take a full set of observations from the patient and ask her to call back when she has these so that you can complete your medical work-up of your current patient.

> How should you deal with confrontation?

Q52. You are the FY1 on call overnight and you are bleeped at 2 am to interpret a patient's activated partial thromboplastin time (APTT) ratio and adjust their heparin infusion accordingly. Unfortunately you normally work on a urology ward and have yet to come across a patient on a heparin infusion during your FY1 year. Consequently you are unable to interpret the result and make any adjustments to the heparin infusion. You have attempted to contact your senior house officer but they haven't responded.

Rank in order the following actions in response to this situation (1 = most appropriate; 5 = least appropriate):

A. Don't interpret the result as you are not comfortable with the management of patients on heparin infusions.

B. Contact the medical registrar on call for their advice.

C. Consult an internet search engine to find advice on the management of patients on heparin infusions.

D. Contact the on-call haematology consultant at home to seek their expert opinion.

E. Speak to the ward sister, who might have experience in managing patients on heparin infusions.

Q53. Owing to having been on call in the previous week and because of annual leave of your fellow FY1 colleagues, your rota has required you to work 12 days in a row. This is your second period of working 12 days in a row in the past 2 months. On day 10 you feel completely exhausted because of work. When bridging the topic of your rota with your consultant previously he remarked that 'you guys have it easy compared with what we went through; I don't know why you complain so much'.

Rank in order the following actions in response to this situation (1 = most appropriate; 5 = least appropriate):

A. Complete hours monitoring to ensure that your rota is compliant with the European Working Time Directive.

B. Discuss your concerns with your educational supervisor.

C. Contact the British Medical Association with your concerns.

D. Write to the medical director of your trust explaining the situation.

E. Arrange annual leave for the rest of the week.

Q54. You are a respiratory FY1 doctor in a busy unit during the winter period. Many of the current inpatients under your care have been diagnosed as influenza A positive. Unfortunately, owing to being very busy during working hours recently, you have not been vaccinated with the flu vaccine this year via the occupational health service at your trust. Owing to on-call commitments, many of your doctor colleagues are not present on your ward this week, leaving yourself and a senior house officer to care for a list of 48 patients. Overnight you have been unwell, feeling generally fatigued and having vomited several times. You correlate your symptoms with a viral illness.

Rank in order the following actions in response to this situation (1 = most appropriate; 5 = least appropriate):

A. Attend work as planned having taken some simple precautions and over-the-counter cold remedies.

B. Contact your rota coordinator first thing in the morning informing them of your illness and request cover for your shift.

C. Make an appointment with your GP in the morning to see whether they think you are able to attend work.

D. Stay at home and recoup from your illness; your SHO is more than capable of looking after the patient list.

E. Contact your consultant informing them of the nature of your illness and how long you anticipate you will be unable to attend work.

> Remember to prioritise patient safety!

Q55. You are the surgical FY1 doctor on call for an evening shift. The main focus of your job is to ensure the safety of patients during the transition between the day and night surgical teams. You respond mainly to pages from nurses and complete reviews of patients as requested by the day team. It is 7 pm and you have just been paged by two nurses from two separate wards; they are both requesting an urgent medical review of separate patients: a 63-year-old man post-laparotomy with a temperature of 37.6 °C and a 82-year-old woman who has become acutely tachypnoeic. As you're leaving the ward to attend to these patients you are asked by a nurse to speak to a patient's relative who has concerns regarding their relative's follow-up post-discharge. You are not on the team who normally looks after this patient and are unfamiliar with their case. The nurse instructs you that the relative is irate that nobody has been available to discuss their concerns.

Rank in order the following actions in response to this situation (1 = most appropriate; 5 = least appropriate):

A. Briefly attend the relative, explain that you are the on-call doctor and as such are unfamiliar with their relative's case. Explain that you understand they have concerns but are needed urgently elsewhere. Explain that you will try to attend them later this evening to address their concerns.

B. Attend the relative immediately to explore their concerns.

C. Ask the nurse to instruct the relative to contact the patient advice and liaison service (PALS) with their concerns.

D. Ask the nurse to contact your SHO, who may be able to attend the relative this evening.

E. Explain to the nurse that you are unable to speak to the relative presently as you have to review these acutely unwell patients. Ask the nurse to explore the relative's concerns and document these in the medical notes for the relative's day team to review tomorrow.

Q56. You are an FY1 doctor working in a urology department. One of your patients has pyelonephritis and is being treated with intravenous gentamicin. You are bleeped by the senior sister in the department; she explains that unfortunately the patient has received two doses of high-dose gentamicin today (having been prescribed only one). The error occurred as the nurse working the morning shift forgot to sign the drug card stating that the drug was administered; the nurse who took over from them assumed the drug had not been given and so re-administered it.

Rank in order the following actions in response to this situation (1 = most appropriate; 5 = least appropriate):

A. Urgently attend the patient informing them of the error and review them for signs of gentamicin toxicity.

B. Complete an adverse incident log for the drug administration error.

C. Email the nurses in question informing them of the mistake.

D. Ask the senior sister to arrange for nursing staff members to undergo extra training in IV antibiotic administration.

E. Complete a reflective entry into your e-portfolio regarding the adverse event.

Q57. You are an FY1 doctor on a very busy orthopaedic surgery unit consisting of four wards. You have just been paged by a nurse from ward 2 to relay an urgent lab result. 'Mr Smith' has had a significant drop in his haemoglobin that will require transfusion. Unfortunately, on looking at your list of patients, you have two patients by the surname of Smith on ward 2 and the result has yet to be posted to the computerised results system. You are currently very busy on ward 3 as there are several patients to be discharged today, all requiring their discharge summaries to be completed. You attempt to call ward 2 back to obtain further information on the patient but nobody is picking up the ward's phone.

Rank in order the following actions in response to this situation (1 = most appropriate; 5 = least appropriate):

A. Stay on ward 3 and complete the urgent discharge summaries on that ward whilst waiting for the formal report for the hemoglobin to be posted to the online results reporting system and then act accordingly.

B. Phone the blood bank to see whether both Mr Smith has a valid group and screens, then attempt to contact the ward again.

C. Attend ward 2 immediately to find the nurse you spoke to in person to identify the correct patient to clinically assess them.

D. Complete the discharge summary you are currently writing before trying to phone the ward back again.

E. Attend ward 2 and take valid group and screen samples from both Mr Smiths, as one of them will need the transfusion.

Q58. You are an FY1 doctor working on the acute medicine unit. You have just attended the morning handover meeting at which the patients to be seen by the consultant on the morning ward round were discussed. Your job for the day is to assist the consultant on call with their ward round. In the handover meeting two patients were discussed who had the same surname but different reasons for their admission. As your consultant begins to see the first of these patients he starts referring to a management plan compatible with the other patient's presenting complaint, but not the one he is currently reviewing.

Rank in order the following actions in response to this situation (1 = most appropriate; 5 = least appropriate):

A. Do not interject; whilst the plan may seem odd, you're sure the consultant understands what he is doing. Complete the jobs requested after the ward round.

B. Say nothing so as to not embarrass the consultant in front of the patient, but switch the patients' management plans after the ward round.

C. Politely and immediately remind the consultant of the current patient's presenting complaint to verify the plan.

D. Do not directly challenge the consultant; wait for him to review the next patient to allow him to realise his error.

E. Wait till after the consultant has finished reviewing the current patient and inform him of the perceived error he has made.

> How should you highlight a mistake?

Q59. You have recently started your second rotation as an FY1 doctor and are currently in your second week working in a busy hepatobiliary surgery unit. Your first FY1 rotation was a supernumerary role within the local psychiatric liaison department. You have certainly noticed the stark increase in your workload since commencing your new role, but thankfully you have another FY1 colleague based on your ward, Mike. You and Mike share equally the work on the ward, looking after two bays of patients each. Mike is very keen to pursue a career in surgery and this is his only surgery-based rotation within his Foundation Programme. You note that you haven't seen Mike on the ward today as he is supposed to be. On enquiring, the surgical matron informs you that they have just seen Mike in theatre with your consultant. You would really appreciate some help on this busy day.

Rank in order the following actions in response to this situation (1 = most appropriate; 5 = least appropriate):

A. Contact Mike's clinical supervisor for his surgical rotation stating that Mike is not adhering to the departmental rota.

B. Go to the other surgical ward and see whether one of their junior doctors is able to assist you today whilst Mike is in theatre gaining surgical experience.

C. Contact the hepatobiliary theatre to request that Mike comes back to the ward.

D. Keep a jobs list of routine jobs that arise for the patients in the bays that Mike looks after during his absence.

E. When Mike returns to the ward around lunchtime after the first case is finished, politely request that he ensures adequate ward staffing prior to going to theatre.

Q60. You currently work for a vascular surgeon, Mr Morris, a well-respected consultant within the hospital who has been working in his current appointment since qualifying as a consultant in 1979. You feel you have formed a good working relationship with him, and have always found him respectful and courteous to colleagues and very knowledgeable about his area of expertise. However, on today's ward round when reviewing Mrs Jones, who had undergone an aneurysmal repair yesterday, you were unable to recall her haemoglobin result from this morning. As a result, Mr Morris, in front of Mrs Jones, called you 'incompetent'.

Rank in order the following actions in response to this situation (1 = most appropriate; 5 = least appropriate):

A. Immediately state to Mr Morris, whilst on the ward round, that his comment was unprofessional and undermines your position.

B. Wait for the ward round to finish before emailing the medical director of the trust informing them of the events.

C. Contact your educational supervisor regarding the incident and ask them to raise your concerns with Mr Morris on your behalf.

D. Discuss the event with the other vascular surgery FY1 doctors to see whether Mr Morris has acted in this way to others.

E. Discuss the incident with another vascular surgeon for their advice.

Q61. You are the medical FY1 on call over the weekend. You are bleeped by the senior sister from the Cavendish Unit, a geriatrics ward. She is requesting that you review a Mrs Du Bois, an 86-year-old woman with advanced dementia currently admitted for treatment of urinary tract infection. Her family is concerned as she 'appears very agitated' today, shouting out frequently and attempting to hit the ward staff and relatives. Some of her relatives are present and are strongly suggesting the use of sedatives to 'calm her down'. On reviewing her medical notes, you note an entry from Dr Jackson, Mrs Du Bois's consultant, from a ward round earlier in the week, which states that Mrs Du Bois became very unrousable on sedation and that this should be 'avoided at all costs'.

Rank in order the following actions in response to this situation (1 = most appropriate; 5 = least appropriate):

A. In view of Mrs Du Bois's clinical deterioration, review her for a cause of this new onset of agitation.

B. Refuse to prescribe anything to sedate Mrs Du Bois.

C. Contact your medical registrar on call to see whether there is anything they can suggest given the situation.

D. Prescribe a very small dose of a sedative to be given as required.

E. Contact Dr Jackson at home to see whether they are happy for you to act against their documented plan.

> Consider the escalation ladder.

Q62. You are working on a cardiology ward. You are looking after Mr Iqbal, a 74-year-old man with end-stage heart failure who is being treated with high-dose diuretics that are unfortunately causing an acute kidney injury. The consultant cardiologist, on discussion with the patient, decided to continue the use of diuretics as they seemed to be improving Mr Iqbal's clinical picture despite the adverse effect. It has also been decided that Mr Iqbal should have careful input/output monitoring and 1.5 litres fluid restriction, despite the acute kidney injury, as this should facilitate the improvement in his clinical picture. You are conducting your morning ward round and note that Mr Iqbal is more symptomatic of fluid overload today with pulmonary oedema and pitting oedema up to his sacrum. On reviewing his medical notes you see that he was seen by the medical FY1 on call overnight who erroneously prescribed aggressive IV fluid replacement despite the documented plan.

Rank in order the following actions in response to this situation (1 = most appropriate; 5 = least appropriate):

A. Inform Mr Iqbal that the likely cause of his clinical deterioration today is due to the 'incompetence of one of your non-cardiology colleagues'.

B. Complete an adverse incident report.

C. Increase Mr Iqbal's dose of diuretics for today to counteract the erroneous prescription.

D. Contact your consultant and ask them to kindly review Mr Iqbal today in view of his clinical deterioration.

E. Ask your consultant to email your FY1 colleague's educational supervisor encouraging your colleague to reflect upon the event.

Q63. You are working on a gastroenterology unit and on the morning ward round your consultant asks you to seek the advice of the on-call general surgery registrar regarding a 72-year-old man who has worsening abdominal pain that he believes may have a surgical origin. After the ward round you bleep the registrar, who is dismissive of your clinical concern and states 'from what you've said to me this just sounds like simple gastroenteritis' and hangs up. You attempt to bleep them again; however, after two attempts they haven't returned your call.

Rank in order the following actions in response to this situation (1 = most appropriate; 5 = least appropriate):

A. Contact your consultant to inform them of the events.

B. Attempt to contact another general surgical registrar to see whether they would be more forthcoming with advice.

C. Contact the on-call general surgical consultant for advice regarding your patient.

D. Continue to bleep the on-call registrar and wait for them to respond.

E. Report the on-call registrar to the clinical lead of surgery for their behaviour to you on the phone.

Q64. You have just finished taking a patient's blood and are just returning your sharps bin to the dirty utility room on the ward. The ward storeroom is next door and through the wall you overhear someone who sounds like your registrar, Suresh, shouting at someone about their 'stupidity and incompetence'. You are unable to identify the recipient of the complaint and do not enter the storeroom immediately to find out. Later on in the day you notice Agnes, a recently qualified staff nurse based on your ward, sitting alone in the staffroom and obviously crying and upset.

Rank in order the following actions in response to this situation (1 = most appropriate; 5 = least appropriate):

A. Go to your consultant's office immediately to report Suresh for his inappropriate behaviour towards Agnes.

B. Confront Suresh about how unprofessional you have found his behaviour to be.

C. Begin to keep a log of incidents regarding Suresh's behaviour towards staff to compile evidence.

D. Enter the staffroom and comfort Agnes; enquire as to why she is upset.

E. Encourage Agnes to speak to her manager, who is the ward sister, about the reasons for her being upset.

Q65. It is 5 pm and your shift is due to finish in 30 minutes. Your registrar and SHO have just gone home for the day. It's been a very busy day so you planned to spend this time checking the blood test results of your patients taken today on the hospital's computer system. Unfortunately on logging into the system you realise it is currently undergoing compulsory maintenance and will be unavailable for another 90 minutes. On realising this predicament, you bleep the on-call FY1 doctor to hand over the job of checking the blood test results, who is very unhappy about accepting 'a job that should definitely be done by someone from the day team' and requests that you stay until 6.30 pm and check the results yourself; you are still on the phone to them.

Rank in order the following actions in response to this situation (1 = most appropriate; 5 = least appropriate):

A. Leave work at 5.30 pm as planned leaving the results unchecked until the morning.

B. Contact the on-call SHO asking them to follow up the results.

C. Discuss your concerns with your consultant on the ward round in the morning asking them to contact the on-call FY1's educational supervisor.

D. Instruct the on-call FY1 that their request for you to stay is 'totally unprofessional'.

E. Acknowledge the on-call FY1's concerns but explain that the situation is the result of a situation out of your control.

Q66. You are the on-call FY1 doctor and are currently attending a cardiac arrest call with the on-call medical registrar and SHO. Whilst there, the registrar is fast-bleeped and asks you to take the call whilst they lead the cardiac arrest. The bleep is from the senior sister from a neighbouring ward requesting an urgent review of a patient who has become acutely unresponsive but has stable observations. You relay this message to the registrar, who asks you to attend this new patient stating that they will join you once they have finished at the cardiac arrest. On attending this patient, your initial thought is that they look critically unwell.

Rank in order the following actions in response to this situation (1 = most appropriate; 5 = least appropriate):

A. Immediately put out a cardiac arrest call for this new patient.

B. Complete an ABCDE assessment and initiate initial management of the new patient.

C. Before reviewing the patient, phone the ward with the initial cardiac arrest call asking the nursing staff to relay to the registrar that you are unhappy at being asked to review someone so critically unwell.

D. Fast-bleep the on-call critical care outreach team.

E. Review the patient but await the registrar's arrival before initiating management.

> What can be expected of an FY1 doctor?

Q67. You are the medical FY1 on call in a small district general hospital that has five medical wards. Joining you on the shift is an SHO, Thom, who is your direct senior. Thom suggests the best way to work through today's jobs is to 'divide and conquer'. He allocates you three wards to attend to whilst he takes the other two, stating 'the work will be even as they tend to be much busier'. Towards the end of your shift you are contacted by Julia, a nurse from one of the wards Thom has allocated himself, saying that none of her ward's patients have been seen today.

Rank in order the following actions in response to this situation (1 = most appropriate; 5 = least appropriate):

A. Ask Julia whether any of the ward's patients are unwell or she has any acute clinical concern.

B. Tell Julia that her ward's patients are not your responsibility and end the phone conversation.

C. Contact Thom and find out why he has not attended Julia's ward today and discuss Julia's concern.

D. Give Julia Thom's bleep number and ask her to contact him.

E. Ask Julia to make a jobs list of the work that needs to be done and explain that one of you will attend her ward shortly.

Q68. At the midpoint review meeting of your second FY1 rotation, your clinical supervisor discusses many potential audits you could complete to satisfy the requirements of your Foundation

Programme. After deliberating your options, he allocates you one to complete prior to the end of your placement with him. After the meeting you note that one day of the proposed data collection period falls within some of your allocated annual leave. Your partner has organised for you to attend a theatre production on that day to celebrate your anniversary.

Rank in order the following actions in response to this situation (1 = most appropriate; 5 = least appropriate):

A. Accept the proposed audit and attend the hospital on your annual leave day to complete data collection. Ask your partner to cancel the tickets for the theatre production.

B. Agree to complete the audit but don't attend on the day of your annual leave to collect data; fabricate the data to hide the fact that the audited period was one day less.

C. Arrange another meeting with your clinical supervisor to re-discuss the possibility of other projects.

D. Agree to complete the audit but don't attend the hospital on the day of your annual leave to collect data; in your analysis acknowledge the shortened audited period.

E. Upon realising the conflict with your annual leave, discuss with your clinical supervisor whether the dates for data collection can be altered.

Q69. You are an FY1 doctor based in a tertiary referral centre for complex urology. The ward-based team consists of two FY1 doctors and two SHOs. Owing to being on call over the weekend you have worked 13 days in a row. As per the European Working Time Directive, this is the maximum number of days you are allowed to work consecutively before having a single day off for rest. Therefore the rota coordinator has allocated you today off. It is 8.30 am and you are woken by your phone ringing. Unfortunately you miss the call, a voicemail is left from your consultant. He tells you that your SHO has called in unwell and he would like you to come in and help out as 'we're extremely thin on the ground'; he is willing to arrange for you to be paid at your trust's locum rates.

Rank in order the following actions in response to this situation (1 = most appropriate; 5 = least appropriate):

A. Contact your rota coordinator and see whether they can arrange for another doctor to cover the shift.

B. Phone your consultant back to inform them that you are unable to attend work today.

C. Do not return your consultant's call but attend work later in the day to help out the team.

D. Attend work at the request of your consultant, but request that you are paid the locum SHO rate.

E. Contact your SHO in person explaining that you have worked the previous 13 days; ask them to attend work to ensure the ward is adequately staffed.

> Is there a legal issue if you work today?

Q70. You have just started your first FY1 rotation. You are an acute medical FY1 and your role is to clerk patients into the medical assessment unit. This involves taking a history and performing a relevant examination, reaching some differential diagnoses and instigating initial investigation and management of the patients prior to their being seen for an initial consultant review. Your hospital adopts a system whereby patients are allocated to clerking doctors to ensure an even spread of the work. It is 10 am and you are 1 hour into your shift; you currently have four patients to clerk. The medical registrar, who allocates patients to clerking doctors, remarks that you are going too slowly. You are presently trying to arrange an urgent echocardiogram for the first patient you clerked, who you believe has worsening heart failure.

Rank in order the following actions in response to this situation (1 = most appropriate; 5 = least appropriate):

A. Immediately begin to clerk your next patient; wait until you have seen a few patients before trying to arrange their investigations together.

B. Meet with your consultant to discuss strategies to speed up.

C. Inform the registrar you've only been working 1 hour and that you're going as fast as you can.

D. Complete arranging the patient's echo before moving on to the next patient.

E. Ask your FY1 colleague whether they would be able to see a couple of patients on your behalf to help you out.

Q71. You are working on a gynaecology unit. Mrs Hopkins is one of your patients; she is a 34-year-old woman admitted for investigations of some post-coital bleeding. The nurse asks you to review Mrs Hopkins as she has developed an acutely tender, erythematous and swollen lower left leg. You suspect a deep vein thrombosis (DVT) and organise a Doppler scan and place Mrs Hopkins on treatment dose low-molecular-weight heparin. On full clinical examination you find a bulky mass in Mrs Hopkins's abdomen that the clerking doctor appears not to have noticed on their examination. You suspect that this is a cancer that has precipitated Mrs Hopkins's DVT.

Rank in order the following actions in response to this situation (1 = most appropriate; 5 = least appropriate):

A. Arrange for Mrs Hopkins to have a CT scan of her abdomen to elucidate the origin of this mass.

B. Document your findings in the medical notes, indicating that you suspect Mrs Hopkins has cancer and that the diagnosis needs discussing with the patient on tomorrow morning's ward round.

C. On Mrs Hopkins's discharge summary, inform her GP of your findings and request that they arrange appropriate investigations to follow this up.

D. Wait for your registrar to return to the ward this afternoon from clinic and discuss your examination findings.

E. Discuss your findings with your SHO and seek their opinion on how the team should proceed.

Q72. You are the urology FY1 doctor on call overnight and are asked to review Mr Benard at 3 am. He is 2 days post-prostatectomy and the nursing staff inform you that he has gone into painful acute urinary retention with a blocked catheter that they are unable to flush. The operation note states that the catheter is to remain in situ for at least 7 days and must not be removed until then. You contact the on-call urology registrar, who is at home. He instructs you to use a needle and syringe to perform a bladder aspiration and that he will attend the ward in the morning to assess the catheter himself. He is reticent to come in to hospital as he is revising for an upcoming exam. You have never seen or performed this procedure before.

Rank in order the following actions in response to this situation (1 = most appropriate; 5 = least appropriate):

A. Attempt the procedure as advised and wait for the registrar to review the patient in the morning.

B. Explain that you have never performed the procedure before and are therefore uncomfortable to do it now without supervision.

C. Remove the patient's currently blocked catheter and attempt to replace it as you are competent in male catheterisation.

D. Contact your on-call urology consultant informing them that the registrar, who is revising at home, is unwilling to review inpatients tonight.

E. Ask the on-call surgical registrar, who you have worked with previously, if they would be happy to attempt the procedure.

Q73. You are the FY1 on call overnight. You attend the night handover meeting to receive a handover from your housemate, Simon, who has been the on-call FY1 this evening. He hands over the pager saying 'I've managed to get everything done so there's nothing to be worried about; there were a couple of unwell patients that I saw but I've sorted them out and the nurses shouldn't trouble you over them'. An hour into your shift you receive a bleep from Janet, a nurse on Cedar Ward; she tells you that one of her patient's was attended by Simon about 90 minutes ago – he left no definite plan in the notes and the patient remains unstable: hypotensive with pyrexia.

Rank in order the following actions in response to this situation (1 = most appropriate; 5 = least appropriate):

A. Attend the patient immediately and perform a clinical assessment.

B. Attend Cedar Ward; as Simon has already reviewed the patient there is no need for you to. Simply ensure the patient is on antibiotics for pyrexia.

C. Instruct Janet that her patient has been seen and you are too busy to review a patient already seen.

D. Submit a clinical incident form about the poor quality of Simon's handover.

E. Call Simon at home to confirm his management plan that was apparently poorly documented.

> Has the clinical context changed?

Q74. You are an FY1 doctor on the renal medicine unit. A patient, Mrs Khan, has just been transferred to the unit from A&E with a diagnosis of acute kidney injury secondary to a urinary tract infection. Susie, the unit's senior sister, bleeps you to ask you to sign the prescription for a bag of fluids she has given Mrs Khan in view of her acute kidney injury. Before doing so, you review Mrs Khan's biochemistry results; it becomes apparent that the A&E doctor must have misinterpreted the blood test results – Mrs Khan does not have acute kidney injury and indeed has normal renal function; thus in your opinion the fluids were not warranted. You instruct Susie that Mrs Khan does not need fluid resuscitation and you are unwilling to sign the prescription. She is in disagreement with you and threatens to discuss your actions with your clinical supervisor.

Rank in order the following actions in response to this situation (1 = most appropriate; 5 = least appropriate):

A. Discuss with Mrs Khan that you don't think she has acute kidney injury.

B. Complete a clinical incident form to investigate how this misdiagnosis occurred.

C. Do not prescribe any further fluids for Mrs Khan.

D. Advise Susie to discuss her concerns with your clinical supervisor.

E. Discuss the incident personally with your clinical supervisor on tomorrow's ward round.

Q75. A final-year medical student, Robert, visits your ward. He is keen to practise IV cannulation and asks whether any of your patients requires a cannula. You advise him that the patient in bay 3, bed 2 needs a new cannula to receive IV antibiotics. However, you are too busy at the moment to supervise Robert's attempt at the procedure and advise him to ask the ward's sister to supervise him. An hour later whilst attending the patient in bay 2, bed 3 you notice that there is a new cannula in situ; on enquiry the patient tells you that a medical student inserted it about an hour ago.

Rank in order the following actions in response to this situation (1 = most appropriate; 5 = least appropriate):

A. Attend the patient in bay 3, bed 2 and cannulate them.

B. Remove the cannula from the patient in bay 2, bed 3.

C. When Robert attends the ward later in the afternoon, discuss the error with him and encourage him to reflect upon the incident.

D. Reflect upon the error in your Foundation Programme e-portfolio.

E. Report Robert to his medical school for his mistake.

Q76. A patient on your ward, Mr Kenworthy, is a 92-year-old man who is registered blind and has advanced dementia. He requires assistance with his feeding from the nursing staff. During afternoon visiting, his family asks to speak to a doctor looking after him. Mr Kenworthy has told his family that he is not being fed and his family is concerned. On speaking to Jane, the patient's staff nurse, she assures you that Mr Kenworthy's feeding is being supported and you are shown food charts documenting the patient's diet. The family is insistent that Mr Kenworthy's claims are formally investigated.

Rank in order the following actions in response to this situation (1 = most appropriate; 5 = least appropriate):

A. Encourage the family to raise their concerns with the ward's senior sister.

B. Explore the family's concerns whilst showing them the food charts as evidence that Mr Kenworthy is actually being fed.

C. Advise Mr Kenworthy's family if they are insistent on the incident being investigated that they liaise with the patient advice and liaison service.

D. Inform Mr Kenworthy's family that their concerns are unfounded as there is irrefutable evidence that Mr Kenworthy's claims are false.

E. Enquire with Jane as to the honesty of her documentation of Mr Kenworthy's diet.

Q77. You are an FY1 doctor in the acute medical unit. On the unit currently you have a final year medical student, Samira, and she is taking a history from Mr English who has presented to the unit with cardiac-sounding chest pain. You happen to overhear Mr English make some perceivably racist comments as you attend to the patient in the next bed. It becomes apparent that Samira, for all intents and purposes, has ignored the comments and is attempting to carry on with her history taking.

Rank in order the following actions in response to this situation (1 = most appropriate; 5 = least appropriate):

A. When Samira is presenting her history to you, raise your concerns about Mr English's comments and explore Samira's thoughts.

B. Immediately interrupt Samira's history and tell Mr English that his comments are inappropriate.

C. Enter Mr English's bed area whilst Samira is completing her history, make no comments initially but observe the remainder of Samira's history. Discuss Mr English's comments away from his bed area.

D. Take no action on the comments you have heard.

E. When Samira is presenting her history to you, inform her that sometimes patients may make comments but that patient care is her upmost priority.

> What is your duty of care to Samira?

Q78. You are a female FY1 doctor. You have been asked to review a male patient who the nurses have observed to have very low urine output for the past 6 hours; a bladder scan reveals that he has acute urinary retention. You want to insert a urinary catheter urgently; however, the patient is requesting this is done by someone of the same sex owing to the intimate nature of the procedure. Unfortunately all of the ward staff members able to insert catheters are also female.

Rank in order the following actions in response to this situation (1 = most appropriate; 5 = least appropriate):

A. Offer to perform a suprapubic catheter as the procedure is less intimate.

B. Attempt to find a male colleague who is competent at urinary catheterisation.

C. Sedate the patient before inserting the catheter yourself.

D. Tell the patient his request is delaying urgent treatment of his condition.

E. Explore the patient's concerns and attempt to persuade him to allow you to perform the procedure.

Q79. You are an FY1 working in a busy orthopaedic surgery department. You have two other FY1 colleagues in the unit. The junior doctors within the department have recently completed compulsory hours monitoring to ensure that their jobs are compliant with the European Working Time Directive. The analysis of the hours monitoring shows that you are working 45 minutes a day more than you are supposed to. Your consultant, Mr Charnley, who is not your clinical or educational supervisor, asks to discuss this with you. You explain that the role is just too busy hence the hours monitoring findings; however, Mr Charnley insists that you must leave on time no matter what. He seems unconcerned by the implications you feel this may have on patient safety.

Rank in order the following actions in response to this situation (1 = most appropriate; 5 = least appropriate):

A. Raise the concerns from your discussion with your educational supervisor.

B. Raise the concerns from your discussion with the British Medical Association.

C. Raise the concerns from your discussion with the medical director of the trust.

D. Raise the concerns from your discussion with the local newspaper.

E. Raise the concerns from your discussion with the clinical lead for orthopaedic surgery.

Q80. You are an FY1 doctor on a cardiology ward. At 3 pm Mr Chakravorty, a patient on the ward, develops chest pain. An urgent ECG taken doesn't show any changes suggestive of myocardial infarction but you deem it best to take a blood test to assess his troponin. The result is reported at 3.45 pm and shows a mildly elevated level – the biochemistry laboratory recommends repeat testing at 3 hours post the initial sample as this would confirm ongoing myocardial damage. The level would therefore need to be taken at 6 pm; your shift is due to finish at 5 pm. You ask the ward charge nurse, Adrian, if he would be happy to take and chase the result of the blood test as his shift is due to finish at 7.30 pm; however, he states he is not willing to do this as he expects the ward will be very busy at that time.

Rank in order the following actions in response to this situation (1 = most appropriate; 5 = least appropriate):

A. Demand that Adrian takes and chases the result of the blood test.

B. Stay behind at work, use the time whilst waiting for the blood test to be taken and the result to come back to catch up on some e-portfolio work.

C. Hand over the job of taking and chasing the troponin result to the on-call FY1 doctor.

D. As the investigations show that Mr Chakravorty's chest pain is probably non-cardiac in nature, go home and await his review on ward round tomorrow.

E. Leave a request for the phlebotomist to take the repeat troponin level on their morning round tomorrow.

> How should you approach confrontation?

Q81. You are an FY1 on an endocrine ward. You are bleeped by the senior sister on your ward. Mrs Jones, a patient on the ward with insulin-controlled type 2 diabetes, has just been administered 180 units of insulin; the prescription was for 18 units. Your fellow FY1, Emma, wrote the prescription as '18u', hence the confusion.

Rank in order the following actions in response to this situation (1 = most appropriate; 5 = least appropriate):

A. Report the drug error via the clinical incident reporting tool.

B. Review Mrs Jones for signs of hypoglycaemia.

C. Report the nurse to your hospital's chief of nursing for her error.

D. Discuss the incident with the patient and apologise for the error.

E. Bleep Emma to attend the ward immediately and notify her how her prescription caused the error.

Q82. You have arranged to watch your local football team with your housemates this evening; it has been booked for you to have seats in a corporate box. It's getting towards the end of your working day and you, your SHO and registrar are still working through today's jobs. It becomes apparent that you probably will not be able to leave in enough time to attend the game.

Rank in order the following actions in response to this situation (1 = most appropriate; 5 = least appropriate):

A. Excuse yourself at the time your shift should end and attend the football as planned.

B. Mention to your consultant on your ward round in the morning that the job is very busy at the moment and see whether further team members can be arranged.

C. Ask a colleague from a neighbouring ward, who happens to be on call this evening, if they wouldn't mind covering your jobs this evening so that you can leave on time.

D. Complete hours monitoring for your current job to ensure that it is compliant with the European Working Time Directive.

E. Negotiate with your SHO and registrar and ask whether they would mind you leaving on time today so that you can attend the football match; agree to stay late to cover them another time.

> How should you negotiate in this case?

Q83. You are an FY1 doctor working in paediatrics. You are spending today clerking patients in the paediatric A&E department. A mother has brought in her child stating that the child has been unwell for the past 2 days and she has noticed a rash on her back this morning. The child is pyrexial and appears very distressed in the lights of the examination room. You would like to admit the child for treatment; however, the mother expresses strongly that she is against admission as her father died in this hospital 2 months ago.

Rank in order the following actions in response to this situation (1 = most appropriate; 5 = least appropriate):

A. Allow the mother to take her child home; instruct her to phone the department if her concerns are ongoing.

B. Ask the mother to complete discharge against medical advice paperwork and allow them to leave.

C. Admit the child for a few hours to take some bloods, initiate some management and observe before letting them go home.

D. Request an urgent review of the child by the paediatric registrar in the department.

E. Explain to the mother the seriousness of her child's presentation and attempt to persuade her to allow you to treat her.

Q84. Your FY1 colleague Patrick is due to work the on-call shift on your ward this weekend. This morning you observe him and Sheila, the SHO for the ward, having a dispute over whose turn it is to assist their consultant in theatre. You are also aware that Sheila is the SHO on call for surgery this weekend. For the rest of the day you note that their attitude to each other is rather frosty and they are avoiding speaking to each other. You are worried that patient safety might be compromised over the weekend if your two colleagues are unable to communicate effectively with each other.

Rank in order the following actions in response to this situation (1 = most appropriate; 5 = least appropriate):

A. Discuss your concerns with your consultant.

B. Arrange to go out for a few drinks on Friday evening and invite them both.

C. Ask Patrick whether he would like to swap this weekend with you to help avoid the confrontation.

D. Ask your educational supervisor for advice as to what to do, given the situation.

E. Discuss with Sheila and Patrick as to why they have fallen out and attempt to mediate their disagreement.

Q85. You are an FY1 in orthopaedic surgery. You are in the ward clinical equipment room talking through the procedure of taking blood with a third-year medical student, Jason. Jason is keen to be observed taking blood. Thankfully there's a patient on the ward, Mr Wildman, who is due to go to theatre this evening for a total hip replacement who needs pre-operative bloods. You are about to observe Jason take Mr Wildman's blood when the ward sister Marie asks you to urgently discuss the knee x-ray results of another patient, Mrs Hurdman, with them. Mrs Hurdman is the mother of an ENT consultant within your hospital. The x-ray was ordered as a routine post-operative follow-up.

Choose the most suitable **three** options from the following list:

A. Rearrange your observation of Jason taking blood and immediately explain the knee x-ray findings to Mrs Hurdman.

B. Explain to Marie that Mr Wildman's blood test is clinically urgent.

C. Observe Jason taking the bloods and then explain the findings of the knee x-ray to Mrs Hurdman.

D. Explain to Marie that relatives of colleagues do not deserve priority over other patients.

E. Contact your SHO to discuss which job should be completed first.

F. Allow the medical student to take the blood test unsupervised whilst you explain the x-ray findings.

G. Explain the x-ray findings to Mrs Hurdman first and then allow Jason to be observed taking Mr Wildman's blood.

H. Provide feedback to Jason on his blood-taking skills after your observation.

Q86. You are an FY1 in haematology. You have just reviewed Mr Jones and owing to an acutely low haemoglobin level decide that he needs a blood transfusion. You send blood samples to the blood bank to allow it to cross-match some units of blood for Mr Jones and you dutifully prescribe the blood to be given. Unfortunately Mr Jones's nurse, Delia, is on her lunch break so you are unable to tell her your plan and you have to leave the ward to attend compulsory teaching. You leave the prescription chart on the nurses' station to ensure that Delia sees it on her return. On your return to the ward 2 hours later you notice that Mr Jones is yet to receive his blood transfusion.

Choose the most suitable **three** options from the following list:

A. Report Delia to the ward sister for not administering the blood.

B. Clinically review Mr Jones again.

C. Do not attend teaching in the future if it is going to interrupt clinical duties.

D. Ensure that your haematology ward has protocols in place to ensure that important tasks are received by the necessary person.

E. Complete an audit for the haematology assessing the time between prescription of blood and the transfusion being started.

F. Ensure in the future that you hand over an urgent task directly to a person who can take ownership of the task.

G. Inform the clinical lead of haematology of the incident.

H. Contact your educational supervisor to inform them that your job does not allow you to fulfil your educational FY1 requirements.

Q87. You are an FY1 working in the acute medicine unit. You and your registrar just reviewed Mr Sanderson who has presented to the hospital today via the emergency department with chest pain. Whilst reviewing Mr Sanderson, your registrar comments that his ECG in the emergency department showed no acute changes. Following your review of Mr Sanderson, your registrar asks you to file Mr Sanderson's ECG in his medical notes. On looking at the ECG you note changes that you feel may represent an ischaemic cardiac event, contrary to your registrar's observation.

Choose the most suitable **three** options from the following list:

A. File the ECG as requested by your registrar.

B. Ask your SHO to review the ECG to obtain a second opinion.

C. Review Mr Sanderson again in view of the observed ECG changes.

D. Repeat the ECG.

E. Arrange for Mr Sanderson to undergo an emergency angiogram to assess his coronary vasculature.

F. Request urgent blood tests in view of the ECG changes.

G. Email the acute medicine unit's clinical director with your concerns regarding your registrar's ability to interpret ECGs.

H. Reflect upon the incident within your e-portfolio.

Q88. You are the FY1 on call today; it is a Saturday and you will be clerking new medical patients as they are admitted to hospital via the emergency department. You will be part of a team including a consultant (who is on call from home), a registrar, two SHOs and one other FY1 doctor. You are due to take over from an FY1 doctor who has been working overnight. You have left home 45 minutes before your shift starts, the commute normally taking about 25 minutes. You are 15 minutes into your drive to hospital and your car breaks down; your team is expecting you to start work in 30 minutes.

Choose the most suitable **three** options from the following list:

A. Call a breakdown service and accompany your car to the garage.

B. Ensuring your car is in a safe place, arrange a taxi to take you the last 10 minutes of your commute to work.

C. Call a breakdown service and obtain their opinion on your car prior to contacting the hospital.

D. Leave a message for the rota coordinator regarding the incident.

E. Attempt to contact your consultant on call to inform them of the incident seeking their advice on how to proceed.

F. Contact your FY1 colleague who is also working today to inform them of the incident.

G. Attempt to contact the overnight FY1 doctor, asking them to stay on until you arrive at the hospital.

H. Attempt to contact the on-call registrar informing them of the incident.

Q89. You are an FY1 on a respiratory attachment over the winter season. Your team has been incredibly busy lately with your consultant being in charge of the care of an average of 35 inpatients for the past 8 weeks. In your spare time you play in a reasonably successful rock band that has a few performances coming up. Owing to having to stay late at work, you have missed three of your last five practice sessions that normally start at 6 pm. Your band mates complain about how your lack of attendance at practice is having a negative impact on the group.

Choose the most suitable **three** options from the following list:

A. Always leave work at 5 pm to ensure you make every practice.

B. Hand over your leftover jobs at 5 pm to your colleagues on the ward to ensure they are completed and to allow you to attend practice.

C. Leave the band; unfortunately it's not compatible with working life.

D. Contact the lead consultant for respiratory medicine explaining that more doctors are needed to help with the current situation.

E. Attempt to rearrange your practice sessions for a later time.

F. Disagree with your band mates; obviously they don't appreciate how busy things are at work at the moment.

G. Discuss your band mates' concerns at the next practice session.

H. Contact your educational supervisor stating that you are concerned that your job may not be compliant with the European Working Time Directive.

Q90. You are an FY1 working on a busy 45-bed hepatology unit. There are three FY1s attached to the unit. Owing to one colleague being on annual leave and the other being on night shifts, you are the only FY1 doctor working on the unit today. You have just completed a ward round with your registrar, who is now in clinic, and have begun to plan the resultant jobs list. At this time, your consultant and educational supervisor, Dr Jackson, walks onto the unit wanting to give you a tutorial now as she has been unable to thus far in your attachment. You are keen to be taught but are anxious as you are currently very busy with your clinical commitments.

Choose the most suitable **three** options from the following list:

A. Ask whether it is possible to re-arrange the teaching session with Dr Jackson.

B. Complete producing the jobs list and then attend Dr Jackson's teaching session before completing your jobs.

C. Contact the medical rota coordinator to see whether another FY1 can cover your ward whilst you receive your tutorial from Dr Jackson.

D. Liaise with Dr Jackson over the junior doctor rota to ensure adequate junior doctor staffing of the unit at all times.

E. Bleep your registrar and ask whether they would be able to complete the jobs list and make a start on them so that you can have a tutorial.

F. Complete your jobs list, prioritising the clinically urgent jobs first.

G. Attend the teaching session with Dr Jackson; you are in a training programme and need time dedicated to your education.

H. Remark to Dr Jackson that the staffing levels of the unit are currently unsafe.

Q91. You have been the FY1 doctor on call for the evening shift this week. Your hospital uses an electronic handover board whereby medical colleagues can post jobs for the evening on-call doctor to do without handing over in person. Throughout your week on call you happen to notice a large number of jobs for one ward in particular. You note that most of the jobs posted are from one colleague, Hassan. A significant number of the jobs that he posts are to chase the results of investigations. Over the week you've noticed that a good amount of these investigation results have been available to view on the computerised investigation reporting system well within working hours. You begin to suspect that Hassan is not chasing the results of the investigations his ward requests, creating a considerable amount of work for the on-call team.

Choose the most suitable **three** options from the following list:

A. Do not chase the results of investigations Hassan hands over to the evening team.

B. Discuss your concerns with your clinical seniors on your shift.

C. Email the Foundation Programme director in your trust informing them of the situation and asking them to remind all FY1s within the trust to use the electronic handover board appropriately.

> Consider the escalation ladder.

D. Contact Hassan directly reminding him that he should be chasing the results of investigations for the patients on his ward.

E. Email Hassan's educational supervisor raising questions as to whether he is coping with his current attachment as he seems to be unable to complete a fair few of his clinical jobs.

F. Hand over the chasing of investigations to the night team on call.

G. Continue to complete the jobs requested of you by your colleagues and hand over to the night team all jobs you were unable to do.

H. Ask the SHO for the evening shift to do all the jobs requiring the chasing of results so that you can address urgent clinical tasks.

Q92. You have been looking after Mrs Green on your ward for the past 11 days and on the consultant ward round this morning she was deemed medically fit for discharge. Whilst an inpatient, Mrs Green was reviewed by the occupational therapists and physiotherapists who identified several unaddressed care needs for Mrs Green and so feel that, although she may be medically fit, she is not fit to return home until these needs have been addressed. The ward's MDT decided that Mrs Green would be well served by being temporarily placed within a care home. However, on discussion with Mrs Green's family later in the day, they 'don't want their mother going to some nursing home!'

Choose the most suitable **three** options from the following list:

A. Allow Mrs Green to be discharged temporarily to a care home.

B. Explain to Mrs Green and family the rationale of the MDT's decision.

C. Allow Mrs Green to remain in hospital until her care needs are met.

D. Ask the nursing staff to discuss the family's concerns and report back.

E. Discharge Mrs Green back to her home at the family's request.

F. Discuss discharge destination preferences with Mrs Green.

G. Inform the MDT the next day of the concerns expressed by Mrs Green's family.

H. Discuss the Green family's concerns regarding Mrs Green's discharge destination.

Q93. You are a geriatric FY1 doctor. You are looking after Mr Roberts, a 92-year-old man who was admitted following a fall secondary to urinary sepsis. Unfortunately as a result of the fall he has fractured his right humerus. This was acutely managed in A&E but has been a secondary issue whilst your medical team has been treating Mr Roberts for his infection. As Mr Roberts has clinically improved, the consultant in charge of Mr Roberts's care has asked you to contact the orthopaedic registrar to request a long-term plan for the humerus fracture. You contacted them this morning and they agreed to review Mr Roberts today; however, at 4.30 pm they have yet to attend.

Choose the most suitable **three** options from the following list:

A. Contact the orthopaedic consultant on call to request a review.

B. Handover to the doctor on call this evening to review Mr Roberts later to see whether the orthopaedic registrar has reviewed your patient.

C. Inform Mr Roberts that the orthopaedic team has agreed to review him today, but there has been some delay with this.

D. Contact another orthopaedic registrar to request a review.

E. Fast-bleep the on-call orthopaedic registrar to remind them that they had agreed to review Mr Roberts today.

F. Attempt to re-contact the on-call orthopaedic registrar and ask whether they will be able to review Mr Roberts today.

113

G. Contact your consultant to inform them that Mr Roberts has yet to be reviewed by the orthopaedic registrar today.

H. Repeat an x-ray of Mr Roberts's right humerus to check on the bone healing.

Q94. You are an FY1 in gynaecology. Mrs Hellenbranth is an inpatient on your ward admitted for investigation of post-menopausal bleeding and longstanding abdominal pain. She was last seen by her consultant, Mr Evans, 2 days ago. She is reviewed by his registrar, Patricia, every day of her admission. You and Patricia meet with Mr Evans in his office at the end of every day to discuss the daily progress of his patients. This afternoon, you attend Mrs Hellenbranth to see how she is; she remarks 'I cannot believe that Mr Evans … it's unacceptable that I have seen him so little!'

Choose the most suitable **three** options from the following list:

A. Ask the ward matron to ensure that Mr Evans conducts a daily ward round.

B. Explore whether Mrs Hellenbranth has any new clinical concerns.

C. Investigate whether patients are entitled to a daily consultant review.

D. Discuss Mrs Hellenbranth's remark with Patricia and Mr Evans at today's afternoon meeting.

E. Inform Mrs Hellenbranth that you agree that Mr Evans should personally review his patients more often.

F. Reassure Mrs Hellenbranth that, although Mr Evans may not see her on a daily basis, he is informed daily of her progress.

G. Inform Mrs Hellenbranth that she should report her concerns to the patient advice and liaison service (PALS).

H. Inform Mrs Hellenbranth that her concerns are unfounded.

Q95. You are the FY1 on the team looking after Mavis Collins, a 93-year-old woman with cognitive impairment and end-stage congestive cardiac failure who presented with severe pulmonary oedema and deteriorating renal function. Your team is finding it very difficult to control Mrs Collins's symptoms; she has clinically deteriorated over the 3 days she has been under your team's care. Your consultant decides that a 'do not attempt CPR' (DNACPR) order is in Mrs Collins's best interests and, on discussion with Mrs Collins's enduring power of attorney, her daughter Sophie, this is put in place. Later in the day the nursing staff explain that the rest of Mrs Collins's family are currently visiting and are in disagreement with the decision regarding the DNACPR.

Choose the most suitable **three** options from the following list:

A. Ask your consultant as to whether the decision made earlier can be reversed.

B. Explore the family's concerns regarding the decision.

C. Explain to the family that a decision regarding DNACPR was made in Mrs Collins's best interests and their concerns are misplaced.

D. Ask Mrs Collins whether she would like the order reversed.

E. Explain the rationale for the decision that was made.

F. Encourage the family to take their concerns up with Sophie as she is Mrs Collins's enduring power of attorney.

G. Explain that the decision was made in discussion with Sophie.

H. Revoke the order yourself as the majority of Mrs Collins's family are in disagreement with it.

Q96. You are an FY1 in respiratory medicine. Earlier in the day you reviewed Mr Blowers with your consultant. He has developed a clinically significant pleural effusion and your consultant would like to have a chest drain inserted under ultrasound guidance, and fills in a request form for the procedure. Later in the day you notice that Mr Blowers remains without his chest drain. You contact the duty radiologist to see whether the chest drain will be inserted today – who informs you that Mr Blowers underwent a computed tomography pulmonary angiogram (CTPA) as your consultant's handwriting was interpreted to read 'pulmonary embolism' rather than 'pulmonary effusion' on the request form.

Choose the most suitable **three** options from the following list:

A. Clinically review Mr Blowers to see whether he has symptomatically worsened and apologise for the unnecessary investigation.

B. Report the duty radiologist, via the clinical incident reporting mechanism, for performing the wrong investigation on Mr Blowers.

C. Contact the clinical lead for respiratory medicine informing them of the incident.

D. Inform your consultant that Mr Blowers has undergone a CTPA.

E. Contact the Care Quality Commission raising your concerns that your hospital needs to update its investigation requesting systems.

F. Contact the medical director of your trust requesting that your trust adopts online investigation requesting.

G. Wait for Mr Blowers to be reviewed by a senior tomorrow to see whether the chest drain is still clinically indicated.

H. Re-request the ultrasound-guided chest drain insertion.

Q97. You are the medical FY1 on call overnight and have been asked by the day team from Huntsman Ward to chase the renal function of Albert Morris, a 78-year-old man who presented with acute-on-chronic renal failure secondary to acute urinary retention. They inform you that the sample was taken at 5 pm. You have had a busy shift so far, being asked to review many unwell patients, but at 2 am you finally have the opportunity to chase the blood test result. However, on looking at the results reporting system, there is no result available and the sample has not been recorded as received by the lab. Mr Morris has completed all of his prescribed IV fluid therapy and is currently asleep.

Choose the most suitable **three** options from the following list:

A. Re-prescribe further IV fluids for Mr Morris and request a repeat renal function sample to be taken in the morning.

B. Wait for Mr Morris's day team to review him later on in the morning as to whether he needs further IV fluid therapy.

C. Leave an entry in Mr Morris's medical notes informing the team that they did not ensure the blood sample was received by the lab.

D. Wake Mr Morris and repeat the renal function blood test overnight.

E. Apologise that, even though the sample was taken earlier in the day, it unfortunately never made it to the lab.

F. Prescribe IV fluid therapy only if clinically indicated.

G. Arrange an ultrasound scan of Mr Morris's urinary tract.

H. Complete a clinical incident form regarding the event.

Q98. Your FY1 colleague on your ward, James, runs a youth group on two evenings a week. The group meets at 5.30 pm in a village hall about a 20-minute drive from your hospital. Recently your team has been very busy and unfortunately the whole team has been having to stay about 20 minutes late most days for the past couple of weeks to ensure that all of the urgent jobs for the day are done. James, however, always leaves at 5 pm on the days his youth group meets, only occasionally explaining that he is doing so. On these days, the rest of the team has to stay even later to compensate for James's absence.

Choose the most suitable **three** options from the following list:

A. Arrange departmental hours monitoring to ensure that the extra time you are all working is compliant with your contracted hours.

B. Encourage your colleagues to all leave at 5 pm every day as these are your contracted hours.

C. Agree an internal rota organising for one person to stay past 5 pm every day.

D. Discuss with your educational supervisor regarding the whole team having to stay late most nights.

E. Ask James tomorrow morning if he would kindly let the team know the days on which he will be leaving at 5 pm.

F. Write a letter to the British Medical Association stating that your job is not compliant with the European Working Time Directive.

G. Email James's educational supervisor regarding his behaviour.

H. Report your trust to the local newspaper for making junior doctors work more hours than they are paid for.

Q99. Your consultant, Professor Chan, oversees a very busy diabetes and endocrine team normally looking after around 50 inpatients. He likes to conduct his ward round accompanied only by the nursing staff to allow his junior doctors to complete the jobs as they arise from his round. He has just reviewed a patient for which he had previously requested that a Doppler ultrasound of the lower limbs be completed. He approaches you annoyed that this has not been organised for his review. However, from your jobs list you note that you are unaware that the investigation needed to be conducted.

Choose the most suitable **three** options from the following list:

A. Explain to Professor Chan that it must be the nursing staff's fault for not informing you of the job.

B. Explain that you were unaware that the investigation needed to be conducted.

C. Ask Professor Chan for more information regarding the jobs he would like completed as a result of his ward round.

D. Explain to Professor Chan that it is common for junior doctors to accompany their consultant on the ward round.

E. Avoid being on the ward when Professor Chan is conducting his rounds.

F. Suggest that he may not have relayed the need for the investigation to you.

G. Ask the nursing staff to give feedback to you if it becomes apparent that jobs Professor Chan requests are not being done.

H. Report Professor Chan to your Foundation Programme director for not allowing you the educational opportunity of attending his ward round.

Q100. You are asked by your ward's nursing staff to review Mrs Craven, a patient who has just been transferred to your ward from the acute medical unit for ongoing care. She appears to be acutely delirious – shouting out and thrashing around in her bed – which is disturbing other patients.

Choose the most suitable **three** options from the following list:

A. Prescribe sedation for Mrs Craven.

B. Allow Mrs Craven to wear herself out.

C. Review Mrs Craven and attempt to calm her down.

D. Review Mrs Craven's medical notes to obtain more background information and the reason for her current admission.

E. Arrange for Mrs Craven to be moved to a side room.

F. Call the hospital's security staff to assist in the restraining of Mrs Craven.

G. Restrain Mrs Craven personally.

H. Ask the nursing staff to contact Mrs Craven's next of kin to gain a collateral history.

> Do you have enough information?

ANSWERS

A51. This question is focusing on your ability to prioritise clinical need in the acute setting. Out of hours it is common for the FY1 doctor to be covering many acute medical wards with many unwell patients. By obtaining more information from the nurse who is calling you, it will be possible for you to begin to determine the clinical urgency for the assessment of this new patient (**answer B**). However, as you have not completed your management of the initial patient you have been called to, it may be appropriate for the new patient to be assessed by one of your colleagues if possible (**answer C**). Having a full set of observations of the new patient will allow you to extrapolate some degree of clinical urgency but has the implication of consuming time (**answer E**). You have stabilised your current patient somewhat, but leaving them before completing your initial management is rather negligent (**answer A**). The least appropriate option would be to respond negatively to the nurse paging you (**answer D**), as if they are concerned with one of their patients you should at least hear their concern.

Ideal order	Your rank choice				
	1st	2nd	3rd	4th	5th
B	4	3	2	1	0
C	3	4	3	2	1
E	2	3	4	3	2
A	1	2	3	4	3
D	0	1	2	3	4

A52. This question is focusing on a scenario when there is clinical uncertainty. You must remember to escalate clinical concern as per the escalation ladder. The best thing to do if your immediate senior (the SHO) is unavailable is to escalate your concern up the ladder; thus speaking to the medical registrar on call is the most appropriate option (**answer B**). The next port of call would be the on-call haematology consultant (**answer D**). Although this might be daunting as an FY1, you must remember that doctors on call regardless of grade should be available to advise others. The next best option would be to discuss the heparin infusion with the senior nurse on the ward; just because you have not come across one in your training doesn't mean to say that they haven't, as they may deal regularly with patients on heparin infusions and so may be able to guide your decision (**answer E**). Consulting the internet for advice is rather risky as you cannot be sure of the source of the advice, so it's always best to use this with caution (**answer C**). It would be least appropriate to do nothing at all about the heparin infusion, as this may put the patient at risk, which is why this is the worst response (**answer A**).

Ideal order	Your rank choice				
	1st	2nd	3rd	4th	5th
B	4	3	2	1	0
D	3	4	3	2	1
E	2	3	4	3	2
C	1	2	3	4	3
A	0	1	2	3	4

A53. This question focuses on your ability to develop resilience in situations that may be personally demanding: in this situation your ability to work many days in a row. Just another tip: in any question that suggests that your job may not be compliant with your contracted hours or the European Working Time Directive a sensible and normally high-ranking option is to complete hours monitoring (**answer A**). The next options require you to escalate your concern along the escalation ladder; therefore discussing the situation with your educational supervisor (**answer B**) supersedes contacting the medical director (**answer D**) and the BMA (**answer C**). Arranging annual leave for the next week (**answer E**) is the worst option as, although it may give you a rest from work, it doesn't address the underlying concern and will in no way lead to a resolution.

Ideal order	Your rank choice				
	1st	2nd	3rd	4th	5th
A	4	3	2	1	0
B	3	4	3	2	1
D	2	3	4	3	2
C	1	2	3	4	3
E	0	1	2	3	4

A54. This scenario is patient safety focused; however, the crux of the issue lies in your ability to put this above the pressure to attend work because of the staffing situation in your unit. The most important thing to appreciate is that if you think that you are unwell and that the condition is potentially transmittable to patients then you should not attend work; therefore the most appropriate action is to contact your consultant in the first instance to inform them (**answer E**), and then your rota coordinator (**answer B**) – this will allow them the best opportunity to arrange cover for your shift. If you are unsure as to the nature of your illness and feel you would benefit from a medical opinion then making an appointment with your GP is a reasonable action (**answer C**). The second least appropriate option from the answer stems is staying at home without informing your team members (**answer D**) as this gives them no opportunity to find cover for your shift. However, the worst option is to attend work whilst potentially infectious (**answer A**) as this jeopardises patient safety.

Ideal order	Your rank choice				
	1st	2nd	3rd	4th	5th
E	4	3	2	1	0
B	3	4	3	2	1
C	2	3	4	3	2
D	1	2	3	4	3
A	0	1	2	3	4

A55. The scenario in this question is one we almost guarantee you will face when you're the on-call FY1 doctor. This scenario is challenging you to prioritise acutely unwell patients alongside an upset relative. Ideally you would want to discuss matters with the relative, but in the face of unwell patients any discussions with relatives drops in priority. What you should do in this situation (and what is the most appropriate answer) is, as the relative is present, acknowledge their concern but urgently attend the unwell patients (**answer A**). The next most appropriate answer is to ask the nurse to contact another doctor (**answer D**) to discuss the relative's concerns to allow you to attend the unwell patients. Following this, asking the nurse to document the relative's concerns in the notes (**answer E**) would ensure that the patient's team was aware of the relative's concerns, albeit this option is unlikely to quell the relative's anxieties. Suggesting that the relative contacts PALS (**answer C**) would ensure their concerns were investigated, but this isn't an appropriate avenue as this service is more for complaints about care issues. The worst option, as alluded to earlier, would be to discuss the relative's concerns immediately (**answer B**) as this should not be prioritised over acutely unwell patients.

Ideal order	Your rank choice				
	1st	2nd	3rd	4th	5th
A	4	3	2	1	0
D	3	4	3	2	1
E	2	3	4	3	2
C	1	2	3	4	3
B	0	1	2	3	4

A56. This scenario is asking you to consider a situation where a mistake has occurred that has the potential to negatively impact a patient's health. In this scenario, the most appropriate response would be to assess the patient urgently for toxicity (**answer A**) as this is the clinical priority. As the error was preventable, and the result of human factors, it is appropriate to report this through the adverse incident log (**answer B**) so that the error can be investigated. As the mistake is the result of a nursing error, arranging additional training for the nurses around the administration of antibiotics (**answer D**) may be a sensible suggestion, but is not an urgent concern. Similarly it would be a reasonable opportunity for you to complete a reflective entry in your e-portfolio (**answer E**), but as you were not implicated in the mistake that occurred this is of a lesser priority. The least appropriate option would be to confront the nurse who forgot to sign the drug chart (**answer C**); although this would inform her of the mistake, it is not your responsibility.

Ideal order	Your rank choice				
	1st	2nd	3rd	4th	5th
A	4	3	2	1	0
B	3	4	3	2	1
D	2	3	4	3	2
E	1	2	3	4	3
C	0	1	2	3	4

A57. If you are on a busy team or working on a large unit it isn't inconceivable that two patients could have the same surname, especially if it's a common name like Smith! This scenario is encouraging you to consider a situation where there is both ambiguity and the pressure of an acutely unwell patient. The theme of communicating with colleagues is also considered. The most prudent and appropriate thing to do would be to attend ward 2 and clarify which patient has the low haemoglobin (**answer C**). If both patients are on an orthopaedic ward it is likely that they will have a valid group and screen blood result in the lab, however clarifying this will reduce delay in treatment once the correct patient is identified (**answer B**). This answer stem is preferential to taking repeat samples from both patients (**answer E**) as it (a) may be unnecessary if a valid sample exists and (b) the incorrect Mr Smith will have an unnecessary procedure; although, it will ensure that there is a valid group and screen for the correct Mr Smith. Although you will feel pressure as an FY1 to complete discharge summaries, they rarely (if ever!) take precedence over a clinically unwell patient, so any answer that gives preferences to completing them will be low ranking. However, completing the discharge summaries whilst looking out for the haemoglobin result (**answer A**) is preferential to attempting to contact the ward as you have already tried this without success (**answer D**). Remember, any option which repeats something already tried in the question caveat is normally inappropriate.

Ideal order	Your rank choice				
	1st	2nd	3rd	4th	5th
C	4	3	2	1	0
B	3	4	3	2	1
E	2	3	4	3	2
A	1	2	3	4	3
D	0	1	2	3	4

A58. This scenario highlights the difficulty of escalating concern in a hierarchical organisation. It's very difficult to tell the consultant they may be making a mistake; however, your priority is to ensure the clinical safety of your patient so politely reminding the consultant of the patient's presenting complaint may subtly correct their error (**answer C**). Challenging the consultant away from the patient (**answer E**) will ensure that the error is addressed, albeit not as timely as possible and so the patient will need re-reviewing, thus delaying a busy ward round. Hoping that the consultant will eventually realise their mistake having reviewed the second patient is a poor option as it does not guarantee the mistake will be corrected (**answer D**). Switching the management plans of the patients without informing your consultant (**answer B**) is very unprofessional, as they are ultimately responsible for the patient's care, not you. The worst option is not to interject when you feel a mistake has been made (**answer A**); you should always feel comfortable to raise your concerns.

Ideal order	Your rank choice				
	1st	2nd	3rd	4th	5th
C	4	3	2	1	0
E	3	4	3	2	1
D	2	3	4	3	2
B	1	2	3	4	3
A	0	1	2	3	4

A59. The most sensible action to take in this situation would be to request that Mike leaves theatre and returns to help you on the ward (**answer C**) as this would remedy the situation acutely. Obviously you can appreciate Mike's predicament in that he wants to gain the most surgical experience from his only surgical job. However, although it is important for him to attend theatre, this shouldn't be to the detriment of the mainstay of his work – looking after ward-based patients – therefore asking him to ensure that the ward is adequately staffed before attending theatre in the future is a prudent response (**answer E**). In his absence, ensuring that all unwell patients are attended to on the ward is your priority, but it seems fairly reasonable to hand over to him the more routine jobs on his return (**answer D**). Requesting help from another surgical team would be an attempt to get you the help you need (**answer B**), but ultimately this doesn't address the underlying issue of the scenario. The worst option would be to contact Mike's clinical supervisor (**answer A**) in the first instance, as this is inflammatory and you have made no attempt to seek Mike's rationale for attending theatre first; maybe he has a legitimate reason to be there?

Ideal order	Your rank choice				
	1st	2nd	3rd	4th	5th
C	4	3	2	1	0
E	3	4	3	2	1
D	2	3	4	3	2
B	1	2	3	4	3
A	0	1	2	3	4

A60. Although Mr Morris and you have forged a good working relationship and this comment is out of character and a one-off, it is still unprofessional. Using the escalation ladder, raising your concern via your educational supervisor (**answer C**) is a better option than another consultant within the same department (**answer E**) and is more sensible than contacting the medical director directly (**answer B**). You should never gossip about a colleague (**answer D**), which is the insinuation of your discussion with your FY1 colleague, however, the least appropriate response would be to confront Mr Morris whilst still on the ward round and in front of patients (**answer A**).

Ideal order	Your rank choice				
	1st	2nd	3rd	4th	5th
C	4	3	2	1	0
E	3	4	3	2	1
B	2	3	4	3	2
D	1	2	3	4	3
A	0	1	2	3	4

A61. This scenario provides you with a very difficult conflict to settle; on one hand you have to manage the concerns of a patient's relatives whilst on the other hand not acting against the wishes of the consultant in charge of her care. Her agitation appears to be acute in onset and so reviewing Mrs Du Bois for a cause of this is a very sensible response initially (**answer A**). You should obtain senior advice if you are considering prescribing Mrs Du Bois's sedation; raising this through the escalation ladder means that you should contact your on-call medical registrar (**answer C**) before attempting to contact Dr Jackson who is not working today (**answer E**). Not prescribing sedation to Mrs Du Bois (**answer B**) isn't the worst option as this action coincides with Dr Jackson's plan but may not reflect the change in clinical picture. The worst option would be to prescribe sedatives (**answer D**) directly against the consultant's advice solely to appease the family's concerns.

Ideal order	Your rank choice				
	1st	2nd	3rd	4th	5th
A	4	3	2	1	0
C	3	4	3	2	1
E	2	3	4	3	2
B	1	2	3	4	3
D	0	1	2	3	4

A62. Remember: Patient safety! Patient safety! Patient safety! The most important response to this scenario is ensuring that Mr Iqbal is clinically reviewed by your senior (**answer D**) despite the aetiology of his clinical deterioration. A mistake has been made and formally reporting this via the adverse incident reporting route (**answer B**) is preferential to it just being a point of reflection for your colleague (**answer E**). Although implicating your colleague in such a manner could be construed as unprofessional (**answer A**), the reason for Mr Iqbal's deterioration is an error made by your FY1 colleague. The least appropriate option is covering up the mistake of your colleague by prescribing medication to simply their actions (**answer C**).

Ideal order	Your rank choice				
	1st	2nd	3rd	4th	5th
D	4	3	2	1	0
B	3	4	3	2	1
E	2	3	4	3	2
A	1	2	3	4	3
C	0	1	2	3	4

A63. This scenario is based on a fairly common occurrence in the FY1 year, with the most junior member of a team being asked to seek the advice of a fairly senior member of another team. As a brief aside, the most important thing to do when giving a handover of information to another healthcare professional is to use a known format like 'situation, background, assessment, recommendation' (SBAR) and to have all the information you think the person will need (current observations, recent results, demographics, past medical history, etc.) to hand. In this scenario, the inference is that the general surgical registrar is now ignoring your attempts to contact him; therefore (using the escalation ladder) the most appropriate step would be to contact the on-call surgical consultant (**answer C**). The next most prudent step would be to discuss the surgical registrar's advice and actions with your consultant (**answer A**). Contacting another general surgical registrar may result in you obtaining the advice you are looking for, but they may be busy with other clinical commitments and are ultimately not on call to respond to requests for clinical advice (**answer B**). It is obvious the surgical registrar is ignoring your attempts to contact him so repeatedly trying this will probably prove fruitless and reduce the amount of time you have to complete your other jobs (**answer D**). Reporting him to his clinical lead is the least appropriate thing to do acutely, as ultimately he has given you his clinical opinion (**answer E**).

Ideal order	Your rank choice				
	1st	2nd	3rd	4th	5th
C	4	3	2	1	0
A	3	4	3	2	1
B	2	3	4	3	2
D	1	2	3	4	3
E	0	1	2	3	4

A64. This question inadvertently assesses your ability to interrogate how a scenario is structured, along with the more domain-specific points about dealing with stressful interactions with staff, coping strategies, seeking support and potentially whistleblowing. Some of the answers within this scenario will be rated higher if you incorrectly assume that your overhearing Suresh shouting at an unidentified person and Agnes being upset are linked events, which the stem itself does not identify. Therefore the most prudent and appropriate response is to comfort Agnes and enquire as to why she is upset (**answer D**). The next most appropriate response would be to encourage Agnes to escalate her concern through her own hierarchical escalation ladder and discuss it with the ward sister (**answer E**). These responses are preferential to the ones that implicate Suresh as the cause for Agnes's upset, although keeping a log of his behaviour towards other staff members would at least form an important step if you were to consider raising your concerns about his behaviour (**answer C**). Discussing your concerns immediately with your consultant (**answer A**) avoids the confrontation of discussing matters with Suresh (**answer B**), which is the least appropriate response.

Ideal order	Your rank choice				
	1st	2nd	3rd	4th	5th
D	4	3	2	1	0
E	3	4	3	2	1
C	2	3	4	3	2
A	1	2	3	4	3
B	0	1	2	3	4

A65. As you are still on the phone to the on-call FY1, the most appropriate action to take would be to reiterate to them the reason for handing over this job (**answer E**) as, although obviously annoyed, their role is ultimately to support the day team's out of working hours. If the on-call FY1's expectation is for you to stay, this is inappropriate and so escalating the job to their immediate senior is the next most appropriate step (**answer B**). Raising the on-call FY1's behaviour with your consultant in the morning seems a sensible thing to do, but is not the most appropriate in this scenario (**answer C**). Although the on-call FY1's request that you stay to check the results is very questionable, confronting them in such a way as to call them 'totally unprofessional' is not a desirable action (**answer D**). The worst option would be to go home leaving the results unchecked (**answer A**) as this has the potential to compromise patient safety.

Ideal order	Your rank choice				
	1st	2nd	3rd	4th	5th
E	4	3	2	1	0
B	3	4	3	2	1
C	2	3	4	3	2
D	1	2	3	4	3
A	0	1	2	3	4

A66. This scenario presents you with clinical uncertainty and assesses how you will cope under pressure. The most appropriate action is to complete an initial ABCDE assessment of the patient and initiate some of the management plan (**answer B**); this is within your competencies as an FY1 doctor and is initially the safest option for the patient in question. The next most appropriate response is to contact the critical care outreach (**answer D**) as this obtains you appropriate senior support given the clinical state of your patient in this scenario. It is preferential to putting out a crash call (**answer A**) as the patient has not arrested (yet!) even though they are unwell and you do require senior medical support; it would also alert the medical registrar of the situation with the new patient. Waiting for the registrar to arrive before initiating management (**answer E**) is a poor option as there may be simple interventions you can make prior to their arrival. Complaining to the registrar that their request for you to attend the new patient is unreasonable (**answer C**) is the least appropriate option listed as the patient remains unreviewed and it is not true; as an FY1 you can carry out an initial acute assessment and initiate basic management.

Ideal order	Your rank choice				
	1st	2nd	3rd	4th	5th
B	4	3	2	1	0
D	3	4	3	2	1
A	2	3	4	3	2
E	1	2	3	4	3
C	0	1	2	3	4

A67. As I'm sure you will gather as you start to form your own ideas about approaching answering SJT questions, any response that hints at ensuring patient safety normally ranks highest; in this scenario seeing whether Julia has any acutely unwell patients (**answer A**) allows you to triage your work and ensures that the most unwell patient is prioritised. Thom has allocated the work and the expectation should be on him to attend the ward in this scenario to review its patients as per his allocation; therefore requesting that Julia contacts him is the next most appropriate response (**answer D**). This ranks above contacting Thom yourself (**answer C**) as your time is better invested in looking after the patients allocated to you. Asking Julia to arrange a job list (**answer E**) would rank next as this is a good way to ensure that the clinically urgent jobs on the ward are done before the end of your shift. Telling Julia that these patients are not your responsibility and hanging up (**answer B**) is the least appropriate response. The method you and Thom have devised to complete today's work is an internally devised strategy; how is Julia to know who's looking after her patients?

Ideal order	Your rank choice				
	1st	2nd	3rd	4th	5th
A	4	3	2	1	0
D	3	4	3	2	1
C	2	3	4	3	2
E	1	2	3	4	3
B	0	1	2	3	4

A68. You have many commitments as an FY1 doctor and throughout your clinical career: your clinical responsibilities, your educational requirements and the need to balance work with your personal life. The most appropriate and sensible action to take in this scenario is to ask your clinical supervisor whether there is a possibility to alter dates for the audit to accommodate your annual leave (**answer E**). The next most appropriate answer would be to re-discuss your options for the audit and complete one that will not coincide with your annual leave (**answer C**). Agreeing to complete the important audit but shortening the audit period (**answer D**) is preferential to agreeing to complete the audit and attending on your annual leave day (**answer A**) as this shows no regard for your need to keep a work–life balance. The worst option is to fabricate data (**answer B**); any response in any question that involves an element of deceit or unprofessional behaviour is likely to be the worst option.

Ideal order	Your rank choice				
	1st	2nd	3rd	4th	5th
E	4	3	2	1	0
C	3	4	3	2	1
D	2	3	4	3	2
A	1	2	3	4	3
B	0	1	2	3	4

A69. This question focuses on balancing expectations from senior colleagues with your personal responsibilities as an employee. The most appropriate action to take in this scenario is to phone your consultant to tell them that you are unable to work today (**answer B**) as it would contravene the European Working Time Directive and hence be illegal. Additionally, one would have to question your ability to be a 'safe doctor' having worked so many days continuously without a break. The next most appropriate thing to do, although not technically your responsibility, would be to inform the rota coordinator to see whether they could arrange alternative cover (**answer A**). The following three answers are, in the main, all inappropriate. Attempting to arrange working the shift for SHO locum rates (**answer D**) supersedes attending work later in the day without contacting your consultant (**answer C**) as not returning the call may prevent your consultant arranging alternative locum for the shift. Contacting your unwell SHO to ask them to attend work (**answer E**) is not helpful and hence the least appropriate answer; it is unreasonable for you to expect an unwell colleague to attend work, in the process jeopardising the safety of current inpatients.

Ideal order	Your rank choice				
	1st	2nd	3rd	4th	5th
B	4	3	2	1	0
A	3	4	3	2	1
D	2	3	4	3	2
C	1	2	3	4	3
E	0	1	2	3	4

A70. This question is assessing your ability to cope when under the pressure of time and expectations of a clinical senior. It further assesses your ability to seek help and prioritise clinical need. It is not uncommon to find yourself with several patients requiring your attention at any given time and it is important that you triage your time to deal with the most important first. In this question, the most appropriate and clinically safe response is to complete requesting the investigations for the first patient you reviewed (**answer D**). Informing the registrar that you have only been working for 1 hour (**answer C**) is the next best option; this response is not worded confrontationally and so should not be avoided, it also informs them of your current progress and complies with the escalation ladder, which is why discussing the situation with your consultant (**answer B**) is the third answer. Asking for help from an FY1 colleague (**answer E**) is the penultimate answer as although it seems like a reasonable solution, the question stem informs you that they are also likely to be busy as patients are distributed evenly. Finally, (**answer A**) is the least appropriate option as waiting until you have cumulated tasks shows a lack of regard for patient safety as certain tasks (e.g. ECG, starting antibiotics, prescribing IV fluids) shouldn't be delayed) – such options will always rank low.

Ideal order	Your rank choice				
	1st	2nd	3rd	4th	5th
D	4	3	2	1	0
C	3	4	3	2	1
B	2	3	4	3	2
E	1	2	3	4	3
A	0	1	2	3	4

A71. This question revolves around your ability to deal with clinical uncertainty and how you choose to escalate clinical concern to your senior colleagues. By following the escalation ladder you should have chosen discussing your findings with your SHO (**answer E**) as the most appropriate answer.

129

Awaiting your registrar to return to the ward in the afternoon (**answer D**) is the next answer as this shows escalation along the ladder; however, waiting until the afternoon introduces a time delay in ordering a further investigation. Requesting an abdominal CT (**answer A**) is the third answer as this scan should aid with diagnosing the mass; it is preferable to documenting your findings in the notes for review tomorrow as there is no guarantee your entry will be read and the information may be missed (**answer B**). The worst option is to hand over your findings to the GP on Mrs Hopkins's discharge summary (**answer C**) – this will introduce a significant time delay in arranging appropriate follow-up and relies on the GP receiving and acting upon your findings.

Ideal order	Your rank choice				
	1st	2nd	3rd	4th	5th
E	4	3	2	1	0
D	3	4	3	2	1
A	2	3	4	3	2
B	1	2	3	4	3
C	0	1	2	3	4

A72. Never do a procedure that you are not competent to do (remember: 'see one, do one, teach one') – any answer that requires this of you should automatically be very low ranking! Explaining your lack of competence at the requested procedure to the urology registrar in a non-confrontational manner (**answer B**) is the most appropriate option. If the registrar is not willing to review the patient, you should escalate your concern to **your** consultant (**answer D**) before a doctor from another team / specialty (**answer E**). Remember, the escalation process involves your direct team (SHO, registrar, consultant) before seeking advice from another doctor. The operation note from the urologist clearly states not to remove the catheter; therefore replacing it is not advisable as this is going against direct instruction, regardless of your ability to insert catheters (**answer C**). Performing the bladder aspirate (**answer A**) is the worst option as it puts the patient at risk as you are not competent in the procedure.

Ideal order	Your rank choice				
	1st	2nd	3rd	4th	5th
B	4	3	2	1	0
D	3	4	3	2	1
E	2	3	4	3	2
C	1	2	3	4	3
A	0	1	2	3	4

A73. This question assesses a broad range of areas within domain 2: dealing with clinical ambiguity, responding to mistakes, coping with pressure, and stressful interactions with staff members. As with any question in the SJT, a response that encourages patient safety and review of an acutely unwell patient is likely to rank highly – the question stem alludes to the fact the patient is clinically unwell requiring medical review, therefore performing a clinical assessment is the most appropriate answer (**answer A**). Simon has informed you that he has reviewed the patient and you should take his word on this; ensuring the patient is on appropriate treatment (**answer B**) is therefore the next best option. (NB. The reason this is not ranked as the most appropriate option is because the patient's clinical picture could have changed since Simon's review.) Ensuring the good quality of information during handover is important – Simon should have given you more information regarding the urgent clinical cases he reviewed (but you could have similarly probed him for more information) – so reporting the poor quality of handover is the next most appropriate step (**answer D**). Calling Simon at home (**answer E**), albeit a logical option, doesn't consider that he may not be available to speak and that he is not currently on duty. The worst option is not to review an unwell patient (**answer C**).

Ideal order	Your rank choice				
	1st	2nd	3rd	4th	5th
A	4	3	2	1	0
B	3	4	3	2	1
D	2	3	4	3	2
E	1	2	3	4	3
C	0	1	2	3	4

A74. This question focuses both on dealing with a mistake and on how it is reported and subsequently discussed with the patient. The question stem tells you that Mrs Khan is not in need of IV fluid therapy and so ensuring that this is not prescribed (**answer C**) is the most acutely concerning issue. The next most appropriate response would be to explain to Mrs Khan her misdiagnosis (**answer A**). All mistakes should be reported and therefore Mrs Khan's incorrect diagnosis should be reported through the clinical incident reporting process (**answer B**). This will ensure that the events that led to it are investigated. The next most appropriate response would be to discuss the incident personally with your clinical supervisor (**answer E**); adverse events are good points for discussion and reflection. Finally, although your non-compliance with Susie's request may be frustrating for her, there's no need to advise she to speak to your clinical supervisor (**answer D**).

Ideal order	Your rank choice				
	1st	2nd	3rd	4th	5th
C	4	3	2	1	0
A	3	4	3	2	1
B	2	3	4	3	2
E	1	2	3	4	3
D	0	1	2	3	4

A75. This scenario assesses your approach to dealing with the mistake of another person – in this case a student; which slightly alters the escalation of reporting the incident. The most important thing to do is ensure that the correct patient has a cannula in situ to receive their necessary therapy (**answer A**) and remove the unnecessary cannula inserted by Robert (**answer B**) – putting in the correct cannula supersedes removing the incorrect one as it has a greater focus on patient safety (i.e. preventing delay in therapy, etc.). Discussing the incident with Robert (**answer C**) is the next most appropriate response; it will be an important point of reflection for him and you will be able to discuss collectively the events that led up to the mistake. Hence, it would be sensible for you to reflect upon the event yourself (**answer D**). The least appropriate response would be to report Robert to his medical school (**answer E**); ultimately you could have given him clearer instructions and found the time to observe him perform the procedure.

Ideal order	Your rank choice				
	1st	2nd	3rd	4th	5th
A	4	3	2	1	0
B	3	4	3	2	1
C	2	3	4	3	2
D	1	2	3	4	3
E	0	1	2	3	4

A76. This question focuses on your ability to cope with a stressful interaction with a patient's relative. Obviously there is a discrepancy between what is documented by the nursing staff and the claims of the patient; you need to take into account that Mr Kenworthy has cognitive impairment, but he may be communicating the truth. What is most important initially is to discuss with the family their concerns (**answer B**). The question stem informs you that the patient's claim is contrary to nursing documentation and so asking the family to discuss their concerns with the ward's sister is the next most appropriate option (**answer A**). Ultimately if the family wishes to pursue their concerns formally then this is best done through the hospital's PALS, who will assess the family's concerns and investigate where necessary (**answer C**). Informing the family that the nursing documentation shows that Mr Kenworthy is being fed (**answer D**) is not necessarily a bad option; however, the wording of the answer stem is fairly confrontational, making it an undesirable action. The worst option is to accuse Jane of falsifying documentation (**answer E**) as you have no real grounds to prove this, other than Mr Kenworthy's claim, and have in no way conducted an investigation into the family's concerns.

Ideal order	Your rank choice				
	1st	2nd	3rd	4th	5th
B	4	3	2	1	0
A	3	4	3	2	1
C	2	3	4	3	2
D	1	2	3	4	3
E	0	1	2	3	4

A77. This question is focusing on your ability to cope with a stressful interaction with a patient and how you choose to support a junior colleague. When you observe any prejudiced behaviour, your immediate response should be to make the individual aware that their actions are inappropriate (**answer B**). The next most appropriate option from the answer stems would be to supervise the rest of Samira's history (**answer C**) – this allows her the opportunity to feel supported whilst she is in a potentially uncomfortable situation. Not providing Samira with immediate support but raising your concerns at a later time (**answer A**) would be the third most appropriate answer as it does provide Samira with the opportunity to discuss any concerns she may have. Normalising wrong behaviour (**answer E**) is totally unacceptable – the Law states that everybody has the right to work in a non-judgemental environment. Patients can sometimes be difficult but there is no place for prejudice in the workplace! That is why completely ignoring Mr English's actions (**answer D**) is the worst option.

Ideal order	Your rank choice				
	1st	2nd	3rd	4th	5th
B	4	3	2	1	0
C	3	4	3	2	1
A	2	3	4	3	2
E	1	2	3	4	3
D	0	1	2	3	4

A78. This question focuses on your ability to strike a balance between clinical necessity and respecting a patient's wishes, thus generating a stressful situation. The best thing to do when presented with situations such as this is to explore the patient's concerns (**answer E**), explaining that you understand them but that clinical necessity may prevent his wishes being adhered to. It is often helpful to explain why a procedure is needed urgently so the patient understands you aren't simply unwilling to consider their request (**answer D**). Trying to find a male colleague from another ward (**answer B**) is a logical solution; however, there is no guarantee that such a colleague exists, hence this answer isn't ranked higher. Ultimately if a patient is competent to make the decision and is unpersuadable, then you have to follow their request; sedating them (**answer C**) is not appropriate. However the worst thing to do would be to put a patient through a procedure that is not warranted, comes with greater risk and you may not be competent to perform (**answer A**).

Ideal order	Your rank choice				
	1st	2nd	3rd	4th	5th
E	4	3	2	1	0
D	3	4	3	2	1
B	2	3	4	3	2
C	1	2	3	4	3
A	0	1	2	3	4

A79. This question is fairly simple but demonstrates nicely how to escalate concern along the escalation ladder. It focuses on a difficult interaction with a senior staff member and potential whistleblowing. In a situation like this you would escalate first to your educational supervisor (**answer A**); failing resolution or action your next most appropriate step would be to approach the departmental lead for orthopaedic surgery (**answer E**) and then to escalate to the medical director of your trust (**answer C**). If resolution or action has not occurred once you have exhausted avenues within your own hospital's managerial structures then this is when you seek support from external agencies. The more appropriate external agency to raise your concerns with would be the doctor's union, the BMA (**answer B**), rather than the local newspaper (**answer D**), as it has the ability to investigate hours monitoring externally.

Ideal order	Your rank choice				
	1st	**2nd**	**3rd**	**4th**	**5th**
A	4	3	2	1	0
E	3	4	3	2	1
C	2	3	4	3	2
B	1	2	3	4	3
D	0	1	2	3	4

A80. This question revolves around coping with a stressful interaction with a healthcare professional, handing over work appropriately and seeking support. Although it would be ideal for Adrian to be able to take and chase the result, if he expects that he will be too busy then the job must be handed over to a medical colleague; therefore the most appropriate action to take would be to hand over to the on-call FY1 doctor (**answer C**). The next best option of the answer stems would be to stay behind whilst being productive with the time in between the sample needing to be taken and knowing the result (**answer B**); however, any option that requires you to stay late rarely ranks highly. The reason it does in this question is because the other three options are confrontational (**answer A**) or have a negative impact on patient safety. Requesting a repeat sample in the morning from the phlebotomists (**answer E**) introduces significant delay in the instigation of treatment should it be shown that Mr Chakravorty has had a myocardial infarction. However, this would confirm the diagnosis and so supersedes ignoring the biochemistry lab's advice and not repeating the sample at all (**answer D**).

Ideal order	Your rank choice				
	1st	**2nd**	**3rd**	**4th**	**5th**
C	4	3	2	1	0
B	3	4	3	2	1
A	2	3	4	3	2
E	1	2	3	4	3
D	0	1	2	3	4

A81. This scenario focuses on your ability to cope with a potential clinical emergency alongside dealing with a mistake made as a result of your FY1 colleague. Mrs Jones has received an insulin dose 10 times that prescribed so will by now almost certainly be hypoglycaemic. In scenarios where a patient is at risk of being acutely unwell, the most appropriate response is always to review them (**answer B**). Once you have ensured Mrs Jones' clinical safety, the first step when dealing with a mistake involving patient care is to inform the patient (or their enduring power of attorney, should they be deemed to lack capacity) and discuss the error (**answer D**). The next step would be to report the mistake via the clinical incident reporting mechanism that exists at your hospital (**answer A**) – this will ensure that the error is investigated and measures are taken to prevent future errors (a potential resolution in this situation would be to ensure that all insulin prescriptions are written out fully, i.e. '18 units'). Requesting Emma attend the ward (**answer E**) is not necessary and the confrontational wording of the answer stem would lead you to rank this response lowly. Indeed, Emma will need to discuss and reflect upon her potential error but it is a discussion best had with her educational supervisor, not an FY1 colleague. The least appropriate action to take would be to report the nurse involved to the chief of nursing (**answer C**) as you have not conducted an investigation or collated evidence to suggest that she is to blame for the incident.

Ideal order	Your rank choice				
	1st	2nd	3rd	4th	5th
B	4	3	2	1	0
D	3	4	3	2	1
A	2	3	4	3	2
E	1	2	3	4	3
C	0	1	2	3	4

A82. This question focuses on the development of resilience amongst junior doctors. A common scenario, especially when in the infancy of your careers, is balancing your work life with your life outside the hospital. Given the answer stems in this question, the most appropriate response is to try to negotiate with your colleagues to leave on time so that you will be able to attend the game as planned (**answer E**) – it's vital that you strike a balance. The next most appropriate stem would be to discuss that the team had to stay late with your consultant the next day. Having more ward staff may negate the need for people to stay late (**answer B**). If you are concerned that you are being required to work beyond your contracted hours, it's advisable to complete hours monitoring (**answer D**). It would be inappropriate to ask one of your colleagues from a fellow ward to complete your jobs (**answer C**), but this option is preferable to just leaving on time without discussing the situation with your colleagues or providing them with support (**answer A**).

	Your rank choice				
Ideal order	1st	2nd	3rd	4th	5th
E	4	3	2	1	0
B	3	4	3	2	1
D	2	3	4	3	2
C	1	2	3	4	3
A	0	1	2	3	4

A83. This question focuses on your ability to deal with a difficult interaction with a patient's relative – in this case the parent of a child. The difficulty in this scenario arises from your duty to ensure the clinical safety of the child – who is obviously unwell – and the expectations of the mother. As an FY1 doctor in this scenario it would be most prudent in the first instance to seek advice from your senior (**answer D**) not only to help manage the unwell child – your immediate priority – but also to help persuade the mother to allow her child to be admitted (**answer E**). All answers beyond this point are suboptimal, but at least initiating some management, and investigation (**answer C**) is a better alternative than letting the mother discharge the child against medical advice (**answer B**) and allowing the mother to take the child home (**answer A**).

	Your rank choice				
Ideal order	1st	2nd	3rd	4th	5th
D	4	3	2	1	0
E	3	4	3	2	1
C	2	3	4	3	2
B	1	2	3	4	3
A	0	1	2	3	4

A84. This scenario focuses on your ability to mediate a dispute between two colleagues and how you cope with the pressure this creates. As you know Patrick and Sheila must work effectively together over the weekend as part of the same team, and so attempting to mediate their disagreement (**answer E**) is the best initial option. Failing that, your next best option is informing your consultant (**answer A**) of the dispute and empowering them to mediate the disagreement. The next rung of the escalation ladder would be to seek advice from your educational supervisor (**answer D**). Agreeing to work the weekend shift for Patrick (**answer C**) is, on face value, a logical resolution as it avoids confrontation; however, it doesn't address or attempt to resolve the underlying issue. The worst option would be to encourage two colleagues who need to work the next day to go out drinking the night before (**answer B**), as this option has the potential to compromise patient safety.

Ideal order	Your rank choice				
	1st	2nd	3rd	4th	5th
E	4	3	2	1	0
A	3	4	3	2	1
D	2	3	4	3	2
C	1	2	3	4	3
B	0	1	2	3	4

A85. This scenario highlights the many roles of the FY1 doctor: you have a clinical commitment to your patients, but you may have students whom you are required to teach and therefore you have an obligation to ensure that they are adequately trained. This may involve supervision of their clinical skills. This question also addresses managing the expectations of and difficult interactions with allied healthcare professionals.

The correct options are to explain to Marie that the job of taking Mr Wildman's bloods is clinically urgent (**answer B**) and so takes precedence over non-urgent tasks. You should then observe Jason's attempt to take the blood sample so that he has the opportunity to develop this clinical skill (**answer C**) and then provide him with timely feedback on your observation of his technique at the skill (**answer H**) to facilitate his development – though this may not be done immediately.

You should not feel pressured into completing non-urgent tasks and so rearranging your observation of Jason taking Mr Wildman's blood (**answer A**) is not appropriate. Being confrontational with Marie (**answer D**) is not appropriate either; you just need to explain that Mr Wildman's bloods are more clinically urgent. Discussing with your SHO (**answer E**) will add unnecessary delay, and allowing the medical student to take the bloods unsupervised (**answer F**) is inappropriate as you have no knowledge of their ability at the skill and will not be in a position to provide them with necessary feedback. Explaining the result of Mrs Hurdman's knee x-ray (**answer G**) is of less clinical urgency than Mr Wildman's bloods and so should not take precedence.

A	B	C	D	E	F	G	H
0	4	4	0	0	0	0	4

A86. This scenario describes a situation where there are communication problems within a team leading to a delay in treatment. The correct options are to clinically review the patient again (**answer B**); this is as there has been a significant time gap since your last review and no treatment has been administered – Mr Jones's clinical picture could have changed. Developing a protocol for the handover of urgent clinical tasks for the unit (**answer D**) is not a pressing concern, but would be an example of how an error results in service improvement. On a personally reflective point, learning from the situation by ensuring that you now hand over a job in person is a positive thing to come from the situation (**answer F**).

The incorrect options are reporting Delia for not administering the blood (**answer A**) as she is not solely culpable for the error. Additionally not attending teaching (**answer C**) will have a negative impact on your professional development and is not an appropriate resolution. Completing an audit (**answer E**) with the question posed by the answer stem will not provide a solution to the error that occurred in this scenario. Informing the clinical lead (**answer G**) is not necessary and does not follow the escalation ladder, and contacting your educational supervisor (**answer H**) is a drastic option in the first instance.

A	B	C	D	E	F	G	H
0	4	0	4	0	4	0	0

A87. This scenario raises the issues of clinical uncertainty and conflict between yourself and a senior doctor; the question assesses your ability to appropriately escalate the concern the scenario instigates. The correct actions to take in this scenario are to escalate your concern along the escalation ladder to your SHO for their opinion (**answer B**), review the patient clinically in view of the new clinical concern (**answer C**), and to repeat the ECG (**answer D**) to ensure the pattern you have observed is definitely that of Mr Sanderson.

The incorrect actions would be to ignore your concern (**answer A**) and file the ECG, arrange for an invasive procedure without seeking a senior opinion on questionable clinical evidence (**answer E**), and request bloods urgently (**answer F**) as this does not acutely address your clinical concern. Emailing the registrar's educational supervisor (**answer G**) and reflecting on the incident (**answer H**) are also both inappropriate, the former as it is unprofessional and neither addresses the urgent clinical problem.

A	B	C	D	E	F	G	H
0	4	4	4	0	0	0	0

A88. This scenario is asking you how you would cope in a situation where you will potentially be late to work, albeit for an unforeseen reason, and how you appropriately seek advice from your senior colleagues. The correct options in this case are to contact the on-call consultant (**answer E**) and registrar (**answer H**) as they will be able to offer you advice on how to proceed with the situation, plus this is in keeping with the escalation ladder. The other correct option is to attempt to arrange alternative transport to the hospital to attend your shift as planned, after ensuring your broken-down car is left in a safe position (**answer B**). Ultimately your responsibility is to attend this shift; it is unfortunate that your car has broken down but you need to provide cover for the shift in the first instance; contacting your FY1 colleague (**answer F**) is inappropriate as they lack the seniority to be able to help you.

Options that involve arranging for your car to be repaired (**answers A & C**) would be appropriate only **after** seeking the advice of your consultant. Contacting the rota coordinator (**answer D**) does not address the acute situation. It is also inappropriate to request that the overnight FY1 covers the shift (**answer G**).

A	B	C	D	E	F	G	H
0	4	0	0	4	0	0	4

A89. This scenario addresses a common problem that foundation trainees face, especially in the infancy of their careers, of striking a work–life balance. This question therefore focuses on developing resilience and coping with the pressure of a busy job.

The correct options in this question are to attempt to arrange your practice for a later time (**answer E**) as this may allow you to attend more practice sessions and will accommodate your busy job, to discuss your band mates' concerns (**answer G**) as this will allow you to appreciate their concerns, and to contact your educational supervisor as your job many not be EU compliant (**answer H**) if you are required to stay past working hours regularly. Remember, any question that alludes to you working past your contractual hours will normally have an answer that suggests you complete hours monitoring.

The incorrect options are to always leave on time (**answer A**), even after handing over your jobs (**answer B**), as this means that your colleagues may have to stay later to cover the work that you would have done; you are all entitled to leave on time! Leaving the band (**answer C**) does not resolve the underlying issue and is a drastic action; you need a life outside of medicine! Contacting the lead consultant (**answer D**) before your educational supervisor does not follow the escalation ladder, and disagreeing with your band mates (**answer F**) is creating unnecessary conflict.

A	B	C	D	E	F	G	H
0	0	0	0	4	0	4	4

A90. This scenario focuses on your ability to recognise that your role as an FY1 is service provision alongside being trained. This question is asking you to prioritise your learning alongside clinical commitments; it also involves a potentially difficult interaction with a senior colleague.

The correct options in this question are to rearrange your teaching session with Dr Jackson (**answer A**) as you are currently short staffed and it would be inappropriate to leave the ward without an FY1 doctor. Therefore, you should complete compiling your jobs list (**answer F**) and discuss your concerns with Dr Jackson (**answer D**) in her role as your educational supervisor to ensure that there is always adequate cover on the unit.

Incorrect options would involve leaving the unit and/or not attending to urgent clinical jobs (**answer B** and **answer G**), it would be inappropriate to expect your registrar to leave clinic (**answer E**) and unprofessional to discuss your concerns regarding staffing levels on the unit (**answer H**). If following the escalation ladder, you should discuss staffing issues with your educational supervisor prior to speaking to the rota coordinator (**answer C**). However, this would not be in the top three responses and therefore is not marked as a correct option.

A	B	C	D	E	F	G	H
4	0	0	4	0	4	0	0

A91. This scenario revolves around highlighting a potentially struggling FY1 colleague by correctly escalating your concern to senior colleagues. The correct options are to discuss your concerns with the senior doctors on your shift (**answer B**), allowing them to escalate matters to Hassan's supervisors as they deem appropriate. You should continue to do the work requested of you (**answer G**) but emailing your Foundation Programme director to ask them to remind colleagues of appropriate handovers (**answer C**) is also a sensible approach; it could be that Hassan is unaware of what is appropriate to hand over?

Incorrect options would be not to chase any of Hassan's jobs (**answer A**) (what if one of them is clinically urgent?) and to contact either Hassan directly with a confrontation (**answer D**) or his own educational supervisor (**answer E**) without discussing the situation with your seniors first. It would be inappropriate to hand over the chasing of all investigation results to the night team (**answer F**) – what if some of the results are clinically urgent and need acting on during your shift? The SHO is also likely to be busy and so, although asking them to help (**answer H**) may be a logical answer, it is an appropriate selection only if they are not busy, which the stem does not imply.

A	B	C	D	E	F	G	H
0	4	4	0	0	0	4	0

A92. This scenario revolves around a difficult interaction with the family of a patient. As an FY1 doctor who is generally based solely on the wards, much of your time will be taken up in informing families of the progress of their relatives, along with discussing management and long-term decisions with them. Sometimes they may not agree or follow the logic of why your team has reached the decision it has. Your role in this situation is to explore their concerns (**answer H**) and explain the reason why the decision was made or recommended (**answer B**). You should always, when the patient is competent, discuss management options and plans with the patient involved (**answer F**), as well as their relatives.

The incorrect options to take here would be to act without discussing the family's concerns (**answer A**), to go against the advice of the MDT without re-discussing matters (**answer C** and **answer E**), not to take responsibility for the planning of a patient's discharge destination (**answer D**) and not to act promptly (**answer G**).

A	B	C	D	E	F	G	H
0	4	0	0	0	4	0	4

A93. This scenario centres on a potentially difficult interaction with another member of the medical team – there is potential that an agreement to review a patient may not occur as promised. Of note, as an FY1 doctor you act very frequently as the interface between your team and the other medical and surgical specialties; many of your jobs will be the seeking of advice from more specialist teams. As you may have discovered from other similar scenarios, communication with a patient is very important and the lack of it is a very common source of complaints. When there is a potential delay in a patient's care it is always good practice to inform them (**answer C**). In this scenario it would be prudent to contact the orthopaedic registrar on call again (**answer F**) to double-check they intend on coming today – it is not the end of the working day and the orthopaedic registrar could still be intending to attend Mr Roberts today. In keeping with the escalation ladder, it would be prudent to inform your consultant (**answer G**) that there may be a delay in Mr Roberts's review – they may be able to make alternative arrangements for the review, etc.

Contacting the orthopaedic consultant on call (**answer A**) would be prudent if Mr Roberts definitely wasn't going to be reviewed, but requesting this ahead of speaking to your own consultant is not in keeping with the escalation ladder. This is not really an acute issue and it is therefore not appropriate to fast-bleep the on-call registrar (**answer E**) or to hand over to the evening team (**answer B**). There is an on-call orthopaedic registrar and contacting another registrar who is not on-call is not appropriate (**answer D**). Repeating the x-ray adds no value to the scenario (**answer H**).

A	B	C	D	E	F	G	H
0	0	4	0	0	4	4	0

A94. This question revolves around a difficult discussion with a patient; there is a query as to the level of involvement of her consultant in her care and she is, by her comment, questioning the professional integrity of Mr Evans. Thus this question is about managing patient expectations. The correct response initially is to enquire as to whether Mrs Hellenbranth has any new clinical concerns that she wishes to discuss (**answer B**), as this may have prompted her comments. In this case you must explain to Mrs Hellenbranth the level of Mr Evans's involvement in her inpatient stay (**answer F**). It would also be appropriate to inform both your registrar and Mr Evans of Mrs Hellenbranth's comments when you meet later today (**answer D**) as this would (a) inform Mr Evans of the patient's concerns and (b) allow him the opportunity to discuss them when he next personally reviews the patient.

Incorrect options would be to ask matron to ensure a daily consultant ward round (**answer A**) as this is not necessarily required and Mr Evans is already well involved in his inpatients' care. Investigating whether a daily consultant ward round is a requirement (**answer C**) may help to justify or refute Mrs Hellenbranth's concerns, but ultimately is unnecessary and time-costly in this case. Agreeing with Mrs Hellenbranth (**answer E**) is not professional in this instance as you know Mr Evans is well involved in his inpatients' care. Asking Mrs Hellenbranth to contact the PALS (**answer G**) may be a sensible suggestion, but it would be prudent to do **this** after exploring her concerns personally, reassuring her regarding Mr Evans's involvement and allowing Mr Evans to explain the situation – if her concerns persist after this then she should be directed down this avenue. Informing the patient that her concerns are unfounded (**answer H**) is not helpful and also confrontational; although you may believe this, it would be unprofessional to challenge her in this way.

A	B	C	D	E	F	G	H
0	4	0	4	0	4	0	0

A95. This is a very challenging scenario that revolves around a difficult interaction with a patient's relatives. What you are having to do here is be a mediator in a disagreement amongst a family regarding the direction of their relative's care. Sophie's position to make this decision is valid; enduring powers of attorney are established to be able to make such decisions as the one this scenario imposes. They are appointed to make best-interest decisions for people lacking the capacity to do so. With the above in mind, you should explore the rest of the family's concerns regarding the decision that was made (**answer B**), and explain to them the clinical reasons for the decision (**answer E**) and that it was done with Sophie's agreement (**answer G**). These actions have the potential to allay their concerns as it explains the process for the decision being reached and reassures them that the decision was made after discussion with Mrs Collins's enduring power of attorney.

In this scenario, incorrect options would be to request that the decision be reversed (**answer A** and **answer H**) as the decision to create a DNACPR order was made appropriately, to allow Mrs Collins the opportunity to reverse the decision (**answer D**) as she lacks capacity, to encourage the dispute amongst the family members (**answer F**) as this is inflammatory, and to dismiss the family's concerns without explaining the rationale for the decision that was made (**answer C**).

A	B	C	D	E	F	G	H
0	4	0	0	4	0	4	0

A96. This scenario presents a situation in which an error leads to a delay in a patient's treatment; as such, the most pressing action to take is to re-review Mr Blowers to see whether there has been a deterioration in his clinical state without the required intervention (**answer A**). It is also prudent to inform your consultant (**answer D**) as this will allow them the opportunity to discuss the mistake with the patient and resolve the problem in relatively good time following the error. The other action to take is to request the correct intervention (**answer H**) as this would reduce the amount of time that Mr Blowers is without treatment.

Urgent clinical concern tends always to supersede incident inquiry; therefore incorrect actions to take before ensuring clinical safety of the patient would be to report the duty radiologist (**answer B**), to contact the clinical lead for medicine (**answer C**), to contact the Care Quality Commission (**answer E**) and to contact the medical director (**answer F**). Additionally, remember the escalation ladder; you should escalate your concern through your chain of command and so contacting senior hospital managers without seeking the advice of your clinical seniors would go against this. Waiting for Mr Blowers to be seen tomorrow (**answer G**) is inappropriate as there is an acute clinical concern that needs addressing today.

A	B	C	D	E	F	G	H
4	0	0	4	0	0	0	4

A97. This is a fairly realistic scenario that you will face as an on-call FY1 doctor; you inevitably will be the only doctor for 300 medical inpatients and if a few become acutely unwell, then all of your routine jobs – like chasing blood test results – are pushed (appropriately!) to the end of your jobs list. Therefore you end up doing these when you have a spare moment, which on a night shift can be any time! The underlying issue in this scenario is that there has been a delay in checking of blood test result, which never made it to the lab. The expectation from the day team is that action needs to occur on the result overnight, even though Mr Morris may not need further fluid therapy; if he does, waiting to repeat the result till later in the day may introduce significant delay in his therapy. Therefore the ideal action to take would be to apologise to Mr Morris (**answer E**) and repeat the blood test overnight (**answer D**).

Any option that has the potential to introduce delay in Mr Morris' therapy is therefore incorrect (**answer B** and **answer C**). With regards to the prescription of the fluid therapy, this should ideally be given on the basis of clinical indication (**answer F**) and not done blindly (**answer A**). Arranging an ultrasound scan (**answer G**) is not an appropriate intervention in this scenario, and submitting a clinical incident form is not necessarily appropriate at this time (**answer H**).

A	B	C	D	E	F	G	H
0	0	0	4	4	4	0	0

A98. This scenario is complicated; obviously working beyond your paid hours is never ideal and it is a realistic expectation of James to be able to attend his youth group outside his working hours. The issue is that leaving on time makes the rest of the team leave even later; therefore there is a potential conflict within the team. As with any question that hints to a job requiring you to work beyond your paid hours, a sensible option would be to arrange hours monitoring (**answer A**). It would be appropriate to raise your concerns additionally with your educational supervisor (**answer D**) as there may be simple interventions, like moving doctors from less busy teams, which could be arranged in the short term. James is entitled to leave on time but he should be courteous about it if that impacts on the rest of his team; therefore asking him politely to inform you when he is leaving at 5 pm is very reasonable (**answer E**).

If everyone left at 5 pm (**answer B**) there is a potential implication for patient safety, so I would avoid this answer. Agreeing for someone to stay late on a rota (**answer C**) is an insufficient solution to the problem. Contacting the BMA (**answer F**), writing to James's educational supervisor (**answer G**) and reporting your trust to the local newspaper (**answer H**) are options that do not follow the correct escalation ladder of concern and so are inappropriate without discussing matters with, say, your educational supervisor first.

A	B	C	D	E	F	G	H
4	0	0	4	4	0	0	0

A99. Every consultant you work with has their own way of doing things in almost every aspect of inpatient care – some do daily ward rounds, some do daily board rounds, some take all the team with them on these including the porter, some go around by themselves, some request their own investigations, whereas others won't write in the notes, and the list goes on. You will find yourself adapting how you work in each foundation job you do and beyond, based on the nuances of your consultant. This is Professor Chan's preferred way of conducting inpatient reviews, and obviously it's not ideal as the educational benefit of being on the ward round is being superseded by service provision and the chance for errors like the one in the question are greater if you are not present to compile your own jobs list. However, in the first instance the best thing to do is explain that you were unaware the investigation was needed (**answer B**), to safeguard similar errors occurring in future by requesting more information from Professor Chan (**answer C**) and to ask Professor Chan whether it is possible to attend his ward round next time (**answer D**) to compile your own jobs list.

Attributing blame to other healthcare professionals (**answer A** and **answer G**) is inappropriate, as is avoiding the situation (**answer E**) and being inflammatory (**answer F**). Obviously if there were a suspicion that Professor Chan's annoyance is potentially bullying then this would need appropriate escalation; annoyance at a task not done is not really justification to report him to the Foundation Programme director (**answer H**).

A	B	C	D	E	F	G	H
0	4	4	4	0	0	0	0

A100. This scenario is posing you an ethical and clinical dilemma – are you potentially sedating Mrs Craven for the benefit of other patients or for the convenience of the ward staff? Is it right to sedate an acutely delirious person? Will this mask her clinical picture inappropriately? Is Mrs Craven posing a potential threat to her own safety and thus would sedation be in her best interest? These are some of the questions we would expect you to be asking yourself on reading the scenario and are the sources of the answer stems given. Acutely delirious patients are very common inpatients and you will find yourself in a similar situation no doubt in your FY1 year. Never prescribe sedation without a clinical review of the patient (**answer C**), their background (**answer D**) and ideally a collateral history (**answer H**); this is why these are the correct three options in this case.

All interventions including prescribing sedation (**answer A**), moving the patient to a side room (**answer E**), and restraining the patient either by yourself (**answer G**) or with the help of hospital security (**answer F**) are all potential options that may be warranted, but only after you have taken the three correct options. As an aside but a tip for your FY1 year, never feel pressurised into making a decision, whether that be by time or another healthcare professional's wishes, and always try to make a decision based on an objective assessment of the clinical picture – you should never do something you are not comfortable with as you are culpable for all decisions actioned by your signature.

A	B	C	D	E	F	G	H
0	0	4	4	0	0	0	4

6. Domain 3 – effective communication

The ability to communicate effectively is without doubt one of the most important qualities a doctor must display. Indeed the UKFPO (2015) states that all doctors must 'have demonstrable skills in listening, writing and speaking in English that enable effective communication about medical topics with patients and colleagues. However, thinking more specifically about the FY1 doctor, you are the most visible member of the medical team on the 'shop floor', you will see all of your team's patients on most days, you will interact with them most frequently, you will often clarify a patient's diagnosis more thoroughly once the ward round has finished, you will explain their discharge plan, you will discuss the patient's progress with their relatives … the list is endless! Additionally, it is normally the FY1 who requests expert opinions from other specialties, discusses investigation requests with the radiology department and communicates medical management with the wider multidisciplinary team (MDT).

Indeed, when the ISFP group began looking into the SJT for FY1 job applications, they determined that the most important domain to assess in the application stage was effective communication. Now, a written test is probably not the best modality to assess your communication skills; it's probably better done through a face-to-face interview, but what a test can assess is your logic and thinking in approaching a communicational task and your knowledge on the key attributes of an effective communicator:

1. Check understanding.
2. Listen effectively and reflect concerns.
3. Communicate in appropriate settings.
4. Be assertive when required.
5. Respond to non-verbal cues.
6. Use non-verbal communication effectively.

When it comes to being assessed on your ability to communicate with patients, the SJT will focus on how you develop and maintain good working relationships through clear, sensitive and precise communication. It should be jargon-free and adjusted to the needs of the patient in terms of style and the amount of information given. It is imperative that you do your best to keep patients updated with their care and answer any of their or their relatives' (providing the patient has given consent) questions in a timely manner.

A significant amount of communication we do as doctors is written (both paper and electronic), whether that be our entries in the medical notes, discharge summaries to GPs, referral letters or investigation requests. You must display high standards of written communication that is legible, concise and clear.

The following practice questions have been developed to provide an opportunity for you to demonstrate how to correctly deal with these topics. Remember, it is what you **should** do, not what you **would** do!

Q101. You are with your registrar, Anil, on a busy ward round. You are currently reviewing Doris, an 80-year-old woman referred to the cardiology unit with worsening of her known heart failure. Whilst discussing Doris's management Anil says 'We're going to check your BNP to see how bad your CCF is'. Doris doesn't appear to understand his plan and looks to you with a confused expression on her face. Anil doesn't seem to have picked up on this and begins to leave Doris' bed area.

Rank in order the following actions in response to this situation (1 = most appropriate; 5 = least appropriate):

A. Tell Anil that you don't think Doris has understood the acronyms he has used and ask him to provide Doris with clarification of his plan.

B. Go back to Doris later to take the brain natriuretic peptide (BNP) blood test yourself; use the opportunity whilst taking the sample to explain the rationale for it.

C. Tell Doris 'don't worry, we've got everything in hand!'

D. Spend a couple of minutes now explaining Anil's plan and re-join the ward round at the next patient.

E. Arrange for the BNP level to be taken as per Anil's plan by the ward phlebotomist.

> Understanding is required for valid consent.

Q102. Mr Kensington was discharged from the ward you work on 2 days ago. He was under the care of another team. He has returned to the ward as he has read his discharge summary and there are some points on it he does not understand; he recognises you as a doctor and holds up the discharge summary showing his diagnosis as 'suspected primary lung Ca' and asks what this means. You notice that the discharge summary was completed by Robert, the registrar for another team.

Rank in order the following actions in response to this situation (1 = most appropriate; 5 = least appropriate):

A. Explain to Mr Kensington that his team suspects he may have a cancer in his lung.

B. Ask Mr Kensington to wait until he is seen by his consultant for his post-discharge follow-up appointment next week and to ask any questions he has then.

C. Ask Anna, the FY1 for the team Mr Kensington was under, to see if she can clarify his concerns.

D. Explain to Mr Kensington that, as you were not on the team looking after him, you are unable to clarify any questions he may have.

E. Contact Robert and ask him to attend the ward to answer Mr Kensington's questions.

> Are you in a position to explain?

Q103. Mr Jensen is a 68-year-old man who looks after a coop of parrots in his spare time. He has been admitted under the respiratory team for which you are the FY1 with increased shortness of breath over the past 2 days. You have been asked to book an urgent high-resolution CT thorax for Mr Jensen by your consultant, Dr Smyth, to exclude pulmonary fibrosis. Later that afternoon the ward clerk tells you that she has received a call from the radiology department. They have declined to perform the scan as the consultant radiologist, Dr Ahmed, notes that Mr Jensen had a CT thorax, abdomen and pelvis scan 4 weeks ago and therefore doesn't feel the scan is indicated.

Rank in order the following actions in response to this situation (1 = most appropriate; 5 = least appropriate):

A. Email Dr Ahmed to reiterate the indications for the scan.

B. Phone the radiology department and insist the scan is performed as per Dr Smyth's plan.

C. Contact Dr Smyth to inform them that the investigation request has been declined.

D. Attempt to contact a different consultant radiologist to discuss the scan request.

E. Go to Dr Ahmed's office in the radiology department to discuss the request with him in person.

Q104. Sarah is a 34-year-old type 1 diabetic who has been admitted under your team with a urinary tract infection requiring IV antibiotics. Dr Johnson, your consultant, advised Sarah to take a higher dose of her insulin whilst on treatment for infection. Sarah did not appear keen on this idea as she said she is 'very prone to hypos' and is scared that increasing her insulin dose will precipitate these. Dr Johnson retorts that it's best for her to increase the insulin dose regardless and continues on with his ward round. You are called back to see Sarah at lunchtime; the nursing staff inform you that Sarah is refusing to take the higher dose of insulin.

Rank in order the following actions in response to this situation (1 = most appropriate; 5 = least appropriate):

A. Instruct Sarah that, although you appreciate her concerns, she really should just take the insulin as prescribed.

149

B. Explore Sarah's concerns further regarding the increased insulin dose.

C. Explain to Sarah clearly the reasons why the increase in insulin dose is needed.

D. Provide Sarah with additional resources on controlling blood sugars in type 1 diabetes during infections.

E. Inform Sarah that she should accept the decision made by her consultant.

> You need to ensure patient understanding.

Q105. You are one of the FY1 doctors on the gastroenterology unit. You are looking after Dr Wilson, a well-respected university lecturer, who has been admitted with symptomatic anaemia. He is due to undergo a colonoscopy to investigate whether there is a lower gastrointestinal cause for his anaemia, namely to rule out malignancy. You have been asked to speak to Dr Wilson as he has some questions regarding the indications for the investigation and what it will entail. You are not competent to perform colonoscopy and have never seen one performed, albeit you attended a teaching session last week where the reasons and method for performing the investigation were discussed.

Rank in order the following actions in response to this situation (1 = most appropriate; 5 = least appropriate):

A. Attempt to answer Dr Wilson's questions to the best of your knowledge.

B. Gather information on the procedure from an internet resource prior to discussing it with Dr Wilson.

C. Explain to Dr Wilson that you will probably not be able to answer his questions but that the registrar will be along later to consent for the procedure and suggest he asks any questions he has then.

D. Explore the questions and concerns Dr Wilson has, answer the ones you confidently know and explain that you will ask your registrar to address the ones you cannot answer.

E. Offer to provide Dr Wilson with the patient information leaflet on colonoscopy now as you are sure it will answer most of his questions; he can discuss any other concerns when he is consented.

Q106. You are an FY1 doctor currently working on a plastic surgery unit. There is another FY1, Lauren, attached to the unit and you both look after all patients. Rebecca Jones is a 22-year-old patient currently on the unit who underwent breast reduction surgery yesterday. You happen to walk past the bay she is in; she appears visibly upset and has no visitors with her at present, although you know her mother and father will visit later.

Rank in order the following actions in response to this situation (1 = most appropriate; 5 = least appropriate):

A. Await her review on the ward round tomorrow morning to discuss the cause of her upset.

B. Approach Rebecca and explore the reason for her emotional state.

C. Wait for Rebecca's parents to arrive so that she has extra emotional support before discussing her emotional state with her.

D. Inform the nurse in charge of the unit that you have observed Rebecca crying and request that she has a word with her and then report back to you her concerns.

E. Ask Lauren if she wouldn't mind discussing with Rebecca why she is upset later on today.

Q107. You work on a busy respiratory ward with 28 patients. There are two FY1s on the ward, yourself and Claire, and you cover half the patients each. Every morning begins with the MDT conducting a board round of all the current inpatients with the purpose of updating each other on the patient's progress – each member speaks in turn and delivers a brief overview of the factors preventing the patient being suitable for discharge. You have noticed that, in comparison with the other members of the MDT, Claire delivers quite extensive medical updates on her patients, which you are sure delays the meeting by at least 10 minutes per day.

Rank in order the following actions in response to this situation (1 = most appropriate; 5 = least appropriate):

A. Politely remind Claire in the doctor's office later that day that her board round updates are supposed to provide a brief overview and not extensively detail a patient's clinical progress.

B. At tomorrow's board round, if Claire's updates are excessive, tell her that she is to present brief overviews.

C. Await the next consultant ward round before letting the consultant know your concerns.

D. Accept that the board rounds will take the time they take; Claire can update the MDT as she wishes.

E. Print off your hospital trust's guidelines on presentations at board rounds and leave a copy in Claire's post tray.

> You need to be assertive when necessary.

Q108. You are one of four FY1 doctors in the cardiology department. As part of your training programme, you rotate through the coronary care unit, the day case angiography unit, the general cardiac ward and the specialist inpatient heart failure service, spending 1 month in each post. As you rotate through each post you take over the role your FY1 colleague Warren has just being performing. You have noticed that Warren's documentation is substandard. You feel it does not reflect patient progress as important results are often omitted and there is very little detail regarding the ongoing plan. Furthermore, his handwriting is generally poor.

Rank in order the following actions in response to this situation (1 = most appropriate; 5 = least appropriate):

A. Discuss your concerns regarding Warren's documentation with your clinical supervisor.

B. Bleep Warren to arrange an informal meeting to discuss your concerns and offer to help him improve.

C. At the next departmental teaching session tell Warren he needs to improve his documentation and legibility.

D. Discuss your concerns regarding Warren's documentation with his clinical supervisor.

E. Accept Warren's documentation style as there isn't a set standard to documentation.

Q109. You are an FY1 working on an endocrine and diabetes ward. Two weeks ago you were looking after Mr Vickers, a 68-year-old man whose GP, Dr Omoyemi, had referred him with poorly controlled type 2 diabetes. Whilst he was an inpatient your consultant and the diabetes specialist nurse altered his insulin regimen, achieving normoglycaemia on discharge. You communicated and clearly documented these medication changes on Mr Vickers's discharge summary so that his GP could alter the repeat prescription. Mr Vickers has just been re-admitted to your ward in a hyperosmolar hyperglycaemic state; you notice on a recent repeat prescription from 1 week ago that Dr Omoyemi had not altered Mr Vickers's insulin regimen.

Rank in order the following actions in response to this situation (1 = most appropriate; 5 = least appropriate):

A. Contact the local clinical commissioning group informing them of Dr Omoyemi's mistake.

B. Contact the medical director for your trust requesting a review of the discharge summary system.

C. Discuss with your consultant your concerns regarding the lack of change of the repeat prescription.

D. Contact Mr Vickers' GP practice to ensure receipt of the initial discharge summary.

E. Ensure that all medication changes are clearly documented on discharge summaries in the future.

Q110. Your SHO, Ken, is reviewing Mr Domingues with the patient's daughter at the bedside. Mr Domingues is in a bay of four patients. He has been receiving treatment for a complicated urinary tract infection but unfortunately has not responded to IV antibiotics and has clinically deteriorated. Your consultant has asked Ken to discuss with the relatives the ceiling of Mr Domingues' care and whether they would be happy for a 'do not attempt resuscitation' (DNAR) order to be instigated. You are at the nurses' station opposite the bay. You can hear clearly the content of Ken's discussion and notice that the other patients in the bay are attentive to his words.

Rank in order the following actions in response to this situation (1 = most appropriate; 5 = least appropriate):

A. Ask the ward matron to intervene in Ken's conversation to ask him to continue his discussion in the ward's relatives' room.

B. Approach the bedside to inform Ken you can clearly hear his discussion from the nurses' station.

C. Approach the bedside, apologise to Mr Domingues' daughter for interrupting and ask to speak to Ken urgently about what you have observed.

D. Approach the other three patients and ask them not to listen in on Ken's discussion with Mr Domingues' daughter.

E. Allow Ken to complete his conversation with Mr Domingues' daughter before informing him of your observations as it would be incorrect to interrupt such a discussion.

Q111. Mr Benson was a patient under the care of your team with a very interesting presentation of right heart failure secondary to a pulmonary embolus. He had an extensive past medical history but your consultant, Dr Hill, is confident about the above cause of death. However, she feels that Mr Benson's case would provide a good learning opportunity for the trainees within the hospital and would like to perform a post-mortem examination so that she can present the findings at an upcoming grand round meeting. She tells you that she has discussed this with the family and they have consented. The following morning, Mr Benson's daughter approaches you in the corridor outside the bereavement office. She tells you Dr Hill was rather persistent with her request for the post mortem and that the family are unsure whether they want it to be performed. She asks you whether it is necessary.

Rank in order the following actions in response to this situation (1 = most appropriate; 5 = least appropriate):

A. Inform Mr Benson's daughter that she should meet with Dr Hill to discuss her concerns further.

B. Tell her that, as the family has consented to the post mortem, it will take place as planned.

C. Contact your registrar and ask them whether they can discuss the family's concerns more thoroughly.

D. Meet with Dr Hill to explore more thoroughly her reasons for requesting the post mortem.

E. Explore Mr Benson's daughter's concerns more thoroughly.

Q112. Mrs Li is to undergo a partial gastrectomy today for a recently diagnosed stomach carcinoma. The operation is planned to take approximately 4 hours. Mrs Li was first on the list and has been nil by mouth since midnight. Unfortunately, two patients with acute appendicitis have presented overnight and a decision has been made by your consultant for your registrar to perform these two relatively simple operations before Mrs Li's. It is now 1 pm and Mrs Li has still not been taken down to theatre. The nursing staff report she is quite obviously distressed.

Rank in order the following actions in response to this situation (1 = most appropriate; 5 = least appropriate):

A. Call your registrar in theatre and ask whether they are able to review Mrs Li as she has been nil by mouth for 13 hours.

B. Instruct the nurse to offer Mrs Li some food as her distress is likely to be secondary to hunger.

C. Apologise for the delay, but tell her you are unsure when her operation will be.

D. Advise her that it is likely that her operation will be cancelled today as there must have been a complication in one of the emergency cases.

E. Advise her that you will contact your registrar in theatre to find out when her operation is likely to happen; keep her updated on the result of your discussions.

> Keep patients updated on their progress.

Q113. You are a care of the elderly FY1 on a ward that is split half and half between your team and a gastroenterology team. Jack is the FY1 for the gastroenterology team. You have noticed over the past couple of weeks that Jack appears quite low and seems very busy with his work. He tells you that he has been staying at least 90 minutes late each day to ensure that all his work is done. Earlier this morning you observed his SHO telling him that his late finishes are due to inefficiencies in his working practice. It just so happens that you take lunch together today; he tells you he doesn't want to bother informing his educational or clinical supervisor of his struggles nor his SHO's comments as he only has 2 weeks left on the job.

Rank in order the following actions in response to this situation (1 = most appropriate; 5 = least appropriate):

A. Reassure Jack that most FY1 doctors struggle with some aspects of practice and discuss how he manages his workload.

B. Encourage him to speak to his educational supervisor as the precipitating factors for his current problems could carry on into his next job.

C. Discuss your concerns regarding Jack with your educational supervisor to seek their advice regarding how you should proceed.

D. Speak to Jack's SHO discreetly that afternoon and inform them that their behaviour towards Jack could be construed as bullying.

E. It's ultimately Jack's choice how he deals with these circumstances; accept his choice not to raise his concerns.

Q114. You are an acute medicine FY1. In your hospital, every Wednesday morning for the medical teams begins with a grand round. This morning you have heard a presentation from the clinical lead for infection control during which they reiterated rules on staff dress in the clinical environment, including the rule that all staff must be bare below the elbows. During your shift you notice Alex, one of the other acute medicine FY1s, has his shirt sleeves rolled down.

Rank in order the following actions in response to this situation (1 = most appropriate; 5 = least appropriate):

A. Remind Alex of the infection control policy that he should be bare below the elbows.

B. Take no action immediately, but observe Alex for a few days to make sure that this is not a frequent occurrence.

C. Inform the senior sister on the ward of your observations regarding Alex's dress.

D. Report Alex to the infection control service for his disregard of their widely accepted guideline.

E. Discuss your observations of Alex's dress with your SHO for their opinion on how to proceed.

Q115. Mr Oliver is an 86-year-old heavy smoker with a 120-pack-per-year history. As a result he has developed chronic obstructive pulmonary disease, which he has managed for the past 30 years. He has required oxygen therapy at home for the past 8 years but, owing to recent chest infections, his oxygen requirement has increased dramatically. He has been admitted to the respiratory unit you work on with increasing shortness of breath. This is his tenth admission in the past 7 months and the fourth whilst you have been an FY1 on the unit. You are conducting your morning ward round of your patients; on review he confides in you that he has 'had enough with this miserable existence' – he cannot cope with being an inpatient so frequently, he claims it's ruining his quality of life and he feels he is too much of a burden on his family. He asks about the possibility of withdrawing active treatment in favour of palliation. You discuss with him the implications of this on the length of his life and he appears to be able to retain and process the information and make a reasoned decision. He requests that this discussion not be raised with his family.

Rank in order the following actions in response to this situation (1 = most appropriate; 5 = least appropriate):

A. Discuss with Mr Oliver's family his wish to stop active treatment.

B. Discuss Mr Oliver's social support with his GP to see whether more care can be instituted to provide the family with support.

C. Inform Mr Oliver that decisions to withdraw active treatment can be made once he is discharged from his current admission.

D. Inform the ward's MDT of your discussion with Mr Oliver.

E. As Mr Oliver has demonstrated capacity, reassure him that your team will respect his wishes on planning his further management.

Q116. You are one of the FY1 doctors working on the acute assessment unit. Miss Johansson is a 34-year-old woman with relapsing–remitting multiple sclerosis who has been admitted this morning with acute visual changes. She has undergone a magnetic resonance imaging (MRI) scan of her head this morning, which has provisionally been reported as demonstrating active lesions in the ocular areas of the brain. The neuroradiology registrar reporting the scan has commented that the findings are likely to be consistent with secondary progressive disease, hence worsening of her disease, but that his report needs to be confirmed by his consultant. You are just about to review the patient in the adjacent bed to Miss Johansson when she asks 'What did that MRI scan show, doctor?' You know that she will be reviewed by the neurologists later this afternoon.

Rank in order the following actions in response to this situation (1 = most appropriate; 5 = least appropriate):

A. Explain that the final report is not available.

B. Re-review Miss Johannson for other symptoms suggestive of progressive disease prior to her neurology review.

C. Inform Miss Johannson that you will chase up the final report of the MRI scan and explain that she will be reviewed by the neurology team later this afternoon.

D. Provide Miss Johansson with the provisional report informing her of the progression of multiple sclerosis.

E. Encourage Miss Johansson not to worry about the MRI.

Q117. You are working on a gastroenterology unit and are reviewing the last patient on the morning ward round. Your consultant asks you to seek the immediate advice of the on-call general surgical registrar regarding a patient. He is a 72-year-old man who has acutely localising abdominal pain on the background of constipation secondary to a colonic tumour. He is haemodynamically unstable. The clinical suspicion is that the patient may have ruptured his bowel.

Rank in order the following actions in response to this situation (1 = most appropriate; 5 = least appropriate):

A. Contact the surgical registrar to inform them that you have a patient who requires a surgical review today.

B. Contact the surgical SHO prior to contacting the surgical registrar to clarify whether the patient requires discussion with their senior.

C. Explain the situation to the surgical registrar, providing relevant background regarding the patient and your assessment. Request an immediate review.

D. Knowing that this patient will take time to manage, try to complete a few of the other jobs from the ward round before contacting the surgical registrar.

E. Contact the medical registrar on call; it is unlikely that the patient will be fit enough for a curative operation so it would be best to manage him conservatively.

Q118. You are in your first week of one of your 4-month FY1 rotations. On your first day your clinical supervisor asked you and the other three new FY1s to submit your requests for annual leave as the rota is arranged internally by the secretary. You have arranged to meet as a team today to discuss everyone's requests. Unfortunately on the 2 days you have requested leave to attend your sister's wedding, two of your other FY1 colleagues have also requested time off. The department's rule is that two FY1s must be working as a minimum at any one time.

Rank in order the following actions in response to this situation (1 = most appropriate; 5 = least appropriate):

A. Explain to your colleagues that you must have these 2 days off as you requested.

B. Explain your reasons for wanting these 2 days off to your colleagues and try to negotiate with them to have this time off.

C. Discuss with your clinical supervisor whether more support could be arranged on these 2 days to allow yourself and your colleagues the time off you have requested.

D. Allow your two colleagues to have annual leave as requested but call in sick on your intended days off.

E. Allow your two colleagues to have annual leave as requested but attempt to arrange study leave for the 2 days instead.

> Consider diplomacy and assertiveness.

Q119. Mr Ali is an 88-year-old patient who was admitted under the care of the orthopaedic team in which you are the FY1 doctor with a fractured right neck of femur that was operatively treated. Following a couple of days of post-operative review he was deemed medically fit for discharge to the local rehabilitation centre for continued supportive care. The centre has been very busy and Mr Ali has been waiting 4 days for his transfer there. It is departmental protocol for patients deemed medically fit for discharge not to be seen by the medical team, but instead to have intensive reviews with the physiotherapists. The ward's physiotherapist informs you Mr Ali is unsure why he is still in hospital and why a doctor has not been to see him for several days.

Rank in order the following actions in response to this situation (1 = most appropriate; 5 = least appropriate):

A. Ask the physiotherapist to explain to Mr Ali the trust protocol and the reason for his delayed transfer.

B. Ask the physiotherapist to explain to Mr Ali that he does not require a medical review.

C. Contact the rehabilitation centre to establish when it is likely that Mr Ali will be transferred to its care.

D. Explain to Mr Ali that, as the medical team is not responsible for the delay in his transfer, he should continue his work with the physiotherapists.

E. Explain the trust protocol to Mr Ali and apologise for the delayed transfer.

Q120. Mrs Aarons is a 72-year-old woman who has been an inpatient many times at your hospital. She has many documented adverse reactions to several classes of antibiotics. She has been admitted this time haemodynamically unstable with pyrexia and has consolidation in the lower zone of her right lung; therefore she is likely to have sepsis secondary to community-acquired pneumonia. Your consultant recommends contacting the microbiology on-call doctor for some advice regarding which antibiotic to use as, from looking briefly through her medical notes, you see that she has an 'itchy rash' reaction to the empirical antibiotic.

Rank in order the following actions in response to this situation (1 = most appropriate; 5 = least appropriate):

A. Quickly review the medical notes for previously used antibiotics and microbiology specimen results prior to contacting the microbiologist.

B. Contact the microbiologist immediately.

C. Discuss with Mrs Aarons the nature of her allergies and complete a summary of Mrs Aarons's previous microbiology specimen results along with the antibiotics used to treat them; document this in the medical notes prior to contacting the microbiologist.

D. Commence the empirical antibiotic, as the reaction is not anaphylaxis, before seeking advice.

E. Speak to the medical registrar on call about which antibiotic they would recommend using.

Q121. You started working in the renal medicine unit 2 weeks ago. Your clinical supervisor is conducting a ward round prior to attending a business development meeting for the department. You have just reviewed a patient with end-stage renal failure with anaemia and your clinical supervisor asks you to prescribe erythropoietin for the patient. You have previously prescribed the drug but are unsure of its indications of use.

Rank in order the following actions in response to this situation (1 = most appropriate; 5 = least appropriate):

A. Ask your clinical supervisor for useful resources for drugs used commonly in renal medicine.

B. Prescribe the erythropoietin. As it is so commonly used in renal medicine you are sure that you will learn about its indications during your renal medicine rotation.

C. Ask the ward pharmacist later on the day about erythropoietin.

D. Use the ward round as a learning opportunity and ask your clinical supervisor to explain the indications for erythropoietin.

E. Email your clinical supervisor later in the day to request a teaching session on the treatment of anaemia in chronic renal failure.

Q122. The nursing staff ask you to speak to the daughter of Mrs McCreath who is angry at the length of her mother's admission. Mrs McCreath is a 92-year-old woman who was admitted initially under your urology team with a blocked suprapubic catheter and acute kidney injury. A new suprapubic catheter was inserted, which resolved matters. Unfortunately Mrs McCreath was found to have a large postural drop in her blood pressure during her admission, which prevented her from being safely discharged. As a result her admission has been prolonged to 3 weeks despite the urological issue being resolved in a couple of days.

Rank in order the following actions in response to this situation (1 = most appropriate; 5 = least appropriate):

A. Establish Mrs McCreath's consent to discuss her inpatient stay with her daughter prior to preparing for your discussion with her daughter.

B. Familiarise yourself fully with Mrs McCreath's case prior to engaging in a discussion with her daughter.

C. Establish the daughter's understanding of the factors prolonging her mother's stay, providing her with information to fill in any gaps in her knowledge.

D. Reiterate to the daughter that the length of her mother's admission is owing to her not being able to be safely discharged.

E. Ask nursing staff members to sit the daughter in the ward's relatives' room and calm her down prior to agreeing to speak to her.

Q123. You are an FY1 doctor on an adult cystic fibrosis unit. A patient with learning difficulties and cerebral palsy in addition to cystic fibrosis presents to the unit with an acute exacerbation, holding their left jaw but reluctant to let you examine their mouth internally. From the brief glimpse you have had inside their mouth it appears that they have a dental abscess, but you would like to examine this further. The patient is unwilling to let you look inside their mouth. The patient has their carer with them.

Rank in order the following actions in response to this situation (1 = most appropriate; 5 = least appropriate):

A. Explain to the patient that you are unable to help them with the 'oral hygiene problem' until you have examined their mouth.

B. Document in the medical notes that you were unable to examine the patient's mouth as they were non-compliant with the examination.

C. Seek the advice of your senior colleague in how best to proceed with gaining the patient's consent to the examination.

D. Ask the carer to help persuade the patient to have the examination performed.

E. Position yourself at the patient's level and explain that 'I can see you're in lots of pain from your mouth, please let me see inside, it will help me understand what is wrong'.

Q124. Mr Jayasuriya has presented to your hospital's A&E department complaining of 'pain, pain, pain' whilst holding his left loin. He has been given analgesia but you are unable to elicit any further history. Whilst attempting to speak to him he presents you with a Sri Lankan passport. You know one of the nurses in the department is Sri Lankan and may be able to translate for you.

Rank in order the following actions in response to this situation (1 = most appropriate; 5 = least appropriate):

A. Continue analgesia for Mr Jayasuriya and organise a CT scan of his abdomen.

B. Use a telephone translation service to help communicate with Mr Jayasuriya.

C. Contact the interpreting services and request an interpreter for your consultation with Mr Jayasuriya.

D. Speak to your senior colleagues for advice regarding the difficulty you are having with your consultation.

E. Ask for help from the Sri Lankan nurse with the consultation.

Q125. You are the on-call FY1 doctor for all medical patients in your hospital overnight. You are called to see a patient who has an anoxic brain injury and is fed by percutaneous endoscopic gastrostomy (PEG). The nurses report that they observed the patient choking during a feed during the day and so they stopped the PEG. They have just performed observations and found the patient to be pyrexial with an increased respiratory rate and decreased oxygen saturations. You believe the patient has aspiration pneumonia and discuss antibiotic choice with the on-call consultant microbiologist. You commence the recommended therapy. The son and daughter of the patient are both GPs and have power of attorney for their mother's care. You receive a call from the nurse on the ward; the son and daughter have visited the ward at 9.30 pm and are unhappy for their mother to have the antibiotic you prescribed.

Rank in order the following actions in response to this situation (1 = most appropriate; 5 = least appropriate):

A. Attend the ward to inform the son and daughter that your decision was made in discussion with the on-call consultant microbiologist.

B. Attend the ward to discuss the son's and daughter's concerns regarding the antibiotic choice.

C. Ask the nurse to inform the son and daughter that the on-call doctor is unable to discuss family concerns with relatives; ask them to raise their concerns with their mother's normal team during the day.

D. Ask the nurse to inform them that the therapy was recommended by a consultant microbiologist.

E. It's their choice as power of attorney to refuse treatment for their mother, and stop the antibiotic prescription.

Q126. You have been looking after Mrs Jones during her very complicated 2-month admission on your ward. Her only daughter lives in Australia and has just arrived in the UK for the first time since her mother has been in hospital. Mrs Jones has asked you whether you would kindly update her daughter on the course of her admission at your earliest convenience.

Rank in order the following actions in response to this situation (1 = most appropriate; 5 = least appropriate):

A. Provide an overview to the best of your current knowledge and instruct the daughter of your plan.

B. Provide only a summary of the current issues affecting Mrs Jones's admission.

C. Arrange a meeting with Mrs Jones's daughter in a few days' time once you've had the opportunity to refresh your knowledge of Mrs Jones's case.

D. Advise Mrs Jones that you are unable to invest the time needed to have such a conversation with her daughter at the present time.

E. Review the medical notes of Mrs Jones's admission prior to discussing her case with the daughter and begin your meeting by asking what the daughter already understands to have happened.

> Relatives should be kept updated.

Q127. You are the on-call FY1 doctor for plastic surgery over the weekend; it is a Sunday evening. Mrs Sweetman was admitted 2 months ago with a breast abscess that was excised and drained. Unfortunately her admission has been prolonged by 'vacant episodes', which the family advises are a new symptom. You are called to see the patient's relatives as they do not feel these symptoms have been adequately investigated. On reviewing the notes, it appears as though they have been well investigated, indeed the patient has had, from what you can discern, a CT and MRI of the head, an electroencephalogram (EEG), confusion screen blood tests and lumbar puncture, all returning normal results. The family would like you to investigate the patient further.

Rank in order the following actions in response to this situation (1 = most appropriate; 5 = least appropriate):

A. Explain that no further investigations are needed as Mrs Sweetman appears to have been very thoroughly investigated.

B. Advise the family that you are the on-call doctor and it would be more appropriate for them to raise their concerns with Mrs Sweetman's normal team tomorrow.

C. Reassure the family that Mrs Sweetman's team is investigating the causes of her vacant episodes actively.

D. Explore the family's concerns regarding their expectations of investigation.

E. Speak to the medical registrar on call regarding the patient and whether any further investigations are warranted at this time.

Q128. You are the on-call medical FY1 doctor overnight. You receive a bleep. On returning the call the person on the other end of the phone says 'I have a patient with a blood pressure of 210/130; you need to attend immediately!'

Rank in order the following actions in response to this situation (1 = most appropriate; 5 = least appropriate):

A. Email your educational supervisor to arrange a meeting to discuss ways of improving handover of information between nursing and medical staff.

B. Email the charge nurse of the ward informing them of the poor quality of information handover you have received.

C. Ask the nurse to provide you first with the details about the patient, including their location and some background for their case.

D. Remind the nurse to use a systematic approach like SBAR when phoning for advice.

E. Ask the nurse to obtain a summary of the patient including their baseline observations and to call you back once they have these.

Q129. You have been asked by your clinical supervisor to arrange teaching sessions for the ward's new medical students amongst the four FY1 doctors on the unit. Your clinical supervisor insists the teaching has to be delivered by the FY1 doctors as it is a compulsory element of your FY1 e-portfolio. They also request that you decide amongst yourselves who's going to teach what. On broaching the subject with your FY1 colleagues, nobody seems keen to teach the students.

Rank in order the following actions in response to this situation (1 = most appropriate; 5 = least appropriate):

A. Ask the SHOs on the ward to see whether they would be willing to do some of the teaching sessions to reduce the burden on the FY1 doctors.

B. Clarify your colleagues' concerns regarding the teaching sessions.

C. Inform your clinical supervisor that you have been unable to persuade your colleagues to teach the students.

D. Arrange the teaching sessions so that the FY1 teaching doctors have their clinical commitments covered by the other FY1s.

E. Allocate the teaching sessions to your colleagues and inform your clinical supervisor who is going to teach each subject.

Q130. Julie, your department's rota coordinator, has just released the rota for the department's six FY1s detailing when you will be working days on the wards, on calls and night shifts or having training days and annual leave. Your deanery, for your educational development, has arranged three training days for FY1s at all hospitals in the deanery for this current rotation. The expectation is that all FY1s should attend at least one day. On looking at the rota you can see that you have not been allocated to attend any of these training days, yet the other five FY1s are able to attend at least two of them.

Rank in order the following actions in response to this situation (1 = most appropriate; 5 = least appropriate):

A. Discuss with Julie whether some changes can be made to the rota to allow you to attend at least one training day as required.

B. Contact the foundation school director at your deanery to inform them that your department has not allocated you to a training day as required.

C. Attend at least one training day against the scheduling of your rota as your department has a responsibility for your continued training and development.

D. Discuss with your FY1 colleagues on the ward whether they would be willing to swap their training days to allow you to attend at least one as required.

E. Contact your educational supervisor to inform them that your rota has not allowed you to attend the mandatory training days.

Q131. The team on your ward consists of a consultant (who is your educational supervisor), a registrar and two FY1s (yourself and James). On the preference of the consultant, you split into two pairs each day with your educational supervisor seeing half the patients with one FY1 and the registrar seeing the other half of the patients with the other FY1. There is no rota to decide who accompanies whom on the ward round. You have noticed that James accompanies your educational supervisor much more frequently than you do and consequently you are worried about missing out on educational opportunities.

Rank in order the following actions in response to this situation (1 = most appropriate; 5 = least appropriate):

A. Mandate that you attend at least three consultant ward rounds a week to ensure you have equal educational opportunities to James.

B. Devise a rota for the ward allocating yourself and James to attend your consultant's ward round on alternating days.

C. Reiterate your concerns to your registrar about the lack of educational opportunities you have through attending very few consultant ward rounds.

D. Discuss your concerns regarding your educational opportunities with your educational supervisor.

E. Raise your concerns with James and discuss whether you could attend more of your educational supervisor's ward rounds.

Q132. Mrs Crankshaw has been a patient on your general medical ward for 4 weeks. She is an 86-year-old woman with a very extensive past medical history including asthma, ischaemic heart disease, previous strokes, hypothyroidism, hypertension and obesity, for which she takes multiple medications. During Mrs Crankshaw's admission your team noted her to be mildly hyponatraemic and hypotensive. A cortisol level taken at 9 am was low and your consultant suspects adrenal insufficiency. The endocrinology registrar on call advises referring Mrs Crankshaw to the endocrinology outpatient clinic on discharge and asks you to arrange this.

Rank in order the following actions in response to this situation (1 = most appropriate; 5 = least appropriate):

A. Ask your ward clerk to arrange an appointment in endocrinology outpatient clinic on Mrs Crankshaw's discharge.

B. Write a referral letter summarising Mrs Crankshaw's inpatient stay, investigation results and clinical background and ensure it reaches the appointment administrator.

C. Forward a photocopy of Mrs Crankshaw's medical notes to the endocrine outpatient clinic including the entry from the endocrinology registrar on call requesting the appointment.

D. Forward a copy of Mrs Crankshaw's discharge summary to the endocrine outpatient department detailing your discussion with the endocrine registrar.

E. In Mrs Crankshaw's discharge summary ask her GP to refer her to the endocrinology clinic on the advice of the endocrine registrar.

Q133. Mr Kenworthy is a 92-year-old man on your ward with community-acquired pneumonia. He is registered blind and has advanced dementia. He normally requires assistance with his feeding from carers but, due to his moribund state, he has been deemed not safe to swallow food or drink. On the advice of the speech and language therapy team, your consultant has asked you to discuss alternative feeding arrangements like total parental nutrition or PEG feeding with Mr Kenworthy's relatives at afternoon visiting.

Rank in order the following actions in response to this situation (1 = most appropriate; 5 = least appropriate):

A. Provide the family with printed out guidelines on many different modalities of alternative feeding to allow them to make an informed decision.

B. Summarise several of the alternative feeding modalities whilst discussing with the family and check the family's comprehension of what has been discussed.

C. Explore Mr Kenworthy's family's understanding of alternative feeding and provide a summary of its use in this patient's case.

D. Ask the speech and language therapist to make a recommendation to the family on the best way to feed Mr Kenworthy alternatively.

E. Make a recommendation to Mr Kenworthy's family regarding which alternative feeding modality would be best for the patient.

Q134. You are the FY1 on a geriatrics ward. Mrs Poppy is a 92-year-old woman with a very extensive neurological history including several strokes, normal pressure hydrocephalus and Parkinson's disease. Unfortunately she has had a fall with a head injury on the ward this morning. Her neurological examination is very difficult to complete owing to her inability to cooperate with the exam and her pre-existing co-morbidities. Therefore your consultant recommends a CT scan of her head. Your hospital uses a computerised system to request imaging, with the clinical information restricted to 500 typed characters. You think it will be difficult to summarise Mrs Poppy's past medical history and presenting complaint to this. CT scans are known to be readily rejected if the request is not detailed enough.

Rank in order the following actions in response to this situation (1 = most appropriate; 5 = least appropriate):

A. Include all of Mrs Poppy's past medical history on the request and attempt to include a brief summary of this morning's fall if space permits.

B. Re-examine Mrs Poppy; if you can find no gross new neurological deficit do not request the CT head scan.

C. Discuss your concerns regarding the information to put on the request with your consultant prior to making the request.

D. Contact the on-call duty radiologist to get their advice on what to include in the request.

E. Include only salient features of Mrs Poppy's past medical history in the request, ensuring that the reason for requiring the CT head scan is made clear to the radiology department.

Q135. Your consultant, Dr Cavendish, has just informed Mrs Livingstone and her family present that the results of her investigations have determined that she has metastatic breast cancer. Mrs Livingstone appears not to be expecting such a diagnosis and appears not to comprehend much of what the consultant has told her following the breaking of the bad news. Dr Cavendish leaves Mrs Livingstone's bedside to continue the ward round after communicating the patient's ongoing management plan. Both the patient and her family appear quite taken aback and upset by the news they have just heard.

Choose the most suitable **three** options from the following list:

A. Apologise to Mrs Livingstone and her family for the way the consultant broke the news to them.

B. Offer to speak to the patient and her relatives and answer any questions they have.

C. Report Dr Cavendish to the GMC with regard to their manner with patients.

D. Refer Mrs Livingstone to the palliative care services.

E. Ask the chaplaincy at the hospital to provide Mrs Livingstone with spiritual support.

F. Ask a nurse whether they are able to spend time with the family to comfort them.

G. Check the patient's and the family's understanding of the news that has been given.

H. Provide the patient and the family with a named contact, like a cancer specialist nurse, who they can contact if they have any further questions.

Q136. Mr Petrescu is a Romanian immigrant who has presented with night sweats and a persistent cough. He has been newly diagnosed with tuberculosis (TB). He speaks very little English. He has been commenced on treatment that requires him to take four tablets once a day for 6 months. He has no other known medical problems and is on no other medications. You happen to observe him this morning with only one tablet in his pill pot and are concerned he is not having his therapy as prescribed.

Choose the most suitable **three** options from the following list:

A. Confirm with Mr Petrescu's consultant the number of tablets he needs to take.

B. Remind Mr Petrescu that he needs to take four tablets once a day.

C. Seek advice from the pharmacist on the ward as to the number of tablets Mr Petrescu needs to take.

D. Review the drug chart to see which nurse dispensed his medication this morning and ask why he has a single pill in his pill pot.

E. Do not allow him to take the medication in his pill pot presently.

F. Await his relatives, who speak better English, to attend this afternoon to instruct them regarding the medication regimen.

G. Allow Mr Petrescu to take the dispensed medication.

H. Obtain a Romanian translator to ensure Mr Petrescu understands how to take his TB medications regimen correctly.

Q137. You have just started your shift taking over from Jennifer as the FY1 doctor to your hospital's clinical decision unit, the short-stay ward. Mrs Bence-Jones presented 3 days ago with cough and fever. You have not yet reviewed the patient but Jennifer tells you that she is objectively improving on oral antibiotics. Fifteen minutes into your shift you are confronted by Mrs Bence-Jones's husband; he appears visibly angry as his wife's cough is still persisting and he 'can't believe nothing has been done to make his wife feel better!' He is requesting different antibiotics and informs you that Jennifer instructed him these are not necessary.

Choose the most suitable **three** options from the following list:

A. Explain to Mr Bence-Jones that you have just started your shift and have yet to review his wife personally.

B. Reassure Mr Bence-Jones that symptoms like a cough can persist despite effective therapy.

C. Answer and address any questions Mr Bence-Jones has after ensuring his wife's consent to such discussion.

D. Arrange for Mr Bence-Jones to meet with the consultant in charge of his wife's care.

E. Ask the nurse in charge of the unit to calm Mr Bence-Jones down before agreeing to speak with him.

F. Review Mrs Bence-Jones for any signs or symptoms suggestive of worsening infection.

G. Ask your SHO to speak to Mr Bence-Jones regarding his concerns.

H. Ask Mr Bence-Jones to calm down prior to speaking to him.

Q138. You are an FY1 doctor on a cardiology ward. At 3 pm Mr Menzies, a patient on the ward, develops chest pain. A blood test is taken to check for myocardial damage. The result is reported at 3.45 pm and shows a mildly elevated level, and a repeat level at 3 hours post the initial sample needs to be taken to assess for ongoing myocardial damage. The level would therefore need to be taken at 6 pm; however, you finish at 5 pm. You ask Mr Menzies' nurse, Meghan, who is phlebotomy-trained, to take the blood test and chase the result as her shift is due to finish at 8.30 pm. She states rudely that she is not willing to do this as she will be very busy at that time.

Choose the most suitable **three** options from the following list:

A. Stay until 6 pm to take the blood test yourself.

B. Ask the FY1 doctor on call for the evening to take the blood test and chase the result.

C. Speak to Meghan tomorrow regarding the way she spoke to you.

D. Discuss with the ward matron regarding procedures for taking essential blood tests at busy times.

E. Ask Meghan to consider the way she addresses other staff members.

F. Explore the tasks Meghan will be performing at the time the sample is required to determine their urgency.

G. Discuss with the nurse in charge about the way Meghan spoke to you.

H. Insist that Meghan finds the time to take the sample.

Q139. You are the FY1 for the cardiology ward and have been looking after Mr Ahktar today. He has decompensated heart failure that is being treated with diuretic therapy. Consequently he has become dehydrated with worsening of his renal function. To compensate this your team has decided to titrate IV fluid therapy closely to his urine output, documenting clear instructions for this in the medical notes. You have arrived in the morning to find the patient delirious with an increased respiratory rate and decreased saturations; he has pulmonary oedema. On reviewing the notes you see he was given 2 litres of IV fluid overnight, not in accordance with the documented plan. You immediately stabilise the patient.

Choose the most suitable **three** options from the following list:

A. Inform the nurse in charge of the unit of the incident.

B. Inform the nurses involved of the error they have made.

C. Explain to Mr Ahktar the mistake that has been made.

D. Offer to write guidelines on the use of IV fluid therapy in acute heart failure.

E. Inform the consultant in charge of the patient's care of their acute deterioration.

F. Reflect on the incident in your Foundation Programme e-portfolio.

G. Find out whether the nursing staff overnight were aware of the documented instructions regarding fluid therapy.

> To whom should you escalate this?

H. Increase Mr Akhtar's observations this morning.

Q140. You and your fellow FY1 doctors are attending mandatory teaching. You are having a teaching session on developing coping strategies for practice as an FY1 doctor. Suddenly Anna, who works on the same ward as you, becomes visibly upset and starts crying. She states that she is not coping well with work and thinks the hospital does not provide adequate support for struggling trainees.

Choose the most suitable **three** options from the following list:

A. Advise Anna to take some annual leave to give her some rest from the post.

B. Ask the team on the ward to offer Anna more support.

C. Offer to assist Anna in seeking support.

D. Encourage her to attend occupational therapy for psychological support.

E. Offer to discuss Anna's concerns with her.

F. Email her clinical supervisor regarding the incident.

G. Offer to assist with Anna's workload.

H. Suggest that she discusses her concerns with her educational supervisor.

Q141. You are the on-call surgical FY1 doctor overnight. You receive a bleep, which you return immediately. The person picks up the phone and says that a post-operative patient has developed a fever and hypotension. The person at the other end of the phone offers no further information.

Choose the most suitable **three** options from the following list:

A. Ask the caller to phone you back once they have more details on the patient.

B. Ask the caller to provide further details of their assessment of the patient and the action they would like you to take.

C. Attempt to locate the patient immediately from the information you have been given.

D. Ask the caller to provide some clinical background of the patient they are calling you about.

E. Contact the matron in charge of the unit during the daytime to inform them of the poor quality of information handover by their nursing staff.

F. Ask the caller to contact your SHO for advice.

G. Ask the caller to identify themselves and their location, in addition to some demographical details of the patient.

H. Ask the caller to check whether the patient is on IV antibiotics; if they are do not attend the patient.

Q142. The nursing staff have noted that Mr Parkinson keeps leaving the ward for extended periods of time and when he returns his speech appears more slurred and his thoughts more disordered. They suspect that he is intoxicated with alcohol at these times and they ask you to discuss these concerns with him.

Choose the most suitable **three** options from the following list:

A. Inform the patient that whilst he is off the ward it is not possible for him to be clinically reviewed.

B. Contact your consultant to inform him of this development in Mr Parkinson's case.

C. Refer Mr Parkinson to the alcohol liaison service.

D. Explore the reasons for Mr Parkinson leaving the ward.

E. Commence Mr Parkinson on alcohol withdrawal therapy.

F. Ask Mr Parkinson whether he has been consuming alcohol when he leaves the ward.

G. Fit Mr Parkinson with an alarm to alert nursing staff when he is leaving the ward to prevent this from happening.

H. Explain to Mr Parkinson that he will not be treated if he is consuming alcohol.

Q143. You are sitting in the doctor's office on your ward. Suddenly you hear a commotion coming from one of the male patient bays on your ward. Mr Brown is a patient who has just been moved to your ward from the admissions unit. He is angry with the nurses as he does not want to be in a bay with 'Asian people'. He is sitting up in bed presently.

Choose the most suitable **three** options from the following list:

A. Tell the patient that his comments are offensive to other patients and will not be tolerated in the hospital.

B. Contact hospital security.

C. Ask the nurse in charge of the ward to contact the police.

D. Move the patient into a side room to appease his concerns.

E. Confidentially talk with other patients to ensure they are well following the commotion.

F. See whether there is another ward to move him to.

G. Explore the patient's concerns and reasoning behind his comments.

H. Instruct the patient that he must leave the hospital immediately.

Q144. You are an FY1 doctor on the vascular surgery unit. There are normally supposed to be two FY1s working on the unit but as your colleague has called in sick you are the only FY1 today. As such, you are very busy. You are approached by a visitor asking about the progress and ongoing management of one of the unit's patients, Mrs Hemingway, who is recovering well following stenting of her right carotid artery. The visitor has been the patient's best friend for many years and, as the patient has no relatives, is the next of kin.

Choose the most suitable **three** options from the following list:

A. Explain to the next of kin briefly Mrs Hemingway's clinical progress.

B. Document your discussion with Mrs Hemingway's friend in the medical notes.

C. Ask the friend to discuss Mrs Hemingway's progress with her nurse, who is likely to have more time to answer the questions.

D. Politely explain that you are very busy and the friend would be better off arranging to meet with Mrs Hemingway's consultant to discuss her progress.

E. Read Mrs Hemingway's medical notes so that you can update her friend correctly.

F. Tell the friend that you do not have the time to discuss patients as you are very busy.

G. Explain that you are happy to meet with Mrs Hemingway and her friend but do not have time at the moment. You will try to come back to the ward later once you are less busy.

H. Ask the friend to wait while you confirm Mrs Hemingway's consent to your discussing her post-operative progress prior to updating them.

Q145. You are an FY1 in haematology. You have just reviewed Mr Bolem and, owing to an acutely low haemoglobin level, decide that he needs a blood transfusion. You have checked with the blood bank and they have valid group and screens for Mr Bolem and so you order 3 units of blood for the patient but it will take 20 minutes to process. You want to ensure the units of blood are given as soon as possible, but you have to attend compulsory teaching in 10 minutes.

Choose the most suitable **three** options from the following list:

A. Inform your senior colleagues of your management plan.

B. Inform Mr Bolem of your findings and gain consent to transfuse.

C. Document your plan in the medical notes before attending your teaching session.

D. Inform the nurse looking after Mr Bolem that his haemoglobin is low, that you would like him to have a transfusion and the blood will need to be collected from the blood bank in 20 minutes.

E. Inform the nurse of the plan and ensure the transfusion is started whilst you are at your teaching session. Inform Mr Bolem of the plan when you return to the unit.

F. Go to the blood bank in 20 minutes to collect the blood for Mr Bolem and then attend the rest of the compulsory teaching session.

G. Inform the nurse in charge of the unit that one of the patients will need a blood transfusion.

H. Wait till your return from the teaching session before prescribing the blood to be transfused so that you can ensure Mr Bolem is transfused.

Q146. You have been looking after Mr Mustard on your ward for a couple of weeks; he is now medically fit for discharge. The occupational therapist has informed you that Mr Mustard has several previously unaddressed care needs and it will take up to 2 weeks to modify his own bungalow. It has therefore been decided that Mr Mustard should spend this time temporarily placed within a care home rather than remain on an acute medical ward. On discussion with Mr Mustard's family later in the day, they state that they 'don't want their father going to some nursing home!'

Choose the most suitable **three** options from the following list:

A. Inform the family that Mr Mustard is to be discharged to a care home and not a nursing home.

B. Ask the family to discuss their concerns with the occupational therapist.

C. Discharge Mr Mustard to the care home as this is the most appropriate place for him to be currently.

D. Instruct the family that the plan is for care home care only temporarily.

E. Explain the rationale for the decision to place Mr Mustard in a care home temporarily to the family.

F. Discharge Mr Mustard to his normal home allowing him to stay there whilst the modifications to his bungalow are made.

G. Explore the family's concerns with Mr Mustard's discharge planning.

H. Ask the family to make an appointment with your consultant.

> Family concerns should be explored.

Q147. The nursing staff ask you to speak to the daughter of Mrs Andrews, who is angry that her mother is being discharged today. Mrs Andrews is a 92-year-old woman who was admitted initially under your urology team with stones occluding her left ureter causing hydronephrosis. A percutaneous nephrostomy tube was inserted and she improved clinically over the course of 3 days. The consultant reviewed Mrs Andrews this morning and plans to review her in his outpatient clinic in 2 weeks to discuss a long-term plan.

Choose the most suitable **three** options from the following list.

A. Reiterate to Mrs Andrews's daughter that her mother's consultant has a plan in place.

B. Allow Mrs Andrews to remain an inpatient for a further day of observation.

C. Allow Mrs Andrews's daughter to ask you questions regarding her mother's care.

D. Ask the nursing staff to instruct the daughter that Mrs Andrews is medically fit for discharge.

E. Reschedule Mrs Andrews's outpatient follow-up to occur 1 week following her discharge.

F. Summarise Mrs Andrews's admission to her daughter, following gaining consent, to ensure her understanding of her mother's clinical course.

G. Encourage the daughter to meet with the consultant today as they are in a position to make decisions regarding her mother's discharge.

H. Explore the concerns of Mrs Andrews's daughter regarding her mother's discharge plan.

Q148. A 17-year-old woman has been admitted to your general medical ward with pyelonephritis requiring IV antibiotics. She has made good clinical progress and is likely to be medically fit for discharge soon. She is currently on the ward unaccompanied and appears very upset. You understand her friends will be visiting the unit later on in the day.

Choose the most suitable **three** options from the following list:

A. Wait for her friends to arrive later in the day to offer her support.

B. Check that the patient understands the current management plan and reassure her that she is clinically improving.

C. Ask the nurse looking after the patient to discuss her concerns.

D. Acknowledge that being in hospital must be difficult and ask whether the patient would like any further emotional support whilst admitted.

E. Ask the patient whether she would like to be referred to hospital chaplaincy services for support.

F. Approach the patient and explore the reason for her emotional state.

G. Continue with your tasks, as being in hospital can be emotional for some people.

H. Recommend that the patient draws the curtains around her bed if she is feeling emotional.

Q149. Mr Morris is a 78-year-old man with a background of multiple cerebrovascular accidents and resultant dysphagia. He has been admitted with a presumed aspiration pneumonia. On the advice of the speech and language therapy team, he has been made nil by mouth but the MDT is unsure whether alternative feeding methods are in the patient's best interest. As Mr Morris has been deemed to lack capacity to make this decision, you have been asked to speak to Mr Morris's relatives to obtain their opinion on whether this treatment should be pursued.

Choose the most suitable **three** options from the following list:

A. Summarise Mr Morris's inpatient clinical course, the decision to make him nil by mouth and the subsequent MDT opinion.

B. Explore their opinion towards alternative feeding options.

C. Inform the family that Mr Morris's clinical state is poor as he is unable to swallow safely and alternative feeding is not appropriate.

D. Delegate the family discussion to the speech and language therapy team to recommend the best alternative feeding option.

E. Ask the family whether they have any questions.

F. Tell the family that you are only the junior doctor and offer to refer their questions to your registrar.

G. Explore whether Mr Morris had expressed any wishes or beliefs regarding his end-of-life care.

H. Discuss DNAR decision planning.

Q150. Mr Peters has been admitted overnight following a fall. You have been asked to review him following his normal CT head scan. As you are reviewing him, his family is escorted to the bedside by the healthcare assistant. Mrs Peters asks you how her husband is doing as this is the third time he has fallen this month.

Choose the most suitable **three** options from the following list:

A. Reassure the family that his investigations have been normal thus far.

B. Politely ask the family to wait outside the curtain until you have completed your review.

C. Refer Mr Peters to the falls clinic following his wife's collateral history.

D. Explain to Mrs Peters that you are very busy and will attempt to update her at another time.

E. Considering the collateral history, ask your clinical senior to update Mrs Peters.

F. Ask Mr Peters whether he is happy for you to discuss his medical information and if so update his family.

G. Explore further concerns that the family has regarding his current health.

H. Inform your clinical seniors about the full history that Mrs Peters has volunteered.

ANSWERS

A101. This question focuses on using communication that is pitched at the patient's level of understanding; ideally Anil should have said something along the lines of 'If it's OK with you, we're going to take a blood test that will help us understand how well your heart is working. Knowing the result will allow us to make sure you're on the right medications to improve your heart failure.' The best option in this case, on identifying that Doris had not understood Anil, would be to ask him to provide clarification (**answer A**). This would allow Doris to consent to an investigation as she would understand the rationale behind wanting to do it. The next best option would be for you to explain the management plan there and then (**answer D**), although you will miss some of Anil's review of the next patient, which may hinder the effective running of the ward round. This is followed by explaining the investigation to Doris when you return to take the blood test (**answer B**); this is not an ideal option as she cannot have truly consented for the investigation without understanding what it was being done for – i.e. explaining to her the rationale for the test whilst taking her blood for it is not valid consent. Ensuring that the test is done by the phlebotomist is a poor choice as Doris still remains unaware of the indication (**answer E**). Finally, blindly reassuring Doris does not address any of the concerns in the scenario at all (**answer C**).

Ideal order	Your rank choice				
	1st	2nd	3rd	4th	5th
A	4	3	2	1	0
D	3	4	3	2	1
B	2	3	4	3	2
E	1	2	3	4	3
C	0	1	2	3	4

A102. This question focuses on breaking bad news, addressing a patient's uncertainty and the content of documentation to which a patient has access. The most appropriate thing to do in this case is to contact Robert (**answer E**) and ask him to clarify Mr Kensington's concerns – he has the seniority to break bad news but also understands the patient's case. Contacting Anna (**answer C**) is less appropriate as she (a) didn't complete the discharge and (b) is an FY1 also and may not be in a position to break bad news (remember: 'know your limitations'). However, the bad news should have already been broken and clarifying the term may be all that Mr Kensington needs; therefore Anna may be able to address the issues. Instructing Mr Kensington to wait until he sees his consultant next week (**answer B**) is not a bad option as it's an opportunity for him to voice his concerns with the person in charge of his care; however, it is not as timely as the other options. Dismissing Mr Kensington as he was not your patient (**answer D**) is legitimate in some respects as you are unaware of the circumstances of his case and is preferential to potentially breaking bad news (**answer A**) to a patient you don't know anything about.

Ideal order	Your rank choice				
	1st	2nd	3rd	4th	5th
E	4	3	2	1	0
C	3	4	3	2	1
B	2	3	4	3	2
D	1	2	3	4	3
A	0	1	2	3	4

A103. The crux of this scenario revolves around your communication with another healthcare professional (i.e. the radiologist) and you should remember that as an FY1 you need to be assertive but courteous. The most appropriate option would be speaking to the radiologist in person about the request (**answer E**) – not only would this give you the opportunity to explain your consultant's rationale for the scan in greater depth but would also offer a learning opportunity through the academic discussion you would have with a senior colleague from a different specialty. The next best option would be to inform your consultant that the request has been declined (**answer C**); this would allow the opportunity to alter the management plan as necessary. You could consider emailing Dr Ahmed but this is not a time-efficient way to resolve the issue (**answer A**). Approaching another consultant radiologist undermines the decision of Dr Ahmed and is thus unprofessional (**answer D**). Finally, demanding that the scan be done is the least appropriate answer as it does not address the reasons for the scan being rejected; furthermore, it has the potential to tarnish working relationships for yourself within other departments (**answer B**).

Ideal order	Your rank choice				
	1st	2nd	3rd	4th	5th
E	4	3	2	1	0
C	3	4	3	2	1
A	2	3	4	3	2
D	1	2	3	4	3
B	0	1	2	3	4

A104. This question is based on your ability to communicate effectively with a patient to clarify your consultant's goal. It is common for patients with chronic conditions to be very knowledgeable with regards to their illness and/or management. Attempting to alter their treatment without

175

understanding their beliefs or fully explaining the reasoning behind the change will often result in conflict. Therefore, the most appropriate option in this scenario is **answer B**; exploring Sarah's concerns further may reveal a misunderstanding that you can clarify to reach a common agreement. The next most appropriate option would involve explaining your consultant's reasoning (**answer C**); this is ranked below answer B because you should always explore a patient's concerns and worries before attempting to explain, otherwise the patient may not be willing to listen to your explanation. Providing written information is always a good idea as it allows the patient the chance to read and consider the information that you have given (**answer D**). Remember though, written information should supplement and not replace your explanation, and therefore answer D is ranked below B and C. Telling a patient that they should simply listen to a doctor's advice is not an acceptable approach to healthcare; patients should be actively involved in their medical management and therefore **answer A** and **answer E** are both inappropriate. However, answer A is marginally better than answer E as it attempts to take Sarah's concerns into consideration.

Ideal order	Your rank choice				
	1st	2nd	3rd	4th	5th
B	4	3	2	1	0
C	3	4	3	2	1
D	2	3	4	3	2
A	1	2	3	4	3
E	0	1	2	3	4

A105. This question is based on your willingness to answer a patient's questions readily; however, this is compounded by your lack of experience with regard to this specific investigation. In this scenario, the most appropriate option is **answer D**. There are likely to be questions that you are able to answer and Dr Wilson will appreciate your willingness to talk with him. However, explaining that you will escalate any questions you are unable to answer will reassure Dr Wilson that his concerns will be addressed appropriately. The next most appropriate option is **answer E**. Patient information leaflets are often very well designed and provide patients with most of the answers. Remember, written information should supplement and not replace your explanation, and therefore answer E is ranked below D. The next most appropriate option would be to explain openly that Dr Wilson should discuss his concerns with the registrar, who will be able to answer all his questions (**answer C**). Answer C is ranked below D because you should always be willing to explore a patient's questions before referring them to a senior colleague. Answer A and answer B are both poor choices. However, attempting to answer Dr Wilson's questions (without an escalation caveat as per answer D) does still show willingness, but will not provide Dr Wilson with much reassurance if your answers are always 'I'm afraid I'm not sure' (**answer A**). Remember,

'I'm afraid I'm not sure but I'll ensure the registrar explains this afternoon' is much better. Clearly, sourcing information from the internet is never an appropriate option (**answer B**).

Ideal order	Your rank choice				
	1st	2nd	3rd	4th	5th
D	4	3	2	1	0
E	3	4	3	2	1
C	2	3	4	3	2
A	1	2	3	4	3
B	0	1	2	3	4

A106. This question is based on the 'softer' communication skills that you should be able to demonstrate when a patient is upset: sensitive use of language, adjusting the style of communication according to a patient's needs, and asking questions to understand the patient. Therefore, the most appropriate action is to explore Rebecca's current emotional state (**answer B**). The next most appropriate option in this scenario is to ask your FY1 colleague, Lauren, to review Rebecca this afternoon to discuss her concerns (**answer E**). Asking the nurse in charge to speak to Rebecca is the next most appropriate action (**answer D**); this would ensure that Rebecca has support and also encourages the nurse to raise any concerns she may have with you. Waiting for the ward round tomorrow before discussing Rebecca's mood with her is the second least appropriate option (**answer A**); if you see a patient is upset you should attempt to help at the time and not delay it until your next routine review. Finally, the least appropriate option in this scenario is to return to Rebecca when her parents are present to discuss her concerns (**answer C**). This would compromise patient confidentiality as you have not asked Rebecca whether she would like to discuss her concerns in front of her parents.

Ideal order	Your rank choice				
	1st	2nd	3rd	4th	5th
B	4	3	2	1	0
E	3	4	3	2	1
D	2	3	4	3	2
A	1	2	3	4	3
C	0	1	2	3	4

A107. This question is focusing on your communication skills with colleagues, in this case another FY1, Claire. You should be able to adapt the style of your communication according to need and situation, use diplomacy and be assertive when necessary. In this scenario the most appropriate option is **answer A**. This is polite, respectful and demonstrates diplomacy. Discussing your concerns with your consultant will enable them to review the situation and if need be to speak to Claire themself (**answer C**). The next most appropriate option would be **answer E**. However, written information should be secondary to resolving the problem in person. Therefore answer E is ranked below A and C. Confronting Claire in front of other colleagues at the board round is not an appropriate option (**answer B**) as it is unprofessional and undermines Claire's position on the ward. However, the least appropriate option is **answer D**. Remember, doing nothing is rarely the correct answer in the SJT. You have identified a problem (Claire is taking too long at the board round) and therefore you should aim to resolve this. Ignoring the problem will not make it go away.

Ideal order	Your rank choice				
	1st	2nd	3rd	4th	5th
A	4	3	2	1	0
C	3	4	3	2	1
E	2	3	4	3	2
B	1	2	3	4	3
D	0	1	2	3	4

A108. This question is based on the importance of clear, detailed and legible documentation allowing for high standards of written communication. In this situation you have noticed Warren's documentation is substandard and affecting the patient care. It is therefore crucial that this concern is addressed sensitively and fairly. The most appropriate action would be to meet Warren in person and discuss your concerns (**answer B**). The next most appropriate response would be to discuss your concerns with your clinical supervisor (**answer A**), who would be best suited to advise you on how to address this problem. The next most appropriate response would be simply telling Warren he needs to improve when you next see him at departmental teaching (**answer C**). This is ranked below answers B and A as you are delaying your action, thus allowing the poor documentation to continue unnecessarily, and this response is also somewhat confrontational. Discussing your concerns regarding Warren's documentation with his clinical supervisor is not acceptable (**answer D**); you should always discuss your concerns with **your** clinical supervisor, who can raise these concerns with the individual's clinical supervisor if it is deemed appropriate. However, the least appropriate option is **answer E**. Remember, doing nothing is rarely the correct answer in the SJT. You have identified a problem (Warren's poor documentation) and therefore you should aim to resolve this. Ignoring the problem will not make it go away.

Ideal order	Your rank choice				
	1st	2nd	3rd	4th	5th
B	4	3	2	1	0
A	3	4	3	2	1
C	2	3	4	3	2
D	1	2	3	4	3
E	0	1	2	3	4

A109. This scenario is focused on sharing of information and ensuring continuity of care between secondary and primary care. As an FY1 you will write many discharge summaries that will communicate medication changes, investigation results and ongoing plans to GPs and you hope that they will be read. When a situation like this arises it is always prudent to begin by gathering information (**answer D**) – if the GP practice didn't receive the discharge summary, or if it was received after the repeat prescription was made, this gives you a better insight when raising your concern. As you are escalating your concern, use the escalation ladder – remember to raise your concerns with your consultant (**answer C**) prior to escalating them to senior management (**answer B**). I am sure some of you will have ranked **answer E** higher in your answer; however, the scenario clearly outlines that the discharge summary was completed correctly and so this is not an issue this scenario identifies. The least appropriate option is to report Dr Omoyemi to the clinical commissioning group as any negligence accusation you raise is currently unfounded (**answer A**).

Ideal order	Your rank choice				
	1st	2nd	3rd	4th	5th
D	4	3	2	1	0
C	3	4	3	2	1
B	2	3	4	3	2
E	1	2	3	4	3
A	0	1	2	3	4

A110. This question is focused on the importance of ensuring your surroundings are appropriate when communicating. Clearly, Ken has failed to appreciate that his current surrounding is not ideal as the patients in the rest of the bay can hear his discussion. Therefore, your immediate action should be aimed at informing him of this and protecting Mr Domingues' confidentiality (**answer C**). Asking the matron to relocate Ken to the relatives' room will also achieve your aims (**answer A**). However, as with all SJT situations it is best to attempt to resolve a problem in person; therefore answer A is ranked below C. The next most appropriate option is **answer B**. This is ranked below C and A because, despite achieving your aim, this approach may undermine Ken's position in front of Mr Domingues and his daughter. Allowing Ken to complete his conversation before informing him of the problem is a poor choice as it does not address the issue. Mr Domingues' confidentiality is still being jeopardised (**answer E**). However, the least appropriate option is **answer D**. It is not realistic to expect patients not to listen to a conversation in the neighbouring bed. This conversation should have taken place in the privacy of the relatives' room.

	Your rank choice				
Ideal order	1st	2nd	3rd	4th	5th
C	4	3	2	1	0
A	3	4	3	2	1
B	2	3	4	3	2
E	1	2	3	4	3
D	0	1	2	3	4

A111. This question is based on your willingness to allow relatives to ask questions. Mr Benson's daughter is clearly concerned about the post mortem and has asked you whether you think it is necessary. This is a challenging position to be in as your consultant has made it clear that they feel it is not necessary to discern a cause of death, but would be a beneficial teaching exercise. However, regardless of your opinion on this matter you should always explore a relative's concerns once they become apparent (**answer E**). The next most appropriate response would be to refer Mr Benson's daughter directly to Dr Hill (**answer A**), who will be able to discuss the daughter's concerns fully. Escalating the daughter's concerns to your registrar is the next most appropriate response in this scenario (**answer C**). However, as Dr Hill was the clinician requesting the post mortem it is unlikely that the registrar will be able to give any additional information and so Mr Benson's daughter really should speak directly to Dr Hill. Arranging to meet with Dr Hill to discuss the reasons behind the post mortem may allow you to gain insight into the request but this will not enable you to answer the daughter's concerns now. Therefore **answer D** is not an appropriate response. However, the least appropriate response is dismissing the daughter's concerns on the basis that the family has consented (**answer B**). Remember, consent is voluntary and can always be retracted.

Ideal order	Your rank choice				
	1st	2nd	3rd	4th	5th
E	4	3	2	1	0
A	3	4	3	2	1
C	2	3	4	3	2
D	1	2	3	4	3
B	0	1	2	3	4

A112. This question is focused on the importance of providing information and keeping patients updated. In this scenario, Mrs Li's elective operation is currently indefinitely delayed owing to two emergency admissions. The most appropriate response is to attempt to contact your registrar for an update and inform Mrs Li of your findings (**answer E**). The next most appropriate option in this scenario is to apologise to Mrs Li for the delay but honestly explain you do not know at what time the operation will be (**answer C**). Asking your registrar to review Mrs Li because she has been nil by mouth for 13 hours is not an ideal response as they are busy in theatre (**answer A**). However, in this scenario this would be your next best option as advising Mrs Li that the operation will be cancelled is not appropriate as the FY1 does not make this decision (**answer D**). Finally, the least appropriate response would involve allowing Mrs Li to eat as this would prevent her from being able to have her operation today (**answer B**).

Ideal order	Your rank choice				
	1st	2nd	3rd	4th	5th
E	4	3	2	1	0
C	3	4	3	2	1
A	2	3	4	3	2
D	1	2	3	4	3
B	0	1	2	3	4

A113. This question is assessing your ability to respond sensitively to cues that your colleague, Jack, is not coping in his current role. The most appropriate response in this scenario is to attempt to reassure Jack and provide support (**answer A**). The next most appropriate response is to encourage Jack to discuss his concerns with his educational supervisor (**answer B**). Remember, it is better not to become directly involved when a colleague is having difficulties. Instead, advise them to act as if you were at the centre of the problem. The next most appropriate response would be to speak to your own educational supervisor to gain advice (**answer C**). This is ranked third as it does not attempt to address the issue immediately. It is not appropriate to challenge Jack's SHO (**answer D**). As with answer B, it is better not to be directly involved. However, the least appropriate option is to accept Jack's discontent (**answer E**). Your colleague is struggling and you should attempt to help him.

Ideal order	Your rank choice				
	1st	2nd	3rd	4th	5th
A	4	3	2	1	0
B	3	4	3	2	1
C	2	3	4	3	2
D	1	2	3	4	3
E	0	1	2	3	4

A114. This question is focusing on your ability to use diplomacy to remind Alex about his infection control responsibilities in clinical areas. Therefore, the most appropriate option is to discuss your concerns with Alex directly (**answer A**). The next most appropriate options respectively would be to discuss your concerns with your SHO (**answer E**), then the senior sister on the ward (**answer C**) and then infection control (**answer D**) as per the escalation ladder. The least appropriate option in this scenario is to do nothing as Alex is putting patients at risk of cross-infection (**answer B**).

Ideal order	Your rank choice				
	1st	2nd	3rd	4th	5th
A	4	3	2	1	0
E	3	4	3	2	1
C	2	3	4	3	2
D	1	2	3	4	3
B	0	1	2	3	4

A115. This question is assessing your ability to communicate and respond appropriately with a patient during a sensitive discussion. In this case, Mr Oliver has demonstrated capacity for this decision and therefore his wishes should be acted upon (**answer E**). This includes not disclosing his request to his family. The next most appropriate response is informing the MDT of Mr Oliver's wishes (**answer D**); this is ranked below answer E as it does not show any regard to reassuring Mr Oliver. The third most appropriate response is **answer B**. However, you should discuss your intention with Mr Oliver as he may not want you to involve his GP or provide further assistance at home. As Mr Oliver has capacity he does have the right to make that request. It is not appropriate to delay a patient's wish to make an advanced directive until they are discharged (**answer C**). Mr Oliver is currently capable of making this plan and therefore it should be acted on during this current admission. In fact, you should consider liaising with his GP, with Mr Oliver's consent, to arrange a community palliation order. Finally, the least appropriate option would be to discuss Mr Oliver's request with his family (**answer A**); this would be a flagrant breach of patient confidentiality.

	Your rank choice				
Ideal order	1st	2nd	3rd	4th	5th
E	4	3	2	1	0
D	3	4	3	2	1
B	2	3	4	3	2
C	1	2	3	4	3
A	0	1	2	3	4

A116. This question is based on your willingness to answer a patient's question readily whilst adjusting the amount of information to provide. In this challenging scenario, the most appropriate response is to explain that you do not have the final report and that she will be seen by the neurology team later that afternoon (**answer C**). This is not because you are trying to withhold information from her, but the diagnosis is provisional and the questions that she is likely to have are better answered by a neurologist. The next most appropriate response is **answer A**. This is a factual statement but doesn't provide much support to Miss Johannson. In this scenario, the next best option would be **answer B** as this would enable you to discuss her case fully with the neurology team reviewing her. Disclosing the provisional diagnosis is not an advisable option and is therefore ranked low (**answer D**). This is a serious diagnosis and, even if provisional, should be delivered by somebody able to fully explain and answer any subsequent questions Miss Johannson may have. Therefore, it is not appropriate for an FY1 to deliver. However, the least appropriate option would be to reassure Miss Johannson falsely. The provisional report demonstrates a potential serious diagnosis and, although you shouldn't deliver that diagnosis yourself, nor should you lead Miss Johannson to believe nothing is wrong (**answer E**).

Ideal order	Your rank choice				
	1st	2nd	3rd	4th	5th
C	4	3	2	1	0
A	3	4	3	2	1
B	2	3	4	3	2
D	1	2	3	4	3
E	0	1	2	3	4

A117. This question is assessing your ability to summarise information accurately and concisely to your colleague in order to request another specialty review. The most appropriate response is **answer C**. When you are referring to a colleague, remember to use an approved handover tool such as SBAR. The next most appropriate option is **answer A**. The surgical registrar will be required to fill in the gaps you have omitted themselves, but at least your request for a review has been made. Contacting the surgical SHO to discuss your patient with them is an unnecessary delay as referrals are accepted directly by registrars (**answer B**). Therefore answer B is below C and A. Delaying your referral to the surgical team as you feel the patient will be complicated and generate several jobs is not appropriate as it will put the patient at unnecessary risk (**answer D**). However, the least appropriate action would be to discuss this patient with the medical registrar as you feel the patient is not fit for a curative surgical procedure; this is a decision a surgical MDT will make and not an FY1 (**answer E**).

Ideal order	Your rank choice				
	1st	2nd	3rd	4th	5th
C	4	3	2	1	0
A	3	4	3	2	1
B	2	3	4	3	2
D	1	2	3	4	3
E	0	1	2	3	4

A118. This question is assessing your ability to appropriately negotiate with your colleagues. Annual leave, study leave, compulsory training days and specialty training post interviews are but a few examples of reasons for needing time off from work. Your colleagues will all be in a similar position to you and so developing negotiation skills is vital. The best method for negotiation is explaining why you need your colleagues to swap (**answer B**). The next most appropriate response would be to discuss the leave clash with your clinical supervisor (**answer C**). They would be able to assess the need of the ward and consider requesting support from other wards to allow all three of you to take leave. Answer C is ranked below B because you should attempt to resolve issues with your colleagues at your own level. The third most appropriate response is **answer A**. However, if you do not attempt to negotiate the swap/call in favours/offer favours, then it is unlikely you will be successful. Attempting to arrange a study day in place of annual leave is not appropriate (**answer E**); this is underhanded and will still leave the ward short-staffed. However, the least appropriate option would be to call in sick (**answer D**).

	Your rank choice				
Ideal order	1st	2nd	3rd	4th	5th
B	4	3	2	1	0
C	3	4	3	2	1
A	2	3	4	3	2
E	1	2	3	4	3
D	0	1	2	3	4

A119. This question is based on your ability to gather information before attempting to resolve a complaint. The most appropriate response is to contact the rehabilitation centre to establish whether it has a transfer date (**answer C**). This will allow you to allay Mr Ali's concerns when you respond to his complaint. The next most appropriate response would be to attend Mr Ali and explain why he has not been seen by a doctor (**answer E**). Asking the physiotherapist who bleeped you to explain the reason for Mr Ali's delay is reasonable as they are seeing him each day (**answer A**). However, as with any complaint it is usually better to review the patient in person. Therefore answer A is below E. **Answer D** is the next most appropriate response in this scenario. It is a factual statement and does encourage Mr Ali to keep working with physiotherapy, which is the main reason for rehabilitation in the first instance. However, a patient that has complained about not being reviewed by a doctor is unlikely to appreciate this response. Finally, the least appropriate response would be to dismiss Mr Ali's complaint (**answer B**).

	Your rank choice				
Ideal order	1st	2nd	3rd	4th	5th
C	4	3	2	1	0
E	3	4	3	2	1
A	2	3	4	3	2
D	1	2	3	4	3
B	0	1	2	3	4

A120. This question is based on your ability to gather information and administer treatment without delay. The most appropriate response in this scenario is **answer A**. Gathering the relevant information will enable you to have a more meaningful discussion with the microbiologist. Remember, gathering information is rarely a poor choice. The next most appropriate option is contacting the microbiologist immediately (**answer B**). This is ranked below answer A as you will not be able to give the microbiologist a full history and so their advice may be less relevant. However, at least this option appreciates the urgency in delivering antibiotics without delay. Taking a full and thorough history, which you clearly document before calling the microbiologist, is a reasonable approach to take but will cause a time delay (**answer C**). It is therefore ranked third. Discussing Mrs Aarons' case with the on-call registrar (**answer E**), who will be poorly equipped to make this decision compared with the microbiologist, is not appropriate. However, the least appropriate option is **answer D**. Empirical antibiotic treatment is unlikely to be effective or well tolerated in a patient with multiple allergies. Furthermore, this is in contradiction to your consultant's recommendation, so is never advisable.

Ideal order	Your rank choice				
	1st	2nd	3rd	4th	5th
A	4	3	2	1	0
B	3	4	3	2	1
C	2	3	4	3	2
E	1	2	3	4	3
D	0	1	2	3	4

A121. This question is based on your ability to ask appropriate questions of colleagues to gain more information. In this scenario, you have a drug which you can prescribe competently but have limited knowledge on its use or benefits. Therefore the most appropriate response is to ask your clinical supervisor for teaching (**answer D**). The next most appropriate option is **answer E** as it still attempts to gather more information; as you did not take the opportunity to learn earlier, answer E is ranked below D. **Answer A** is an indirect method for gathering more information about renal drugs and is therefore ranked below direct methods (i.e. D and E). Asking the ward pharmacist is a reasonable approach to learning more about a medication (**answer C**). However, they may know less with regards to clinical application and practicalities and so your clinical supervisor should be your first point of contact for teaching. The least appropriate option is to assume you'll learn about erythropoietin another time (**answer B**). You have identified a learning deficit in your knowledge and you should attempt to resolve it as soon as possible.

Ideal order	Your rank choice				
	1st	2nd	3rd	4th	5th
D	4	3	2	1	0
E	3	4	3	2	1
A	2	3	4	3	2
C	1	2	3	4	3
B	0	1	2	3	4

A122. This question is based on your ability to adjust your style of communication and the amount of information given according to a relative's need. In this situation, the most appropriate action is first to gain Mrs McCreath's consent to discuss her admission with her daughter (**answer A**). Always remember: patient confidentiality! The next most appropriate option is **answer B**. It is important that you are as informed as possible so that you can alter the level of information you are providing according to Mrs McCreath's daughter's need. Discussing Mrs McCreath's admission with her daughter without familiarising yourself with her case is not advisable (**answer C**); you may be unable to answer the daughter's questions, which could further antagonise her. **Answer D** is unlikely to appease Mrs McCreath's daughter as this response gives no information as to why she is unsafe currently; therefore it is ranked fourth. However, the least appropriate option is **answer E**. Mrs McCreath's daughter is understandably upset and discussing her mother's admission calmly with full explanations and plans is what will appease her, and not being asked to wait in a relatives' room until she calms down.

Ideal order	Your rank choice				
	1st	2nd	3rd	4th	5th
A	4	3	2	1	0
B	3	4	3	2	1
C	2	3	4	3	2
D	1	2	3	4	3
E	0	1	2	3	4

A123. This question is based on the challenges involving patients who are unable to communicate verbally and how you can present information in a way they can understand. Poor non-verbal communication such as standing over a patient or speaking above a patient to their carer can impair the patient's trust in you. Therefore the most appropriate option is **answer E**. The next most appropriate option would involve asking the carer, who knows the patient better than you, to communicate on your behalf (**answer D**). Discussing this problem with your senior colleague is a sensible approach (**answer C**). However, if you are able to tell them you have attempted direct communication and with the assistance of their carer, it will enable your senior colleague to advise you more appropriately; therefore answer C is ranked third. Telling a patient you are unable to help them unless you can examine them is necessary as you cannot treat something unless it can be diagnosed (**answer A**). However, this approach is ranked fourth as you should try every verbal and non-verbal technique to help a patient who has difficulty communicating. Finally, the least appropriate response is to refuse to help the patient (**answer B**).

Ideal order	Your rank choice				
	1st	2nd	3rd	4th	5th
E	4	3	2	1	0
D	3	4	3	2	1
C	2	3	4	3	2
A	1	2	3	4	3
B	0	1	2	3	4

A124. This question is based on your response to a language barrier and the methods used to ensure adequate communication with the patient. In this scenario, the most appropriate response is to arrange an urgent interpreter (**answer C**). The next most appropriate option would involve a telephone interpretation service (**answer B**). This is ranked below answer C as an interpreter should be present in person to allow a fluid conversation. The next most appropriate response is **answer E**. Remember, another healthcare professional can assist with interpretation but as they are not formally trained this should be only after all interpretation services have failed. The next most appropriate option would involve discussing your inability to gather a history with your senior colleague (**answer D**). This answer is ranked fourth as they will be in a similar position to you unless they also speak Sri Lankan. Therefore it would be appropriate to attempt to arrange translation, escalating to your senior colleague. Finally, the least appropriate option would be to continue the patient's analgesia and arrange a CT scan to attempt to diagnose the cause of the pain (**answer A**). This would not solve the communication problem and the patient would be unable to consent.

Ideal order	Your rank choice				
	1st	2nd	3rd	4th	5th
C	4	3	2	1	0
B	3	4	3	2	1
E	2	3	4	3	2
D	1	2	3	4	3
A	0	1	2	3	4

A125. This question is based on your willingness to meet with relatives in order to keep them updated. However, as both relatives are healthcare professionals you would also be expected to demonstrate an ability to adapt the language chosen in your discussion. In this scenario the most appropriate choice is **answer B**. It is important to explore the concerns relatives may have as this allows you to explain why a decision has been taken, thereby appeasing their concerns. The next best choice is **answer A**. This still keeps the relatives updated but demonstrates less willingness to explore their concerns; instead this response is more matter of fact and therefore ranked below answer B. Delegating this responsibility to the nurse is an option but is not ideal (**answer D**). As with all communication, the fewer individuals involved the less is the chance of miscommunication. Therefore this option has been ranked below explaining in person (i.e. B and A). **Answer C** is not an appropriate response. Even as an on-call doctor you should be willing to spend time with concerned relatives. However, the least appropriate option would be **answer E**. In this scenario the relatives are concerned about a specific antibiotic chosen, not that antibiotics have been given at all. Therefore, to stop the antibiotic because the relatives are appearing 'difficult' is not appropriate. Remember, your concern is always the patient's wellbeing.

Ideal order	Your rank choice				
	1st	2nd	3rd	4th	5th
B	4	3	2	1	0
A	3	4	3	2	1
D	2	3	4	3	2
C	1	2	3	4	3
E	0	1	2	3	4

A126. This question is based on the importance of preparing for a planned discussion, updating relatives, gathering information and your willingness to answer questions readily. In this situation the most appropriate option is **answer E**. With any discussion it is important that you know as much information as possible. Therefore it is advisable to refresh your memory by reading the patient's notes. A good communication tip is to clarify what a patient or their relative already knows before giving any information. The next most appropriate option is **answer A** as this still demonstrates a willingness to meet with a relative and provide them with an update. However, you may not be providing the most up-to-date information and therefore it is ranked below answer E. There will be occasions where a summary is appropriate (**answer B**). Patients or their relatives may not be interested in detail and may prefer less information. However, you should always clarify this first and not simply assume as per answer B, and therefore it is ranked third. Delaying your meeting with Mrs Jones' daughter is not appropriate (**answer C**). You should be willing to meet with relatives to provide an update regarding their loved one. However, the least appropriate option is to decline Mrs Jones' request (**answer D**).

Ideal order	Your rank choice				
	1st	2nd	3rd	4th	5th
E	4	3	2	1	0
A	3	4	3	2	1
B	2	3	4	3	2
C	1	2	3	4	3
D	0	1	2	3	4

A127. This question is based on gathering more information about relatives' understanding, ensuring you have relevant knowledge before communicating, communicating information clearly and demonstrating sensitive use of language. In this scenario Mrs Sweetman's family is understandably upset by their mother's deteriorating health. However, the medical team has been unable to illicit a cause for her symptoms despite a thorough investigation. Therefore, the most appropriate response is **answer D**. This will clarify what the family has understood regarding the investigations and will allow you to simplify any misunderstandings they may have. The family's main worry is that their mother is not being adequately investigated. Therefore, you should try to reassure them that this is not the case (**answer C**). Normally, informing a family that it would be better to raise their concerns with the regular doctors as you are on call is not ideal. However, in this scenario where there are no acute medical problems with Mrs Sweetman this is the next most appropriate option (**answer B**). As Mrs Sweetman is clinically stable it is not necessary to discuss this case with the on-call registrar and therefore **answer E** is ranked fourth. However, the least appropriate response is to dismiss the family's concern (**answer A**).

190

Ideal order	Your rank choice				
	1st	2nd	3rd	4th	5th
D	4	3	2	1	0
C	3	4	3	2	1
B	2	3	4	3	2
E	1	2	3	4	3
A	0	1	2	3	4

A128. This question is assessing your ability to gather more information in order to clarify your own understanding. In this situation you require more information about the patient before you can take action. Therefore **answer C** is the most appropriate response. The next most appropriate response is **answer D** as reminding the nurse to use an approved communication tool (e.g. SBAR) will reduce future miscommunication. However, as this response does not gather information about this patient, it is ranked below answer C. Asking the nurse to complete additional observations and then bleep you again it not an ideal response (**answer E**). A patient is potentially unwell and, as frustrating as poor handovers are, your priority should be to that patient. Therefore you should ask for the information whilst you are on the phone (e.g. answer C). However, this response is still more appropriate than answer A and answer B, which are the final two responses respectively. Remember, in the SJT it is better to act now, and report later. Although it is important to discuss your concerns regarding handover with your supervisor (**answer A**) and the nurse in charge (**answer B**), this can be done after you have reviewed the patient.

Ideal order	Your rank choice				
	1st	2nd	3rd	4th	5th
C	4	3	2	1	0
D	3	4	3	2	1
E	2	3	4	3	2
A	1	2	3	4	3
B	0	1	2	3	4

A129. This question is based on your negotiation and diplomacy skills. In this scenario, the most appropriate response is **answer B**. Discussing your colleague's concerns may reveal a problem that you can overcome as a team. The next most appropriate option is **answer D**.

Ensuring that each other's clinical commitments are covered will encourage your colleagues to participate in the teaching programme. This is ranked below answer B because without exploring your colleagues' concerns they will be unlikely to agree to teach. **Answer C** would be the next most appropriate option as your colleagues are currently declining to take part; however, as you should be able to demonstrate diplomacy and negotiation skills as an FY1, both B and D should be attempted before you escalate to your supervisor. Arranging a teaching session under duress is not advisable (**answer E**); if your colleagues are unwilling to agree to teach a session you need to raise this with your supervisor as per answer C. Finally, in this scenario asking your SHO colleagues to teach some of your programme is not appropriate (**answer A**). It does not attempt to resolve the fundamental issue in this scenario of FY1s not cooperating.

Ideal order	Your rank choice				
	1st	2nd	3rd	4th	5th
B	4	3	2	1	0
D	3	4	3	2	1
C	2	3	4	3	2
E	1	2	3	4	3
A	0	1	2	3	4

A130. This question is based on your negotiation and diplomacy skills. In this scenario, the most appropriate response is **answer A**. Discussing your scheduling concern directly with the rota coordinator Julie may reveal a solution to your lack of training days and resolve this issue. The next most appropriate option is **answer D**. Attempting to negotiate with your fellow FY1s would be a worthwhile effort as you may be able to agree a local swap. This is ranked below answer A because study leave should be agreed with your rota coordinator initially. **Answer E** would be the next most appropriate option as your educational supervisor may be able to persuade your team to rearrange the training schedule. However, as you should be able to demonstrate diplomacy and negotiation skills as an FY1, both A and D should be attempted before you escalate to your educational supervisor. Contacting the foundation school director is the fourth most appropriate option as per the escalation ladder (**answer B**). However, the least appropriate option would be to attend a teaching session without regard for your clinical commitments as this would potentially risk patient safety (**answer C**).

Ideal order	Your rank choice				
	1st	2nd	3rd	4th	5th
A	4	3	2	1	0
D	3	4	3	2	1
E	2	3	4	3	2
B	1	2	3	4	3
C	0	1	2	3	4

A131. This question is based on your negotiation and diplomacy skills. In this scenario, negotiating directly with your colleague James through explaining your reasoning should be your first action (**answer E**). **Answer B** would be the next most appropriate option as this is a diplomatic method to resolve your concern. However, without attempting to negotiate with James first he may simply ignore your rota. Therefore answer E should be attempted initially. The next most appropriate option is **answer D**. As per the escalation ladder, your educational supervisor would be next in this scenario, but this option is ranked after E and B because exploring James's understanding of your situation and attempting a rota may negate the need to speak with your educational supervisor. **Answer C** is an immature response to a fairly simple misunderstanding and is not appropriate behaviour. However, the least appropriate option is **answer A**. James and you are peers and attempting to mandate his workload is unlikely to be successful.

Ideal order	Your rank choice				
	1st	2nd	3rd	4th	5th
E	4	3	2	1	0
B	3	4	3	2	1
D	2	3	4	3	2
C	1	2	3	4	3
A	0	1	2	3	4

A132. This question is based on written communication and providing only relevant information when referring to another specialty. In this scenario the most appropriate response is **answer B**. This ensures that the relevant information regarding Mrs Crankshaw reaches the right individual who can arrange an appointment. The next most appropriate response is **answer D**. The discharge summary will contain the relevant information required but, as you have not forwarded it to the correct individual, Mrs Crankshaw's appointment may take time to arrange. **Answer A** is a perfectly suitable response to ensure an appointment is arranged but, as this is not accompanied by a referral letter, the endocrinologist will not have any background about Mrs Crankshaw when she is seen in outpatients. Therefore this response is ranked third. Forwarding a copy of Mrs Crankshaw's inpatient medical notes is not appropriate (**answer C**). Medical notes are ordered and transferred by medical records and to send a photocopy is not protocol. However, the least appropriate option is **answer E**. It is your responsibility to arrange Mrs Crankshaw's outpatient appointment as it has originated from a secondary care source. Asking her GP to make a referral risks delaying Mrs Crankshaw's follow-up.

Ideal order	Your rank choice				
	1st	2nd	3rd	4th	5th
B	4	3	2	1	0
D	3	4	3	2	1
A	2	3	4	3	2
C	1	2	3	4	3
E	0	1	2	3	4

A133. This question is based on your ability to clarify relatives' understanding and summarise information clearly, and willingness to update relatives. In this scenario, the most appropriate option is to meet with Mr Kenworthy's family to explore their current understanding (**answer C**). This enables you to clarify any misunderstanding and attempt to resolve their concerns. The next most appropriate option is to provide summarised information to the family about feeding options (**answer B**). This is ranked after answer C as it presumes Mr Kenworthy's family has no prior knowledge. You should always confirm a patient's or relatives' understanding so that you can adapt the amount and type of information provided. Providing the family with printed information is always recommended (**answer A**). However, this should be in addition to your discussion and not in place of it. Therefore answer A is ranked below C and B. It would not be appropriate for you to make a recommendation at this stage as Mr Kenworthy's family has not been given the chance to make an informed decision (**answer E**). However, the least appropriate option is **answer D**. Asking another specialty to discuss a family's concerns before you have attempted to do so demonstrates a lack of willingness to meet with relatives. Referring Mr Kenworthy to speech and language is a sensible idea, but this should be raised with the family during your discussion with them.

Ideal order	Your rank choice				
	1st	2nd	3rd	4th	5th
C	4	3	2	1	0
B	3	4	3	2	1
A	2	3	4	3	2
E	1	2	3	4	3
D	0	1	2	3	4

A134. This question is based on your ability to communicate relevant information concisely and clearly. In this scenario you are required to summarise Mrs Poppy's salient medical history and clearly state the indication in a request to arrange an urgent CT scan. Therefore, the most appropriate option is **answer E**. The next most appropriate response, as per the escalation ladder, is to escalate your concerns initially to your consultant (**answer C**) followed by another specialty – i.e. radiology (**answer D**). Failure to summarise Mrs Poppy's medical history, thereby leaving an inadequate space for your CT request, is not an appropriate response as the scan will probably be rejected (**answer A**). However, the least appropriate response is cancelling the CT scan as this would be contradicting the consultant, who is ultimately responsible for Mrs Poppy (**answer B**).

Ideal order	Your rank choice				
	1st	2nd	3rd	4th	5th
E	4	3	2	1	0
C	3	4	3	2	1
D	2	3	4	3	2
A	1	2	3	4	3
B	0	1	2	3	4

A135. This question focuses on empathetic communication and the communication of management plans to a patient and their relatives. Ideally all discussions where such bad news is broken should be done sensitively and patients should be given adequate time to reflect on the news they have heard. Obviously sometimes news isn't broken in the most ideal settings and patients may not be adequately supported. You should initially ensure that the family has taken away from Dr Cavendish's discussion the relevant information (**answer G**). You should also provide them with

195

the opportunity to ask further questions (**answer B**). Longitudinally you should provide them with a named contact for them to ask questions that may arise in the coming days (**answer H**).

It is not appropriate to apologise for the way Dr Cavendish broke the news (**answer A**); it undermines the position of the consultant in charge of Mrs Livingstone's care and it may be the nature of the news being broken rather than the way it was delivered that has caused the distress. Therefore it is inappropriate to report Dr Cavendish to the GMC (**answer C**). It would be inappropriate to refer Mrs Livingstone to palliative care services (**answer D**) as these sorts of management decisions should be made in conjunction with your senior colleagues. You should refer patients to a service such as the chaplaincy (**answer E**) only after ensuring that this is an option they would like explored. On seeing that a patient and family are distressed, it is your duty to attend to them initially to explore their concerns and not immediately delegate this discussion to the nursing staff (**answer F**).

A	B	C	D	E	F	G	H
0	4	0	0	0	0	4	4

A136. This question focuses on your ability to ensure that a patient understands the treatment through providing information in an appropriate way. It also focuses on your communication with colleagues. You should initially prevent the patient from taking the drug if you have concerns that it is not being taken as prescribed (**answer E**), prior to discussing with the nurse who dispensed the medication whether it was given as prescribed (**answer D**). If you have concerns with compliance with therapy then it is appropriate to provide the patient with instruction in a way that will be understood. As Mr Petrescu is Romanian, providing a Romanian translator (**answer H**) will allow you to communicate how to take the medication effectively to the patient.

Confirming the dosage with the consultant and attempting to converse with the patient (**answer A** and **answer B**) are not suitable options as you know the latter probably will not understand, hence your conversations are likely to be fruitless. If you are concerned that the patient is not taking medication as prescribed, you should not let him take it (**answer G**). You are breaching the patient's confidentiality by using his relatives as translators (**answer F**); this should be done only if professional translation services are unavailable. Seeking the advice of the pharmacist (**answer C**) does not necessarily address the issues highlighted in this case.

A	B	C	D	E	F	G	H
0	0	0	4	4	0	0	4

A137. This question focuses on your allowing relatives to ask you questions and your answering them in a timely fashion. It also focuses on your ability to check relatives' understanding and listen effectively. The most suitable thing to do would be to state to Mr Bence-Jones your unfamiliarity with his wife's case (**answer A**) as this would inform him that you need the opportunity to review both the patient and her medical notes prior to entering a discussion with him. Therefore, you are currently not prepared to have a discussion with the patient's husband as the only information you have on the patient is from your handover from Jennifer, and so you need to review the patient personally (**answer F**). As with any discussion with a relative, you should ensure that the patient has first consented to it (**answer C**).

Reassuring a relative without personally reviewing a patient is not safe or best practice (**answer B**). As an FY1 you should be in a position to discuss a patient's progress with relatives without immediately deferring this conversation to a senior colleague (**answer D** and **answer G**). It may be that speaking to the relative will calm him down and so asking other staff members to get involved at this point (**answer E**) or asking the husband personally to calm down (**answer H**) may not be productive.

A	B	C	D	E	F	G	H
4	0	4	0	0	4	0	0

A138. This question focuses on your ability to use diplomacy when dealing with colleagues. In this scenario, you are attempting to hand over a clinical task to another colleague and are met with 'rude' resistance, hence the focus of the question. The blood test needs to be taken and so this should be handed over to the FY1 cover for your ward out of hours (**answer B**) if you are unable to recruit the nurse to do the task. As a result of the incident it would be sensible to discuss your conversation with Meghan later (**answer C**) as her response may have been secondary to an underlying issue separate to your request. It would also be advisable to strategically plan with the matron a way in which such blood requests are dealt with (**answer D**) to avoid such a situation in the future.

It would be inappropriate for you to stay late to take the blood test yourself (**answer A**) as there should be another doctor covering your ward at that time. It would also be inappropriate to confront Meghan immediately with your concerns (**answer E**) or to interrogate Meghan about the tasks she has to complete (**answer F**). It may be appropriate to discuss with Meghan's seniors (**answer G**) should the issue not be resolved, but this should be following your own attempts to address these. It would be inappropriate also for you to insist that Meghan takes the blood test (**answer H**) as she may legitimately be busy and not be able to perform the task at the required time.

A	B	C	D	E	F	G	H
0	4	4	4	0	0	0	0

A139. This question focuses on your ability to ask questions to gain more information, to clarify information to check your own understanding and to be assertive when necessary. The scenario describes an incident where a clearly documented plan has not been followed, for an unknown reason, resulting in the clinical deterioration of a patient who has now been clinically stabilised. In such an incident you should find out whether the nurses who did not follow the plan were aware of it (**answer G**) – obviously if they were aware of it and acted against it then that is negligence. If they were not aware of it then they are not as implicated in the negative patient outcome. Regardless, it is appropriate to inform the nurse in charge (**answer A**) so that a thorough investigation can be carried out. Additionally it is good practice and suitable to inform the consultant in charge (**answer E**) that the incident has occurred and that one of their patients is unwell.

It would not be suitable to advise a nurse involved initially that they have made an error (**answer B**) without an investigation. Mr Ahktar is currently delirious and so discussing the incident with him at this time is not appropriate (**answer C**). Offering to write guidelines (**answer D**) or writing a reflection on the incident (**answer F**) may be sensible in the long term, but is not relevant acutely. Increasing Mr Akhtar's observations (**answer H**) may be a reasonable step, but is not a suitable option when resolving the issues identified by the scenario.

A	B	C	D	E	F	G	H
4	0	0	0	4	0	4	0

A140. This scenario focuses on your ability to respond to non-verbal communication, listen effectively and sensitively to a colleague's concerns and communicate empathetically in response. The most suitable action to take is to offer Anna support (**answer E**) and suggest that she raise her concerns with her educational supervisor (**answer H**) as they will be the person in the best position to offer Anna guidance. This would obviously be quite daunting for Anna and offering her help in seeking support is a very suitable option (**answer C**).

Advising Anna to take annual leave (**answer A**) may give her the opportunity to rest from what is inducing her stress but in no way addresses the underlying cause for her concern. Similarly, offering to assist Anna with her workload (**answer G**) masks underlying issues. It would be against Anna's confidentiality to share her concerns with the wider ward team (**answer B**) and if this is an avenue she would like explored it should be initiated by her, as should any discussions with her clinical supervisor (**answer F**). Psychological support (**answer D**) may be a route Anna wishes to take but this should ideally take place following a discussion with her educational supervisor and be organised through the proper support networks for foundation trainees.

A	B	C	D	E	F	G	H
0	0	4	0	4	0	0	4

A141. This relatively short scenario is apt because it gives you very little information on the clinical case; it focuses on your ability to obtain more information from a colleague to help you triage clinical information. It also focuses on your ability to comprehend what a clinical colleague is asking you for and why. In the scenario, the handover of information from your colleague is poor; the most suitable answers have therefore been focused on your obtaining more information in a structured manner. The person phoning you has not identified either themselves or the patient and you need to obtain this information (**answer G**). Similarly, to help contextualise the information you require, it is useful to have some clinical background on the patient (**answer D**) (i.e. what operation they have had, their past medical history, etc.). It would additionally be useful to obtain the rest of the patient's observations and how well they are clinically, in addition to what the nurse would like to do with the information they are phoning you about (**answer B**). You should be given a request like 'and I would appreciate your review of the patient in the next 20 minutes' or 'please can you come and take blood cultures?'

It is not appropriate to ask the person to call you back (**answer A**) as careful questioning may elucidate the information you require. It would be impossible to locate the patient based on the information you have been given (**answer C**). The person phoning may not be aware of a structured communication tool and so reporting them to the matron is not necessary instantly (**answer E**); again, you just need to ask the right questions! It is within your competencies to deal with a pyrexial patient (**answer F**) and you need more clinical information than you currently have for **answer H** to be a clinical safe approach.

A	B	C	D	E	F	G	H
0	4	0	4	0	0	4	0

A142. The crux of this scenario revolves around your ability to ask insightful questions to gain understanding from patients and listening effectively to their response. When investigating such accusations regarding a patient, it is appropriate to deal with matters sensitively. You should begin your discussion in an exploratory way that is non-accusing (**answer D**); this is a compassionate approach that will allow you to gain the trust of a patient and ask more insightful questions. It is important to ratify your concern about Mr Parkinson being absent from the ward, as if he is not there you cannot review him (**answer A**). Ultimately, however, you should ask the patient directly whether he has been consuming alcohol (**answer F**).

It is inappropriate to contact your consultant (**answer B**) or refer Mr Parkinson to alcohol liaison services (**answer C**) without first investigating yourself whether the claims may be true. Nor is it appropriate to commence him on withdrawal treatment (**answer E**). With any question that is asking you to investigate a claim, you should generally investigate the situation to some extent before doing anything reactionary. As long as Mr Parkinson has capacity, it is against his rights to fit him with an alarm (**answer G**) and his leaving the ward does not necessarily impact on his right to be treated (**answer H**).

A	B	C	D	E	F	G	H
4	0	0	4	0	4	0	0

A143. This scenario revolves around your ability to be assertive when required. The patient in this scenario is exhibiting views loudly that are unacceptable and intolerable in a public organisation. Your first priority would be to tell the patient in an assertive way that these views are unacceptable (**answer A**), but you should nevertheless explore their concerns in an effort to placate them (**answer G**) – this in no way implies agreement with Mr Brown's views. Your duty of care should extend to other patients on the ward and you should communicate effectively with them to ensure that they are content and not offended by the views expressed by Mr Brown (**answer E**).

It is inappropriate at this stage to contact security (**answer B**) or instruct the police to be called (**answer C**) as the situation has not escalated to the point that the patient is violent or out of control; you should in the first instance try to 'talk Mr Brown down'. In some ways attempting to move him immediately to a side room (**answer D**) or to another ward (**answer F**) would seem like a sensible thing to do, and in the long run may be what happens, but if this is allowed it gives a degree of acceptance to his views, which should not be complied with. Even though you may not agree with his expressed views, it would be inappropriate to ask Mr Brown to leave the hospital immediately (**answer H**).

A	B	C	D	E	F	G	H
4	0	0	0	4	0	4	0

A144. The scenario revolves around divulging information to next of kin. In the scenario the person identifies themself as a friend of Mrs Hemingway but also her next of kin. As with any discussion with family members, the patient has to have consented to you sharing their medical information (**answer H**), this includes such comments as 'she is doing well' and not just diagnoses, medication, etc. In the absence of relatives it is important to keep the next of kin updated on a patient's progress. It is also important when sharing information to update yourself with the information regarding the case being discussed (**answer E**); this is good preparation and an outcome the UKFPO has deemed necessary to assess. It is good practice to document discussions with relatives in the patient's medical notes (**answer B**) – this is important as, should you generate any useful information from the collateral history, it will then be available to other people within the MDT.

You should not discuss a patient's care with other people without a patient's prior consent (**answer A**). You should aim to have discussions regarding clinical progress yourself (**answer C**) and in a timely manner (**answers D, F and G**) as this is good practice and implicated in your responsibilities as a doctor.

A	B	C	D	E	F	G	H
0	4	0	0	4	0	0	4

A145. This scenario revolves around the communication of a management plan in an acutely unwell patient. The rules do not change – if you are instigating management you should first seek consent from the patient and discuss the plan with them, therefore you should update the patient with your plan immediately (**answer B**). It is also imperative that you inform members of the MDT who would be involved in implementing your plan, in this case the nurse looking after Mr Bolem (**answer D**). You should immediately document your management plan in the medical notes (**answer C**).

This takes precedence over informing your senior colleagues acutely (**answer A**). It is also inappropriate to delay the discussion or prescription (**answer E** and **answer H**). In this scenario, it is more important that the nurse looking after the patient knows the management plan than the nurse in charge of the unit (**answer G**) as the former will ensure the blood transfusion happens. It is not necessary for you to collect the blood from the blood bank yourself (**answer F**); other staff members have had training to do this and it is unnecessary for you to miss your compulsory teaching solely for this.

A	B	C	D	E	F	G	H
0	4	4	4	0	0	0	0

A146. A recurring theme you will have identified throughout these questions is that, with scenarios that involve relatives questioning decisions, it is always prudent to explore the family's concern and address any questions that arise; these are indeed themes identified by the UKFPO for you to be assessed on as applicants to the Foundation Programme. In this scenario it would be prudent to understand the concerns of Mr Mustard's family with regard to his being placed temporarily in a care home (**answer G**). It is always helpful to explain to relatives why a particular decision has been made (**answer E**) as this allows them the opportunity to understand why a particular option has been recommended and may persuade them to change their opinions. In this regard it is always important to clarify understanding (**answer D**) – you should explain fully the recommendation you are making so that the family can make an informed decision.

It is inadvisable to be confrontational with the family (**answer A**) and you should take responsibility for discussions with the family revolving around discharge planning (**answer B**) – remember: the clinical team is ultimately responsible for the care of a patient and services like occupational therapy in the main provide advisory and planning roles. You should always try to make decisions in agreement with the family and so discharging Mr Mustard to a situation the family is not currently in agreement with should be avoided (**answer C**), as would discharging a patient to a situation that has been deemed unsafe (**answer F**). Again, as the FY1, you should try to have preliminary discussions with the family to explore their concerns prior to escalating them to your senior colleagues (**answer H**).

A	B	C	D	E	F	G	H
0	0	0	4	4	0	4	0

A147. As an FY1 doctor your role is mainly ward-based and you tend to have many discussions with relatives of patients. To maintain effective working relationships with families you should always listen to and address their concerns (**answer H**), be readily available to answer their questions (**answer C**) and keep them updated on their relative's progress by summarising the clinical course thus far (**answer F**).

In this scenario, the relative has concerns and either not listening to these (**answer A**) or acting on them without exploring them (**answer B**) is poor practice. It would be inappropriate to alter the follow-up plan as set out by her consultant (**answer E**) to falsely appease the daughter. You, as an FY1, are able to meet with relatives to address their concerns initially (**answer G**), so it's inappropriate to escalate these without first exploring them as you may be able to address the issue yourself. As with previous scenarios, you should not delegate relative discussions inappropriately (**answer D**); the daughter's concern is in regard to a clinical decision and so this should be addressed by the clinical staff.

A	B	C	D	E	F	G	H
0	0	4	0	0	4	0	4

A148. This scenario revolves around your ability to act and speak sensitively towards patients, particularly when breaking bad news or when they are upset. The most suitable thing to do with upset patients is to be empathetic (**answer D**) and offer them emotional support. It is useful to reassure them with the management plan (**answer B**) so that they can rationalise their clinical progress. A patient may be upset for a variety of reasons and exploring the cause of the current emotional state may be appropriate (**answer F**) as the patient may volunteer new information.

It would be inappropriate to leave the patient upset until her friends arrive (**answer A**), as would delegating speaking to the patient about the cause of her state (**answer C**). Referring a patient to the chaplaincy service is not immediately the most suitable thing to do (**answer E**) as there are alternative sources of emotional support within a hospital and it may be the patient's preference to explore these first. You should not ignore an upset patient (**answer G**), and asking her to draw the curtains whilst upset (**answer H**) is insensitive and does not attempt to address the underlying issue causing the distress.

A	B	C	D	E	F	G	H
0	4	0	4	0	4	0	0

A149. This question revolves around your ability to involve relatives in decisions surrounding a patient's ongoing care, called 'shared decision making'. To have effective discussions in this regard you need to provide the relatives with an overview of the patient's clinical course and the medical opinion (**answer A**). The reason we involve the family in decision making is the thought that they will make decisions in the patient's best interests. Additionally the family may have had discussions regarding ongoing care previously at a time when the patient was well and so it's helpful to explore this (**answer G**). With this information in mind, it is then prudent to explore the family's view to alternative feeding (**answer B**) thus demonstrating your ability to be an effective listener.

You should allow the family to reach their own conclusion regarding the decision and not enforce your opinion on them (**answer C**). You should not delegate these decisions to other members of the MDT (**answer D**); it is your responsibility as part of the medical team to assist the family with decisions regarding ongoing care. You should ask the family for questions (**answer E**) but this would be the 'fourth best answer', as summarising and exploring their and the patient's wishes all precede this as suitable options. You are in a position as an FY1 to have these discussions and should not shy away from them (**answer F**). Resuscitation decision planning (**answer H**) is not the focus of this current discussion but may be useful if you are deciding upon a patient's ceilings of care.

A	B	C	D	E	F	G	H
4	4	0	0	0	0	4	0

A150. This question revolves around the need to keep relatives updated on a patient's clinical progress and how to gather information, from alternative sources like collateral histories, to clarify your own understanding. With this in mind you should gain consent from Mr Peters and update his family accordingly (**answer F**). With regard to the collateral history that has been provided, you should explore this further (**answer G**). In clinical practice, information from alternative sources like GPs who know the patient well, relatives, friends and nursing homes can be extremely useful in clinical decision making. It would also be prudent to inform your seniors of this information (**answer H**) to guide their decisions surrounding this patient's care.

It is inappropriate to update the family of Mr Peters without his consent (**answer A**) and you should always obtain this in a competent patient. Reviewing Mr Peters without the benefit of a collateral history (**answer B**) is not particularly sensible; additionally obtaining it at the same time as your review is time-efficient. Referring Mr Peters to specialist services without discussing the case with your senior colleagues (**answer C**) is not advisable; there may be further investigations you can make without introducing a delay in time by referring the patient elsewhere. You should always strive to keep a family updated and this is an expectation of you as an FY1 doctor; you should not try to put off these discussions (**answer D**). It is within the competency of an FY1 doctor to take a full history and utilise collateral information; it is not necessary to immediately ask your senior to review (**answer E**).

A	B	C	D	E	F	G	H
0	0	0	0	0	4	4	4

7. Domain 4 – patient focus

This domain focuses on attributes that all foundation doctors should have when caring for patients. *Good Medical Practice* (GMC, 2013a) makes it clear that all doctors have a duty to treat patients with respect, dignity and without discrimination. However, the FY1 job analysis that was carried out by the Work Psychology Group further described a candidate as being able to 'demonstrate an understanding and appreciation of the needs of all patients, showing respect at all times. Takes time to build relationships with patients, demonstrating courtesy, empathy and compassion, and works in partnership with patients about their care' (Patterson et al, 2013).

Although the overriding theme of this domain is patient-centred care, there are many subcategories on which questions can be based. These can broadly be grouped into four areas:

1. Patient safety, patient safety, patient safety!
2. Developing patient relationships
3. Patient's ideas, concerns and expectations
4. Patient-centred care.

Patient safety has been a constant theme throughout many SJT questions so far. This is because everything we do as doctors should be with patients at the centre of our minds. However, this domain focuses specifically on patient-centred care. This involves being aware of patient safety at all times, working jointly with patients to reach a mutually agreed plan and recognising that patients may have different values and beliefs to you.

An important factor towards achieving patient-centred care is understanding that a truly successful doctor will achieve this by developing relationships with their patients and listening to their concerns and expectations. You will be expected to build and maintain a rapport with patients (and their relatives); be polite, empathetic and show compassion, and be respectful towards patients at all times.

You are expected to instil confidence in your patients, and show a genuine interest in each individual patient. Remember, each patient is different and will have different needs. You will need to make yourself available to patients and their relatives and be willing to speak with them to explain what is happening. Finally, a professional doctor will be able to maintain an appropriate distance from patients and their relatives too.

The following practice questions have been developed to provide an opportunity for you to demonstrate how to deal with these topics correctly. Remember, it is what you **should** do, not what you **would** do!

Q151. You are the FY1 for urology in a large tertiary referral centre. Mrs Molyneux, a 66-year-old woman with a ureteric stricture, is due in theatre in 1 hour for an elective laparoscopic pyeloplasty. Jane, the ward sister, has asked you to speak with Mrs Molyneux this morning as she has told Jane she doesn't understand what the operation will involve. You have never observed this type of surgery and are unsure of exactly what it will involve. Your consultant and registrar are currently in theatre and there are several patients after Mrs Molyneux scheduled for procedures.

Rank in order the following actions in response to this situation (1 = most appropriate; 5 = least appropriate):

A. Meet with Mrs Molyneux and explain the procedure to the best of your ability.

B. Ask your SHO colleague, who has observed and assisted with this procedure several times before, to speak with Mrs Molyneux.

C. Bleep your registrar and ask for advice.

D. Go to theatre and discuss the situation with your registrar directly.

E. Telephone the theatre matron and delay Mrs Molyneux's procedure until the consultant is available to speak with her.

Q152. You are the FY1 on a general surgical ward. Mr Williams is awaiting an elective cholecystectomy and has been nil by mouth (NBM) since midnight as his procedure was scheduled for 9 am. It is now 11 am and Mr Williams has still not been operated on owing to several emergencies this morning. He demands to speak with a doctor and you are asked to see him.

Rank in order the following actions in response to this situation (1 = most appropriate; 5 = least appropriate):

A. Apologise to Mr Williams for the delay and explain that, owing to emergencies, you are unsure what time his operation will be.

B. Tell Mr Williams you will arrange for your registrar to speak with him.

C. Tell Mr Williams that you will call theatre and try to find out what time his procedure is likely to happen.

D. Tell Mr Williams that his operation is likely to happen tomorrow now owing to emergencies and he can eat lunch.

E. Tell Mr Williams that emergencies always take priority and, although you are sorry, he should accept there is nothing you can do.

> What is the best way to appease Mr Williams' anger?

Q153. You are the FY1 on anaesthetics. Your consultant, Dr Georgiou, asks you to administer intrathecal antibiotics to Mrs Levy on Damson Ward. She has been diagnosed with meningococcal meningitis and your consultant feels that, owing to her instability, intravenous antibiotics will not take effect quickly enough. You have never seen this done before and your consultant is busy in theatre.

Rank in order the following actions in response to this situation (1 = most appropriate; 5 = least appropriate):

A. Bleep your registrar and ask them for advice.

B. Ask the staff nurse on Damson Ward for advice.

C. Research how to administer intrathecal antibiotics on the trust intranet.

D. Ask your SHO colleague, who has administered intrathecal antibiotics before, to help you.

E. Wait until your consultant is free from theatre and ask him to show you how to administer intrathecal antibiotics.

Q154. Sarah, a 23-year-old student with insulin-dependent diabetes, has been admitted to the acute medical unit with pyelonephritis. On the ward round this morning your consultant Dr Jacobs decided to increase Sarah's insulin temporarily owing to her infection. After the ward round, Sarah asks to speak to you. She explains that she is not happy to take the higher dose of insulin and asks that you change the prescription back to her normal dose.

Rank in order the following actions in response to this situation (1 = most appropriate; 5 = least appropriate):

A. Call Dr Jacobs and explain that Sarah is not willing to increase her insulin.

B. Discuss Sarah's insulin regimen with the ward pharmacist.

C. Discuss Sarah's concerns about increasing her insulin whilst in hospital.

D. Refer Sarah to the diabetes nurse specialist.

E. Alter Sarah's insulin dose as per the consultant's request.

Q155. You receive a phone call from a good friend of yours, Richard. He tells you that he has been suffering from repeated episodes of diarrhoea and has been to see his GP. He is concerned that his GP is not taking his concerns seriously because he is young. You are aware that Richard's uncle has Crohn's disease and recently underwent an elective colectomy.

Rank in order the following actions in response to this situation (1 = most appropriate; 5 = least appropriate):

A. Reassure Richard that the GP's advice will be fine.

B. Give Richard the number of a gastroenterologist that you know and suggest he calls them for advice.

C. Tell Richard you are not allowed to treat family and friends.

D. Ask Richard for more information about his symptoms.

E. Ask Richard to make another appointment with his GP to discuss his concerns further.

Q156. You are the FY1 on general surgery. Jenifer, a staff nurse, asks you to speak to Mr Lewis, as he has become aggressive. You can hear him shouting from the doctor's office and he seems very angry. You ask Jenifer what the matter is and she explains that he won't tell her but is demanding to see the consultant. You are aware that your consultant is in clinic all afternoon. You are very busy and have three patients who are being discharged and require their discharge paperwork completed urgently.

Rank in order the following actions in response to this situation (1 = most appropriate; 5 = least appropriate):

A. Tell Mr Lewis that the consultant is not available this afternoon.

B. Ask Jenifer to call your consultant explaining that Mr Lewis is requesting a consultation.

C. Inform the discharge coordinator that the discharge paperwork will be delayed as you are needed by Mr Lewis.

D. Review Mr Lewis urgently and explore his concerns.

E. Call your consultant and explain the situation. Ask him what he thinks you should do.

Q157. You are the FY1 on the neurology ward. You are asked to see Miss Barons, a 41-year-old female with end-stage multiple sclerosis. You know Miss Barons well as she has previously been admitted to your ward. On this occasion, she has been admitted with urosepsis. She has been started on intravenous fluids and antibiotics and is improving. While you are completing her ward admission, she tells you that she cannot go on any longer and begs you to give her an overdose of pain relief so that she can die peacefully. She is clearly upset and you are unsure of what to do. You strongly disagree with euthanasia or assisted dying.

Rank in order the following actions in response to this situation (1 = most appropriate; 5 = least appropriate):

A. Tell Miss Barons that you think her request would upset her family and she should consider their situation as well as her own.

B. Ask Miss Barons to discuss her thoughts with her family.

C. Discuss Miss Barons's concerns further.

D. Refer Miss Barons to the palliative care nurse.

E. Call Miss Barons's next of kin and inform them of her current frame of mind.

Q158. Mrs McDonnah has been diagnosed with metastatic breast cancer and has been advised by oncology that she is likely to have less than 3 months left to live. She has been on your ward for 2 weeks currently and you enjoy speaking with her each morning. She seems remarkably calm about her prognosis. She is preparing to be discharged with a home help package and has been seen by the community palliative team. She has agreed an end-of-life care plan that involves being treated at home and not being admitted to hospital. She is not for resuscitation. Today Mrs McDonnah is due to be discharged. You see her on the ward round for the final time and she tells you that you have made all the difference to her admission and have made it easier for her to come to terms with her terminal diagnosis. She asks if you would be able to visit her at home for a cup of tea and chat from time to time.

Rank in order the following actions in response to this situation (1 = most appropriate; 5 = least appropriate):

A. Tell Mrs McDonnah that her words are very kind and you'll visit her at home.

B. Explore Mrs McDonnah's social situation and suggest you refer her to the community voluntary service.

C. Write to Mrs McDonnah's GP and ask them to arrange regular home visits.

D. Explain to Mrs McDonnah that you aren't allowed to do home visits as a hospital doctor.

E. Tell Mrs McDonnah that you have enjoyed getting to know her but do not think it would be appropriate to visit her at home.

Q159. You are on call covering the medical wards. You are bleeped by Aiva, a staff nurse on the cardiology unit. Mr Patel has been admitted overnight and his wife has not been able to meet a doctor yet. She is currently on the ward and is very anxious. She has asked to speak with a doctor about her husband. You do not know Mr Patel's case but you are currently free of other tasks.

Rank in order the following actions in response to this situation (1 = most appropriate; 5 = least appropriate):

A. Familiarise yourself with Mr Patel's case notes and meet with Mrs Patel.

B. Ask Aiva to speak to Mrs Patel about her husband.

C. Ask Mrs Patel to arrange a meeting with Mr Patel's regular doctor during the week to discuss her husband's progress.

D. Meet with Mrs Patel, but explain that you will be able to give only general information as you are not Mr Patel's regular doctor.

E. Tell Aiva that you do not have time as the on-call doctor to meet with family members.

> Are you as informed about Mr Patel's admission as you can be?

Q160. You are the FY1 on rheumatology. You are seeing Mrs Lemont, a 78-year-old woman who has presented with a non-traumatic thoracic vertebral fracture. Your consultant, Dr Lisk, explains that this is very likely to be the result of osteoporosis and asks you to commence Mrs Lemont on bisphosphonate therapy. He explains that as she is over 75 we do not need to bother with a DEXA-scan. He tells you to prescribe alendronic acid, 70 mg, once daily. You recall from medical school that this specific bisphosphonate therapy should be once-a-week administration. Dr Lisk has a reputation for chastising junior doctors who question his decisions.

Rank in order the following actions in response to this situation (1 = most appropriate; 5 = least appropriate):

A. Ask Dr Lisk to clarify his prescription request.

B. Prescribe the alendronic acid as requested.

C. Ask the ward pharmacist to confirm the prescription for alendronic acid.

D. Ask another consultant if the prescription is correct.

E. Prescribe alendronic acid once-weekly as you were taught at medical school.

Q161. You are on call providing ward cover when you receive a bleep from Dipthi, a staff nurse on the stroke rehabilitation unit. She tells you that Mr Edwards, a 97-year-old man, was admitted to the ward this afternoon following a minor stroke. He has told Dipthi that he does not want any aggressive treatment, including resuscitation, as he has had a good life. Apart from his stroke Mr Edwards does not have any other medical conditions and is generally fit. Dipthi asks whether you can attend the ward to discuss this with Mr Edwards. You have not been involved in a DNAR discussion before and you are not sure of how to proceed. However, you feel that based on Mr Edwards's lack of co-morbidities a DNAR would be inappropriate.

Rank in order the following actions in response to this situation (1 = most appropriate; 5 = least appropriate):

A. Attend the ward and complete the DNAR form.

B. Discuss this request with the on-call registrar.

C. Attend the ward and discuss Mr Edwards's comments.

D. Refuse to sign the DNAR form as Mr Edwards is fit and healthy.

E. Ask the on-call registrar to see Mr Edwards and whether you can observe the discussion.

Q162. You are the FY1 on the respiratory ward. One of your patients, Mr Williams, who was admitted this morning, has presented with a 4-week history of dry cough and corresponding weight loss. He has been a smoker for 40 years. Your consultant asks you to arrange a CT scan of his chest to exclude cancer as the chest x-ray that Mr Williams had on admission was inconclusive. It has now been 5 hours since Mr Williams has returned from the radiology department and your consultant has not returned to the ward. You can see that Mr Williams is clearly anxious and has asked you several times whether the scan result is back yet. You read the CT scan report and can see that Mr Williams has a lesion highly suggestive of cancer, but bronchoscopy has been recommended to confirm the diagnosis.

Rank in order the following actions in response to this situation (1 = most appropriate; 5 = least appropriate):

A. Reassure Mr Williams that the consultant will discuss the results with him when he returns to the ward.

B. Tell Mr Williams that the scan is highly suggestive of cancer but he will require further investigation to confirm the diagnosis.

C. Discuss Mr Williams' concerns and explain that you are not experienced enough to conclusively interpret the CT scan.

D. Tell Mr Williams that the delay in finding out the result is not indicative of the outcome.

E. Call your consultant and explain the results of the CT scan. Ask whether they are available to meet with Mr Williams to discuss the diagnosis.

Q163. You are working on the general surgery ward in a small community hospital. Your registrar is discussing the recent diagnosis of cancer with Mr Sheik and his family on the ward. They are very upset as the prognosis is poor owing to the progression of the cancer. You happen to notice that several other patients are listening to the conversation.

Rank in order the following actions in response to this situation (1 = most appropriate; 5 = least appropriate):

A. Express your concerns to the registrar that other patients are listening to his conversation.

B. Suggest that the registrar continues his discussion in the relatives' room.

C. Ask the nurse in charge to suggest that the registrar relocates to the relatives' room.

D. Ask to speak to the registrar urgently.

E. Close the curtains around the other patients who are listening.

> Should other patients be able to hear this conversation?

Q164. You are working on the medical admission unit when your consultant asks you to book a CT scan of Miss Archer's head. You telephone the radiology department but the radiologist is unwilling to authorise the scan as you are not sure of the indication for Miss Archer's CT scan. You try to explain that you are requesting the scan on your consultant's behalf but the radiologist still refuses to arrange the CT scan. Your consultant has since left the ward and you do not know when they will return.

Rank in order the following actions in response to this situation (1 = most appropriate; 5 = least appropriate):

A. Ask to speak with a different radiologist.

B. Read Miss Archer's medical notes to determine the indication.

C. Call your consultant on their telephone and ask what the indication is.

D. Leave the scan until tomorrow when you can discuss the indication with the consultant on the ward round.

E. Demand that the radiologist authorises the CT scan.

Q165. You are on call in A&E. You are asked to see Charlie, an 18-month-old child, who has been brought to A&E by his mother, Jessica. Charlie is pyrexial, very drowsy and has a rash on his trunk. You suspect Charlie has meningitis and you tell Jessica that he is very unwell and will need immediate antibiotics. You explain that he will be admitted to the paediatric ward whilst he has treatment. Jessica tells you that she does not want Charlie admitted as she has heard that a child recently died at this hospital owing to a mistake by the medical team.

Rank in order the following actions in response to this situation (1 = most appropriate; 5 = least appropriate):

A. Ask Jessica to sign a disclosure form if she is insisting on taking Charlie home.

B. Suggest that Jessica allow you to start treatment in A&E and you can discuss admission once you have observed Charlie for a few hours.

C. Explore Jessica's concerns and explain why Charlie needs to be admitted.

D. Call your registrar and explain the situation.

E. Allow Jessica to leave with Charlie.

Q166. You are the FY1 working on the oncology ward. Your team has been caring for Susan, a 58-year-old woman, with end-stage metastatic lung cancer. On the ward round this morning Susan asked your consultant to sign a DNAR. As she was deemed to have capacity, your consultant agreed and the form was completed. Later that afternoon you are called to see Susan who is very anxious about the level of pain she will experience. She tells you that she doesn't want to die yet and is worried the pain will increase.

Rank in order the following actions in response to this situation (1 = most appropriate; 5 = least appropriate):

A. Offer to sedate Susan so that she doesn't experience any pain.

B. Ask the specialist pain team to review Susan to ensure she is receiving optimal pain management.

C. Discuss the DNAR discussion she had earlier with the consultant to ensure she understands what that means.

D. Discuss Susan's concerns with your consultant.

E. Explore Susan's concerns further regarding her end-of-life care.

Q167. You are asked to see Mrs Brown, who has attended A&E today with a fever and productive cough. When you introduce yourself to her she tells you that her brother is a GP and she will be checking everything you say with him. You examine her and explain that her complaint is most likely the result of a community-acquired pneumonia. She tells you that she would like you to speak to her brother before prescribing her anything because she wants to make sure you're right.

Rank in order the following actions in response to this situation (1 = most appropriate; 5 = least appropriate):

A. Politely decline her request and reassure her that you are confident with your diagnosis.

B. Explain why you have reached your conclusion and discuss the treatment options available to Mrs Brown.

C. Tell Mrs Brown that she will also be reviewed by the consultant on his post-take ward round.

D. Discuss your management plan with Mrs Brown's brother as per her request.

E. Tell Mrs Brown that her brother is contravening GMC guidance by getting involved with her medical treatment.

Q168. You are the FY1 on the respiratory ward. On the ward round this morning, Mr Xavier was told that he has lung cancer. The consultant explained what was going to happen next and arranged for the lung cancer nurse to review Mr Xavier this afternoon. Mr Xavier has asked to speak to you as he has some questions since the ward round this morning. You discuss this with your registrar who recommends you discuss Mr Xavier's concerns about his new diagnosis. As you are talking with Mr Xavier one of the ward nurses rushes over to you and asks you to review a patient in the next bay who has deteriorated over the past 15 minutes.

Rank in order the following actions in response to this situation (1 = most appropriate; 5 = least appropriate):

A. Attend to the unwell patient with the nurse immediately.

B. Ask the nurse whether there are any other doctors available to review the deteriorating patient.

C. Attend to the emergency but tell Mr Xavier you will return to answer his remaining questions.

D. Attend to the emergency but ask the nurse to sit with Mr Xavier until you return.

E. Attend to the emergency but ask the nurse to bleep your FY1 colleague to continue your discussion with Mr Xavier.

> Have you considered the needs of all your patients?

Q169. You have been caring for Mr Wassleflaw on your ward since you started your rotation. He has been admitted for more than 2 months owing to complex co-morbidities and recurring infections. You have become very fond of him and his family who visit him regularly. You often find yourself having a lengthy conversation with a member of the Wasseflaw family. Mr Wasseflaw is finally nearing discharge when his daughter, Julie, asks whether she and her husband Peter can take you for a drink one evening to thank you for everything you have done for her father.

Rank in order the following actions in response to this situation (1 = most appropriate; 5 = least appropriate):

A. Tell Julie that the GMC guidance advises against socialising with patients or their relatives.

B. Accept Julie's offer for a thank-you drink; you have worked very hard over the past 2 months.

C. Politely thank Julie for the kind offer but explain that you don't think it would be appropriate.

D. Thank Julie but suggest she buy a box of biscuits that the entire ward team can enjoy.

E. Explain to Julie it was your pleasure to treat her father and her gratitude is thanks enough.

Q170. You have been asked to review Mrs Toulet's prescription before she is discharged. She was admitted following a myocardial infarction and has been started on secondary preventative therapy, including a statin. She has also been counselled for smoking cessation as she is currently smoking 30 cigarettes per day. As you are speaking with Mrs Toulet, she explains that she doesn't want to take the atorvastatin that has been prescribed but would prefer pravastatin. She tells you that she won't take the statin if it is atorvastatin. Unfortunately, atorvastatin is your hospital formulary and the pharmacy will be unable to supply pravastatin.

Rank in order the following actions in response to this situation (1 = most appropriate; 5 = least appropriate):

A. Explore Mrs Toulet's concerns about taking atorvastatin.

B. Tell Mrs Toulet that you can prescribe only atorvastatin as it is your hospital's choice of statin.

C. Suggest Mrs Toulet starts taking atorvastatin and explain that her GP can change her prescription to pravastatin once she has been discharged.

D. Write to Mrs Toulet's GP and ask them to alter the prescription from atorvastatin to pravastatin once she is discharged.

E. Explain to Mrs Toulet that it doesn't matter which statin she takes.

Q171. You are the FY1 working on the acute medical unit. You are always very busy and believe that there should be more doctors on your rotation. You are asked by Jasmine, a staff nurse, to insert a cannula into Ellie Persons in bed 24. She has been admitted with pyelonephritis and is due intravenous antibiotics in 45 minutes. She did previously have a cannula but Jasmine removed it as it had been 72 hours since it was inserted. You attempt to insert a new cannula but are unsuccessful. You tell Jasmine that you will try again in 30 minutes to allow Ellie to have a break from your repeated attempts. Before you are able to re-cannulate Ellie you are called to see a very unwell patient elsewhere on the ward. It has come to the end of your shift and as you are about to leave Jasmine reminds you about the cannula. Ellie is now several hours overdue for her antibiotics.

Rank in order the following actions in response to this situation (1 = most appropriate; 5 = least appropriate):

A. Ask Jasmine whether Ellie has a temperature and if not tell her you'll do the cannula first thing tomorrow.

B. Bleep the on-call doctor covering the wards and ask whether they would be willing to cannulate Ellie on your behalf.

C. Prescribe oral antibiotic therapy so that Ellie does not require a cannula.

D. Ask Jasmine to bleep the on-call doctor covering the wards this evening to insert the cannula as your shift has ended.

E. Immediately attend to Ellie and attempt to re-insert a cannula.

Q172. You are the FY1 on gastroenterology. Your consultant invites you to join him for an endoscopy list this afternoon. He suggests that you speak to Mrs Bekir in bed 17 who is due to have an oesophagogastroduodenoscopy (OGD) this afternoon owing to an episode of haematemesis over the weekend. As you are speaking with Mrs Bekir about her presentation she tells you that she is scared to have the OGD this afternoon as she is worried she will choke or stop breathing during the procedure. Your consultant joins you at the bedside and tells you it is time for you both to start the afternoon list.

Rank in order the following actions in response to this situation (1 = most appropriate; 5 = least appropriate):

A. Ask your consultant whether you could have more time with Mrs Bekir to explore her concerns as she is nervous about her OGD.

B. Ask your consultant whether you can have a quiet word and explain what Mrs Bekir has told you. Ask your consultant to discuss Mrs Bekir's concerns with her.

C. Tell Mrs Bekir that she will be sedated during the OGD and will not remember any unpleasantness from the procedure.

D. Reassure Mrs Bekir that an OGD is a routine procedure and she will be fine.

E. Excuse yourself from Mrs Bekir and join your consultant as requested.

Q173. You are on call in the surgical admissions unit. You overhear your colleague Peter talking to Mrs Beecham about her abdominal pain. It clearly sounds like irritable bowel syndrome (IBS) and Peter is trying to explain this to Mrs Beecham. She is unwilling to believe him and is demanding he seek a senior opinion. She is being very rude and asking Peter whether he is 'even a real doctor' as he 'looks too young to be qualified'. Peter's next remark to Mrs Beecham is very impolite and bordering on offensive. You are shocked as you have never heard Peter speak to a patient in such a manner.

Rank in order the following actions in response to this situation (1 = most appropriate; 5 = least appropriate):

A. Politely interrupt Peter and suggest he take a short break before returning to Mrs Beecham to apologise for his comment.

B. Interrupt the consultation and tell Mrs Beecham that she should show more respect toward doctors. If she is unhappy with the opinion she has received she can always attend another hospital.

C. Politely interrupt Peter and ask to speak with him urgently away from Mrs Beecham. Tell him that his comment was unprofessional.

D. After Peter has finished with Mrs Beecham, remind him that he should always be polite and courteous when dealing with patients, even when they are as difficult as Mrs Beecham.

E. Ignore what you heard as you probably would have said the same thing in his position.

> How can you prevent Peter from making this situation worse?

Q174. You are an FY1 on a busy respiratory ward in a large tertiary referral centre. You have been looking after Juliet, a young patient with cystic fibrosis. She has been an inpatient on your ward for 4 weeks and her parents, Janet and Larry, visit daily. During her admission Juliet has been making good progress and the team is planning her discharge for the end of this week. Unfortunately, today Juliet has deteriorated and your consultant has decided that she should be moved to the respiratory high-dependency unit (HDU). Janet and Larry arrive on the ward and ask to speak with you about Juliet's condition. They have already met with your consultant who explained the need for HDU. You still have several jobs to finish before the end of your shift.

Rank in order the following actions in response to this situation (1 = most appropriate; 5 = least appropriate):

A. Tell Janet and Larry that you are unable to speak to them as Juliet has been moved to HDU. She is under a different team now.

B. Apologise to Janet and Larry but explain that you are too busy to speak with them currently. If they are able to come back to the ward after 5 pm you will be free to talk to them.

C. Suggest Janet and Larry wait until Juliet has settled in HDU before asking for further information.

D. Offer to call the consultant as Janet and Larry clearly have unanswered questions.

E. Take Janet and Larry into the relatives' room to discuss their concerns about Juliet.

Q175. You are on call providing ward cover over the weekend. You have been asked to review Mrs Brown, who has been complaining of vomiting and stomach pain since she was admitted last night. You arrange for blood tests to be taken and an erect CXR to exclude a bowel perforation. The blood test results indicate an infective process but little else. You ask the ward nurse to bleep you once the CXR has been done. The rest of your shift is very busy and you forget about Mrs Brown's CXR. As you return home you remember that this outstanding result needs to be checked.

Rank in order the following actions in response to this situation (1 = most appropriate; 5 = least appropriate):

A. Review the CXR first thing tomorrow when you return to work.

B. Telephone the ward nursing staff and ask them to get the night FY1 to check the x-ray and escalate as necessary.

C. Contact the on-call registrar through switchboard and explain the situation.

D. Contact the night FY1 through switchboard and explain the situation.

E. Return to work that evening to check the x-ray result personally.

Q176. You are working on the day surgery unit (DSU) and your consultant has performed a left knee arthroscopy for Mrs Bunton following repeated episodes of her knee 'giving way'. Your consultant tells you that Mrs Bunton can be discharged this evening if occupational therapy (OT) feels that she is safe to go home. Later that afternoon, Julie, the occupational therapist, tells you that Mrs Bunton is safe to go home. It is now 5 pm and John, a staff nurse, tells you that Mrs Bunton is refusing to leave until she is seen by a doctor as she does not feel safe to be at home alone. Mr Patel, a patient due for an examination under anaesthesia (EUA) tomorrow, is already waiting in the admission lounge and has been allocated to the bed that Mrs Bunton is currently refusing to leave.

Rank in order the following actions in response to this situation (1 = most appropriate; 5 = least appropriate):

A. Politely explain to Mrs Bunton that there is already a patient expecting to use her bed tonight and she will have to leave.

B. Contact Julie and explain the situation. Enquire whether Mrs Bunton is able to have any support at home.

C. Review Mrs Bunton and explore her concerns about her discharge.

D. Ask Mr Patel to return early tomorrow morning so that Mrs Bunton can stay for another night.

E. Ask Julie to re-assess Mrs Bunton to ensure it is appropriate for her to be discharged.

Q177. You are working as the FY1 on care of the elderly. Overnight Mrs Greenberg passed away as expected with her family present. This morning you have received a call from the bereavement office asking you to complete her death certificate urgently as Mrs Greenberg's family has explained that her religious beliefs require her to be buried within 24 hours of death. You are on the consultant ward round and still have more than half the ward to review.

Rank in order the following actions in response to this situation (1 = most appropriate; 5 = least appropriate):

A. Tell the bereavement office that you are busy and you will complete the death certificate if you have time this afternoon.

B. Politely excuse yourself from the ward round and complete Mrs Greenberg's death certificate as a matter of urgency.

C. Explain the situation to your consultant and ask whether you should stay on the ward round or go to the bereavement office.

D. Visit the bereavement office immediately to complete Mrs Greenberg's death certificate.

E. Ask the bereavement office whether there are any other doctors able to complete Mrs Greenberg's death certificate.

Q178. You are working on the adult assessment unit (AAU). This morning you have been asked to clerk Siobhan, a 19-year-old female, who has been admitted following an unresponsive episode. The ambulance crew found Siobhan at a disused warehouse and although she was unresponsive she was maintaining her airway and did not require any intervention. She is now alert and responsive. Her investigations are normal. You suspect she may have been under the influence of an illicit substance.

Rank in order the following actions in response to this situation (1 = most appropriate; 5 = least appropriate):

A. Discuss your concerns with Siobhan and explore her social situation.

B. Arrange for a urinary opiate test to be conducted on the urine sample sent to the laboratory for culture.

C. Ask Siobhan's nurse to increase the frequency of her observations.

D. Discuss your concerns with your consultant.

E. Offer to refer Siobhan to the hospital drugs and alcohol services.

Q179. You are one of two FY1s for healthcare services for the elderly at a small district hospital. Your colleague Jessica informs you that Mrs Lewis has been re-admitted following another fall at home. You know Mrs Lewis well as she was admitted following a fall for 3 weeks last month and you spent a lot of time with her. She is very demanding and constantly refuses any package of care. You are relieved that Jessica is overseeing her care this time. This afternoon Jessica tells you that Mrs Lewis has asked if you can look after her again.

Rank in order the following actions in response to this situation (1 = most appropriate; 5 = least appropriate):

A. Agree to oversee Mrs Lewis's care as you already know her well.

B. Tell Jessica that you are unwilling to oversee Mrs Lewis's care.

C. Speak with Mrs Lewis and explain that Jessica is going to be overseeing her care during this admission.

D. Tell Mrs Lewis that Jessica will be overseeing her care but you will help when needed.

E. Discuss Mrs Lewis's request with your registrar.

> Are you considering the importance of continuity of care?

Q180. Elsie, a 16-year-old female, presented to A&E in status epilepticus. She has been treated in A&E and has been moved to your ward for observation. You are reading Elsie's medical notes and you see that she is known to suffer from epilepsy. She is prescribed valproate following several unsuccessful regimens of levetiracetam. You also note that she has been admitted repeatedly with seizures and you suspect she does not adhere to her medication.

Rank in order the following actions in response to this situation (1 = most appropriate; 5 = least appropriate):

A. Write to Elsie's GP and ask them to monitor her compliance in the community.

B. Offer to refer Elsie to an adolescent support group for chronic conditions.

C. Discuss your concerns with Elsie focusing on why she isn't taking her medication.

D. Explain to Elsie that it is very dangerous and irresponsible to stop taking anti-seizure medication.

E. Explore Elsie's social support network.

Q181. You are waiting to start the ward round when you receive a call from your registrar who tells you that they are running 30 minutes late this morning as their car has broken down. They suggest you begin the ward round but leave any new admissions until they arrive. Your consultant will review the plans this afternoon but is in clinic this morning. You begin to review Mr Higgins, who informs you that he was told yesterday afternoon by your registrar that he would be discharged early this morning. He has to take his mother to a hospital appointment at 9.30 am. You can see he is clearly agitated.

Rank in order the following actions in response to this situation (1 = most appropriate; 5 = least appropriate):

A. Call your registrar and ask whether they can authorise Mr Higgins's discharge over the phone.

B. Explain to Mr Higgins that your registrar is delayed and it is advisable for him to inform his mother.

C. Complete Mr Higgins's discharge paperwork yourself.

D. Find another senior member of your team and ask them to review Mr Higgins's suitability for discharge.

E. Apologise to Mr Higgins but explain that a more senior doctor is needed to make this decision.

Q182. You are the FY1 on the cardiology ward. Mr Leeming, an 87-year-old patient, is admitted with worsening breathlessness and is suspected of being in acute heart failure. He is deteriorating and your registrar decides to transfer him to the coronary care unit (CCU). Whilst on the ward you receive a telephone call from the patient's wife asking for an update. She is currently on her way to the hospital and you can tell she is anxious. She tells you that she is approximately 45 minutes away from the hospital. You explain that, owing to patient confidentiality, you are unable to disclose information over the telephone. You are due to attend mandatory teaching in 30 minutes. The session is anticipated to last 2 hours.

Rank in order the following actions in response to this situation (1 = most appropriate; 5 = least appropriate):

A. Arrange for the on-call SHO to meet with Mrs Leeming when she arrives to give her a brief update.

B. Tell Mrs Leeming that you will speak to her once you return from your mandatory teaching session.

C. Explain the situation to the doctor running your teaching session and apologise for leaving when Mrs Leeming arrives.

D. Ask the ward clerk to bleep you when Mrs Leeming arrives so that you can meet with her immediately.

E. Suggest that Mrs Leeming aims to visit her husband tomorrow morning when the consultant will be on their ward round. They will be able to give Mrs Leeming a better update.

Q183. You are the surgical FY1 on call in the surgical admission unit (SAU). Miss White, a 25-year-old patient, has been admitted to the SAU following A&E attendance with acute abdominal pain. She told the triage nurse that she fell into the kitchen counter and hurt her side. When you examine Miss White you feel that her history is not consistent with her injuries. You are worried that she is suffering from domestic violence. She is in a hurry to be discharged because she needs to go home to cook her boyfriend dinner before he returns from work. You are concerned for the safety of Miss White.

Rank in order the following actions in response to this situation (1 = most appropriate; 5 = least appropriate):

A. Reassure Miss White that you are here to help her.

B. Sensitively raise your concerns with Miss White.

C. Explore Miss White's social support network.

D. Ask Miss White how long her boyfriend has been abusing her.

E. Contact your hospital's domestic advice advisor.

Q184. You have just started your final shift on the inpatient psychiatry ward. You have really enjoyed your training and one patient in particular, Neil, has made a real impact on you. He has been an inpatient for 7 weeks owing to a complex eating disorder and several attempts to discharge him have failed. He is aware that today is your last day as his FY1 and he has arranged for his mum to bring in a gift for you. You open the gift and are surprised to find a framed photograph of yourself. He asks if you would be able to visit him occasionally in the evenings.

Rank in order the following actions in response to this situation (1 = most appropriate; 5 = least appropriate):

A. Agree to visit Neil as you do not want to impair his progress by upsetting him.

B. Tell Neil you will not be able to visit him socially as you were part of his medical team.

C. Inform Neil's psychiatrist about the photograph in case he has developed an attachment disorder.

D. Explain that you are very flattered but as Neil will have a new team you do not think it will be appropriate to visit.

E. Thank Neil for the gift but explain that the GMC has clear guidance on forming inappropriate relationships with patients.

> What are the boundaries for patient–doctor relationships?

Q185. Your registrar asks you to file an ECG taken in A&E for Mr Patel into his medical notes. As you are doing this you notice that there are changes consistent with an ischaemic event. You haven't seen Mr Patel this morning as you have been on the other half of the ward. Your registrar has gone to clinic and you are on the ward by yourself. You are aware that blood tests to exclude an ischaemic event are routinely taken if ECG changes are detected.

Choose the most suitable **three** options from the following list:

A. Ignore the ECG changes as the registrar will have seen them.

B. Review Mr Patel immediately.

C. Ask your FY1 colleagues on the adjacent ward for their opinion on the ECG.

D. Ask the nursing staff to take urgent blood to test for ischaemic changes.

E. Arrange for urgent angiography as the patient is having an ischaemic event.

F. Arrange for the nursing staff to repeat the ECG.

G. Call your consultant and explain that the registrar did not see ischaemic changes on the patient's ECG.

H. Call your registrar in clinic and explain the situation.

Q186. You are on the ward round reviewing Mrs Barrons. She has been under investigation for abdominal pain and had a colonoscopy 3 days ago. Your consultant abruptly tells Mrs Barrons that the biopsy taken during her colonoscopy has confirmed that she has bowel cancer. Mrs Barrons was not expecting such a diagnosis. The consultant leaves to continue his ward round and you can see that Mrs Barrons is visibly upset.

Choose the most suitable **three** options from the following list:

A. Apologise for the consultant's insensitive method of breaking the diagnosis.

B. Offer to speak to Mrs Barrons and answer any questions she may have.

C. Report the consultant to the GMC.

D. Arrange for the cancer nurse specialist to review Mrs Barrons urgently.

E. Arrange for the chaplaincy to visit Mrs Barrons.

F. Ask one of the ward nurses to sit with Mrs Barrons and explore why she is upset.

G. Ask the consultant whether you can leave the ward round for a short time to speak with Mrs Barrons.

H. Continue the ward round.

Q187. Mr Robin, a 67-year-old man, has been admitted to your ward this afternoon with delirium. The staff nurse looking after him asks whether you would be able to review the patient as he is screaming out and disturbing the other patients.

Choose the most suitable **three** options from the following list:

A. Call Mr Robin's next of kin and suggest they visit him as recognising his family may calm him down.

B. Apply soft restraints so that Mr Robin cannot hurt himself.

C. Call security.

D. Suggest the staff nurse talks to Mr Robin to try to calm him down.

E. Review Mr Robin's medical notes to ensure he is being adequately treated for his delirium.

F. Review Mr Robin and attempt to calm him down.

G. Refuse to see Mr Robin as his delirium will settle down eventually.

H. Prescribe sedation as required.

Q188. You are working on the oncology ward and have noticed that two of your patients have the same name: Patricia Brown. This morning, the night FY1 has handed over that he was called to review one of your patients as they were 'spiking a temperature'. He tells you it was Patricia Brown. When you ask which Patricia Brown your FY1 colleague appears confused and tells you he did not realise there were two patients called Patricia Brown on your ward. He is unsure which Patricia he reviewed as he does not have the date of birth (DOB) or hospital number to hand. When you review both patients, you realise that he has prescribed antibiotics to the wrong Patricia Brown. No medication has been given yet as the nurse has just started her drug round.

Choose the most suitable **three** options from the following list:

A. Discuss your concerns with the night FY1's educational supervisor.

B. Design a protocol for identical patients on the same ward.

C. Correct the prescription immediately.

D. Complete an incident form.

E. Inform the ward manager of this incident and discuss methods to deal with two patients having the same name in the future.

F. At handover tomorrow morning, tell the night FY1 about their mistake and the corrective actions you took.

G. Raise awareness on the ward to ensure all staff members have noticed two patients have the same name.

H. Call the night FY1 and inform him of the mistake he has made.

Q189. You are working on the trauma and orthopaedic ward. James, a 34-year-old man, has been admitted overnight for observation following reduction with sedation of his dislocated left shoulder. His injury was caused by a fall earlier that afternoon. He has recovered well with no complications and has been discharged by your consultant. You are preparing his discharge summary when one of the nurses tells you she is worried James may have an 'alcohol problem'.

Choose the most suitable **three** options from the following list:

A. Discharge James as planned.

B. Discuss the nurse's concerns with James regarding his alcohol consumption.

C. Ask the nurse why she is concerned about James.

D. Call James's GP to obtain an alcohol use history.

E. Discuss the nurse's concerns with your consultant.

F. Offer to refer James to the community alcohol and drugs service.

G. Delay James's discharge to review for clinical signs of alcohol withdrawal.

H. Write to James's GP and ask them to monitor James's alcohol intake.

Q190. You are the FY1 working on the oncology ward. Sarah, a staff nurse, has asked you to review Mrs William's DNAR status as Sarah feels she is likely to pass away shortly. Sarah informs you that Dr Jacobs, the on-call consultant, confirmed yesterday that Mrs William is not for resuscitation owing to progressive ovarian cancer. The family was in agreement with this decision and believed Mrs William would have been too. Unfortunately, Dr Jacobs did not have a DNAR form available at the time and so it wasn't completed. You can see from the post-take ward round entry yesterday evening that Mrs William is not for escalation of care or resuscitation. When you briefly assess Mrs William she is unresponsive and appears comfortable. You acknowledge that she is likely to pass away shortly.

Choose the most suitable **three** options from the following list:

A. Sign the DNAR form.

B. Call your registrar and explain the situation. Ask them to sign a DNAR form urgently for Mrs William.

C. Ask Sarah to speak to the registrar directly.

D. Call Mrs William's NOK and inform them of her current clinical state.

E. Call your consultant and explain the situation.

F. Call the ITU registrar and ask them to assess Mrs William as she is unresponsive and currently for resuscitation as the DNAR form is unsigned.

G. Ensure end-of-life analgesia, antiemetic and sedation are prescribed as required to ensure Mrs William remains comfortable.

H. Ask Sarah to call Mrs William's NOK.

> What are the components of a 'good death' compared with a 'bad death'?

Q191. You are an FY1 on paediatrics. Susy McKay has been admitted for an elective bone marrow transfer as she has been diagnosed with leukaemia. You are asked by your registrar to complete the admission clerking. As you review Susy's blood results you notice that she is neutropenic. You discuss this with your registrar and they recommend starting the neutropenic sepsis protocol. You give Susy immediate intravenous penicillin as per the trust policy; 10 minutes later you receive a bleep from the nurse looking after Susy explaining that she appears to be having a reaction to the penicillin. You don't recall Susy having an allergy during your clerking.

Choose the most suitable **three** options from the following list:

A. Explain to Susy and her parents that you didn't realise she had an allergy and apologise for not asking beforehand.

B. Ask the nurse to give some fluids and say you will assess Susy soon but will need to finish the task you are currently doing.

C. Update Susy's drug chart and medical notes with her allergy status.

D. Tell the nurse that she shouldn't be bothering you unless she has a full set of observations available.

E. Destroy Susy's drug chart. Re-write it with the allergy clearly stated and a non-allergic antibiotic prescribed.

F. Inform your registrar of what has happened.

G. Immediately return to the ward and assess Susy.

H. Ask the nurse to call the cardiac arrest team so that you have help when you arrive.

Q192. You are the FY1 on the breast surgery unit. Mrs Harris is an inpatient on your ward admitted for investigation of a painless breast lump post menopause. Your unit is very busy and Mr Carey, the consultant, is often operating daily so asks his registrar, Patricia, to conduct the morning ward round. Mrs Harris was last seen by Mr Carey 2 days previously. You and Patricia meet with Mr Carey in his office at the end of every day to discuss the progress of his patients. This afternoon, you attend Mrs Harris to see how she is doing. She expresses a concern that Mr Carey is not reviewing her and is worried she is receiving suboptimal care.

Choose the most suitable **three** options from the following list:

A. Explore whether Mrs Harris has any new clinical concerns.

B. Reassure Mrs Harris that, although Mr Carey may not see her on a daily basis, he is informed daily of her progress.

C. Inform Mrs Harris that Mr Carey will review her tomorrow.

D. Discuss Mrs Harris's remark with Mr Carey at today's afternoon meeting. Politely ask whether he can review her tomorrow.

E. Ask the ward matron to ensure Mr Carey conducts daily reviews.

F. Inform Mrs Harris that you agree that Mr Carey should personally review his patients more often.

G. Inform Mrs Harris that she should report her concerns to the PALS.

H. Inform Mrs Harris that her concerns are unfounded.

Q193. Julie, a staff nurse, has informed you that one of your patients, Ivanov, repeatedly leaves the ward for prolonged periods of time. When he returns he seems intoxicated and becomes unwilling to cooperate with the ward staff. He is currently being treated for a community-acquired pneumonia and is known to your hospital's alcohol and drugs service.

Choose the most suitable **three** options from the following list:

A. Tell Ivanov that you are unable to treat him if he continues to leave the ward.

B. Explore the reason behind Ivanov's behaviour.

C. Ask Ivanov whether he is drinking alcohol when he leaves the ward.

D. Discuss your concerns about Ivanov with your consultant.

E. Explain to Ivanov that you are unable to review him if he is not at his bedside.

F. Call the alcohol and drugs service and discuss your concerns with them.

G. Discharge Ivanov on oral antibiotics so that he doesn't have to stay in hospital any longer.

H. Discuss inpatient detoxification with Ivanov to help him abstain from alcohol.

Q194. You are on call providing ward cover for surgical patients. You have been called to AAU to review Mr Xiou, a 67-year-old Chinese man, who has been admitted with suspected acute pancreatitis following an alcoholic binge. The patient is no longer intoxicated but is refusing to be given IV fluids as he doesn't believe in Western medicine. The patient is shouting profanities and threatening to assault the nurse if they attempt to treat him. The patient is in bed but is disturbing other patients.

Choose the most suitable **three** options from the following list:

A. Tell Mr Xiou that he is disturbing other patients and upsetting the nurse. Explain that this will not be tolerated and if he continues to be disruptive he may not be treated.

B. Call security.

C. Call the police.

D. Prescribe a sedative so that you and the nurse can carry on with your duties.

E. Ensure that the other patients are not upset.

F. Assess Mr Xiou's capacity to make this decision.

G. Explore Mr Xiou's concerns and reasoning behind his comment. Try to calm him down by explaining that everyone is trying to help him.

> What function must a patient have in order to make this decision?

H. Tell Mr Xiou to leave the hospital immediately.

Q195. You are on call and are reviewing Mr Archer, a 65-year-old man with severe heart failure secondary to ischaemic heart disease. The day team has asked you to review his CXR and implement any necessary management. You discuss his CXR with your registrar as you believe he is still in extensive pulmonary oedema. When you assess Mr Archer he is very unwell. Your registrar recommends starting a furosemide infusion, which you do; 45 minutes later your cardiac arrest bleeper goes off and you arrive to find that Mr Archer has gone into cardiac arrest and did not survive. The registrar tells you that it was probably secondary to his heart failure. Mr Archer's NOK is waiting in the relatives' room and has been informed.

Choose the most suitable **three** options from the following list:

A. Offer to sit with Mr Archer's NOK.

B. Ask the registrar whether there was anything else you could have done.

C. Suggest the ward nurse sits with Mr Archer's NOK.

D. Ask your registrar if you can have your bleep transferred to his bleeper for 30 minutes so you are not disturbed with Mr Archer's NOK.

E. Confirm whether the furosemide infusion had been started.

F. Turn your bleeper off so you are not disturbed with Mr Archer's NOK.

G. Ask Mr Archer's NOK whether they would like any additional support such as chaplaincy or if you can call anybody on their behalf.

H. Return to your job list as you are on call.

Q196. You are an FY1 in acute medicine. You have just reviewed Mrs Sweeny and discovered she has a markedly reduced haemoglobin level secondary to an upper gastrointestinal (GI) bleed. You have arranged for Mrs Sweeny to undergo blood transfusion while she awaits her urgent OGD. You prescribe the blood to be given on Mrs Sweeny's prescription chart and attempt to hand over to Peter, Mrs Sweeny's nurse. Unfortunately Peter is helping another patient to use a commode and so you leave the prescription chart on the nurses' station to ensure that Peter sees it. On your return to the ward 3 hours later you notice that Mrs Sweeny is yet to receive her blood transfusion.

Choose the most suitable **three** options from the following list:

A. Report Peter to the ward manager for not administering the blood.

B. Clinically review Mrs Sweeny.

C. Prescribe iron tablets for Mrs Sweeny whilst she is awaiting transfusion.

D. Ensure that your ward has a protocol in place so that important tasks are received by the necessary person.

E. Complete an audit assessing the time between prescription of blood and the transfusion being started.

F. Ensure that you hand over urgent tasks correctly in the future.

G. Inform Mrs Sweeny's consultant of the incident.

H. Speak to Peter urgently to ensure the blood transfusion can begin.

Q197. You have been asked to review Noah Jenson, a 39-year-old man who has presented to the acute medical team with haematemesis. He has a known medical history of peptic ulceration and has been admitted twice previously for active bleeding. As you are clerking Noah he explains that he is a Jehovah's Witness and does not believe in receiving blood products of any description, including fresh frozen plasma (FFP) and platelets. You have seen Noah's blood results and his haemoglobin level is dangerously low. He is clinically unwell and isn't able to undergo OGD until he is haemodynamically stable. Your registrar is on their way to help you manage Noah but while waiting you have started the trust's severe haematemesis protocol.

Choose the most suitable **three** options from the following list:

A. Offer to call Noah's NOK to inform them that he is critically unwell.

B. Monitor Noah's condition and if he becomes unresponsive arrange a blood transfusion under the 'Good Samaritan' principle.

C. Arrange for Noah to be given a blood transfusion as he currently lacks capacity.

D. Contact your hospital's Jehovah's Witness advisor urgently.

E. Plead with Noah to allow you to arrange a blood transfusion as he is critically unwell.

F. Tell Noah that he will die without a blood transfusion.

G. Explore Noah's religious beliefs explaining the differences between the blood products.

H. Accept Noah's views and support him with IV fluids and proton-pump inhibitor (PPI) as per the trust's protocol.

> Does a patient lack capacity if the choice they make is deemed unwise by their doctor?

Q198. You are the FY1 working in the endocrine and diabetes team. The ward is very busy and there are two nurse consultants who specialise in diabetes management. You have been seeing Liam, a 19-year-old patient with insulin-controlled diabetes. He was diagnosed at 6 years of age and has had multiple admissions throughout his childhood. Owing to poor parental compliance when Liam was younger, he has been left with an element of brain injury. This is his third admission this year owing to poor compliance with his insulin.

Choose the most suitable **three** options from the following list:

A. Complete an adult safeguarding referral as Liam's parents may be abusing him.

B. Arrange for the diabetes nurse specialist to review Liam.

C. Tell Liam that he needs to try harder to comply with his insulin regimen to reduce his admissions to hospital.

D. Suggest a family meeting with Liam to discuss managing his diabetes.

E. Discuss stopping insulin with your consultant as Liam is non-compliant anyway.

F. Discuss your concerns with Liam and explore his beliefs regarding his diabetes.

G. Call Liam's parents and discuss your concerns with them.

H. Ensure that Liam understands the risks of poor compliance to insulin.

Q199. You are the FY1 working on medical care for the elderly. Your team has been caring for Mrs Dudley who was admitted unresponsive earlier this week. Today, Mrs Dudley has deteriorated and your consultant has referred her to ITU. Unfortunately, owing to her co-morbidities it is decided that ITU would not be suitable escalation. The decision is taken to withdraw active treatment and to ensure that Mrs Dudley remains comfortable. Your consultant has informed Mrs Dudley's daughter, but when she arrives on the ward she asks to speak to you about her mother.

Choose the most suitable **three** options from the following list:

A. Ask Mrs Dudley's daughter to wait in the relatives' room.

B. Explain to the daughter that you won't know any further information other than what the consultant has already provided.

C. Ask the staff nurse looking after Mrs Dudley to speak to her daughter.

D. Discuss the daughter's concerns at her mother's bedside.

E. Arrange for a palliative care nurse to join you in the relatives' room with Mrs Dudley's daughter.

F. Apologise to Mrs Dudley's daughter but explain you are too busy with other patients to speak with her at the moment.

G. Review Mrs Dudley to ensure she is comfortable before her daughter sees her.

H. Offer your condolences to Mrs Dudley's daughter and answer any questions she may have.

Q200. You are the FY1 working on the acute admission unit. You have been very busy throughout the day when a patient's relative approaches you and asks whether you could spare a moment to discuss Mr Couldridge in bed 13. You ask what relation he is to Mr Couldridge and he explains that they have been close friends for many years and live next door to each other. As you are discussing bed 13 your bleeper goes off and as you're answering your bleep Jane, the ward sister, asks whether you have completed today's patient discharge summaries.

Choose the most suitable **three** options from the following list:

A. Explain why Mr Couldridge has been admitted.

B. Document your discussion with Mr Couldridge's friend in his medical notes.

C. Arrange for the staff nurse to speak with Mr Couldridge and his friend as she is likely to know the case better.

D. Ask Jane whether the relatives' room is available for you to use.

E. Read Mr Couldridge's medical notes so that you are familiar with his case.

F. Tell the friend that you do not have the time to discuss Mr Couldridge at the moment.

G. Explain that you are happy to meet with Mr Couldridge and his friend but do not have time at the moment. You will try to come back to the ward later once you are less busy.

H. Ask the close friend to wait while you confirm whether Mr Couldridge is happy for you to speak to them about his medical condition.

ANSWERS

A151. This question is focusing on your ability to ensure that patients are adequately reassured. In this scenario, Mrs Molyneux is unsure of what is involved in the procedure she is undergoing. She is likely to be anxious and the most appropriate course of action is to reassure her by explaining the procedure and answering her questions. However, this is complicated by the fact that you are not competent to do this as you are unsure of the details yourself. Therefore the most appropriate choice is **answer B**. The SHO is competent to discuss this procedure, answer Mrs Molyneux's questions and (hopefully) allay her concerns. The next most appropriate choice would be to ask your registrar for advice; they will be assisting with the procedure and will also be able to suggest a plan for you. Bleeping the registrar (**answer C**) is more appropriate than visiting theatre directly (**answer D**) as the registrar may be busy and unable to answer your questions in person at that time. Therefore bleeping the registrar will allow them to reply to the bleep once free. At this point, you would have no option but to cancel Mrs Molyneux's slot in theatre (**answer E**). Remember: in order for a patient to have valid consent they must understand the risks and benefits of the planned procedure. In order for Mrs Molyneux to do this she would need to understand what is going to happen in the procedure. Finally, the least appropriate answer would be to attempt to explain the procedure as you are not competent to do so and could cause further anxiety to Mrs Molyneux (**answer A**).

Ideal order	Your rank choice				
	1st	2nd	3rd	4th	5th
B	4	3	2	1	0
C	3	4	3	2	1
D	2	3	4	3	2
E	1	2	3	4	3
A	0	1	2	3	4

A152. This question is assessing your proclivity to make yourself available to patients to discuss their concerns. In this scenario Mr Williams has been NBM for longer than anticipated owing to unpredictable conditions. The most appropriate course of action is to speak with Mr Williams and apologise for the delay (**answer A**). You can then attempt to call theatre (**answer C**) but there is every chance that if the team is dealing with an emergency they will be unsure of the time as well. Arranging for the registrar to speak with Mr Williams (**answer B**) is the third most appropriate answer in this scenario. However, the registrar will not be able to provide any additional information and should not be your first port of call in this case. You should be willing to meet with patients and attempt to discuss their concerns. **Answer E** is a realistic situation but will not ease Mr Williams' grievance and is therefore a poor choice in this scenario. Finally, the least appropriate choice would be allowing Mr Williams to eat (**answer D**). He may be taken to theatre soon and eating would certainly delay his operation until tomorrow – an outcome that neither Mr Williams nor your consultant will want forced upon them.

Ideal order	Your rank choice				
	1st	2nd	3rd	4th	5th
A	4	3	2	1	0
C	3	4	3	2	1
B	2	3	4	3	2
E	1	2	3	4	3
D	0	1	2	3	4

A153. This question is focusing on patient safety. Administering intrathecal antibiotics should not be attempted unless you are competent in this skill. There have been several cases of paralysis or cerebral damage from incorrect use of intrathecal medication. In this scenario you are not competent in intrathecal administration but have a very unwell patient. Therefore your priority must be to ensure that Mrs Levy is given the intrathecal antibiotics promptly and safely. The most appropriate option is **answer D**. Your SHO colleague, who is competent, would be able to assist you. Remember: see one, do one, teach one. The next most appropriate option is seeking advice from your registrar (**answer A**). The antibiotics do need to be given urgently and your registrar would be able to give you appropriate advice. The next most appropriate option is **answer C**. Mrs Levy requires her antibiotics urgently; the trust intranet will have approved guidelines for most medical problems and you can consult them if you are unsure. Asking the staff nurse (**answer B**) is not an appropriate choice in this situation. Although ward nurses are highly experienced with administering medications they will not normally be competent with the intrathecal route. Remember, always consult with colleagues according to the escalation ladder. Finally, the least appropriate option is to wait for your consultant to return from theatre (**answer E**). This delay in administering antibiotics could result in Mrs Levy dying. If in doubt, seek help! Waiting is rarely the correct answer.

Ideal order	Your rank choice				
	1st	2nd	3rd	4th	5th
D	4	3	2	1	0
A	3	4	3	2	1
C	2	3	4	3	2
B	1	2	3	4	3
E	0	1	2	3	4

A154. This question is focusing on your ability to work jointly with Sarah about her care. Patients with chronic conditions are often highly knowledgeable and rightly have their own views about their management. These should be listened to and your aim is to work with the patient to come to a mutual agreement. Therefore, the most appropriate option is to explore Sarah's concerns (**answer C**). The next most appropriate option is **answer A**. Any decision that alters the management plan of a patient should be discussed with the consultant. The next best option would be to refer Sarah to the diabetic nurse specialist (**answer D**). They will often be able to spend more time with a patient and can offer additional support. The ward pharmacist will be able to advise you on an insulin regimen best suited for Sarah whilst in hospital (**answer B**). However, this answer is not ranked highly in this scenario as it does not address the primary concern, which is Sarah's unease at changing her insulin regimen. Finally, the least appropriate option is to change Sarah's insulin despite her concerns (**answer E**). Sarah has the right to decide on her treatment and your role is to provide her with the relevant information to facilitate this.

Ideal order	Your rank choice				
	1st	2nd	3rd	4th	5th
C	4	3	2	1	0
A	3	4	3	2	1
D	2	3	4	3	2
B	1	2	3	4	3
E	0	1	2	3	4

A155. This question is focusing on your willingness to provide reassurance as a doctor. However, this is complicated by the 'patient' being your friend. It is not an uncommon occurrence for a friend or family member to ask for your professional advice once you become a doctor. Of course, the GMC has clear guidance about treating family or friends and it is generally frowned upon. However, you are still expected to act in that individual's best interest and if you do give advice it should be congruent with your daily practice. The most appropriate option is to advise Richard returns to his GP to seek further medical attention (**answer E**). The GP is best suited to investigate his complaint. The next most appropriate option would be to reassure Richard that the GP is acting correctly (**answer A**). At this point, it would be wise to advise Richard that you shouldn't be treating family or friends (**answer C**). This option is not ranked higher as it is very impersonal and you should always show empathy towards an individual with a medical complaint, even if you are not planning on treating the individual concerned. Asking Richard about his symptoms (**answer D**) is not appropriate. This is clearly not an emergency and you should avoid treating, or even advising, family or friends. They should be referred to their GP first and foremost. The least appropriate option is supplying a gastroenterologist's telephone number (**answer B**). If there is something seriously wrong with Richard it must be coordinated through his GP.

Ideal order	Your rank choice				
	1st	2nd	3rd	4th	5th
E	4	3	2	1	0
A	3	4	3	2	1
C	2	3	4	3	2
D	1	2	3	4	3
B	0	1	2	3	4

A156. This question is focusing on your readiness to make yourself available to Mr Lewis. Although you are clearly busy with discharge paperwork, you should be able to balance this workload with responding to patient needs. There may be several reasons why Mr Lewis has become agitated and aggressive towards staff. Therefore, the most appropriate option is to review him urgently and explore why he is demanding to see the consultant (**answer D**). Following this, you would be wise to seek advice from your consultant (**answer E**). Whilst your consultant will be busy in clinic they are normally able to provide telephone advice as an interim. Although Mr Lewis's needs are important, you also have the needs of the other patients and the ward to consider. You are likely to be delayed in your discharge paperwork whilst reviewing Mr Lewis and so the next most appropriate option would be informing the discharge coordinator (**answer C**). The next most appropriate answer would be to ask the nurse to call your consultant (**answer B**). However, this is ranked low as you should always seek advice in person to minimise any miscommunication. Finally, the least appropriate option would be to dismiss Mr Lewis's request (**answer A**).

Ideal order	Your rank choice				
	1st	2nd	3rd	4th	5th
D	4	3	2	1	0
E	3	4	3	2	1
C	2	3	4	3	2
B	1	2	3	4	3
A	0	1	2	3	4

A157. This question is based on your ability to appreciate that patients will have differing needs and views, and these may not be in accordance with your own personal views. However, you need to be able to support your patient to the best of your abilities whilst remaining respectful and non-judgemental. As euthanasia/assisted dying is illegal in the UK, the answer to this question is not going to focus on the practicality of Miss Barons's request, but instead on how you can attempt to understand it. The most appropriate option in this scenario is **answer C**. In such an alarming and distressing situation, discussing Miss Barons's views with her in an open and non-judgemental manner will allow you to understand what she must be feeling to make such a request. The next most appropriate action would be to refer Miss Barons to the palliative care team (**answer D**) as they will be trained to manage this type of situation, and importantly have the community team to support Miss Barons once she is discharged home. It would be wise for Miss Barons to discuss how she is feeling with her family (**answer B**), but all you can do is suggest she does so. You would be in breach of confidentiality to discuss what Miss Barons has told you with her family – even if your intention is to protect her. Sharing your personal opinion on the matter with Miss Barons is unprofessional (**answer A**). The guideline *Good Medical Practice* (GMC, 2013a) states that all doctors should treat their patients in a non-judgemental manner. Finally, the least appropriate option is **answer E** as this is breaking patient confidentiality.

Ideal order	Your rank choice				
	1st	2nd	3rd	4th	5th
C	4	3	2	1	0
D	3	4	3	2	1
B	2	3	4	3	2
A	1	2	3	4	3
E	0	1	2	3	4

A158. This question is assessing your ability to maintain a professional distance from your patient. Mrs McDonnah is clearly fond of you and it may seem harmless to accept this type of offer. However, it is the role of Mrs McDonnah's GP to arrange home visits and the appropriate community support for her to manage her new diagnosis. Developing a balance between caring for patients and becoming too emotionally involved can be challenging, but in this situation the most appropriate option would be **answer C**. The next most appropriate option would be to attempt to arrange a support network for Mrs McDonnah (**answer B**). Many hospitals have voluntary services from which patients can benefit. There are also charities (e.g. Age UK) that assist with providing social support for patients. Ultimately, you need to ensure you do not blur your professional boundaries and, as callous as it may seem, the next most appropriate option is **answer E**. Tell Mrs McDonnah openly that as much as you have enjoyed getting to know her it would not be appropriate to visit her at home. You should try to avoid statements such as **answer D** as they will seem impersonal and are not well received by patients. Finally, the least appropriate option would be to accept Mrs McDonnah's invitation (**answer A**).

Ideal order	Your rank choice				
	1st	2nd	3rd	4th	5th
C	4	3	2	1	0
B	3	4	3	2	1
E	2	3	4	3	2
D	1	2	3	4	3
A	0	1	2	3	4

A159. This question is focusing on your willingness to spend time with a patient's relatives (i.e. Mrs Patel). Remember, your role as an FY1 is often to bridge the gap between patient, or in this case the relative, and the health profession. At times, it may not be appropriate to meet with relatives as the on-call doctor – for example, if you have unwell patients to review, or in complex matters regarding a patient you know nothing about (e.g. DNAR status). However, in this scenario, you would have sufficient time to read Mr Patel's notes to familiarise yourself with his admission and discuss this with his wife (**answer A**). The next most appropriate option would be to meet Mrs Patel to attempt to allay her concerns, but with the caveat that as the on-call doctor you have not been dealing with Mr Patel directly (**answer D**). The next most appropriate option would be to ask Aiva to discuss Mr Patel's care with his wife (**answer B**). She will be familiar with his current condition and will be aware of his treatment plan. The penultimate option is to encourage Mrs Patel to arrange a meeting with Mr Patel's regular team of doctors (**answer C**). This option is fair but does not solve the current issue and so has a low ranking. Finally, the least appropriate option is to dismiss Mrs Patel's request simply because you are the on-call doctor (**answer E**). If time allows, you should be willing to meet with relatives out of hours as this may be the only time they visit their family member.

Ideal order	Your rank choice				
	1st	2nd	3rd	4th	5th
A	4	3	2	1	0
D	3	4	3	2	1
B	2	3	4	3	2
C	1	2	3	4	3
E	0	1	2	3	4

A160. This question is focusing on patient safety with regards to the incorrect prescription of alendronic acid. In this scenario, the situation is compounded by the reputation that Dr Lisk has for chastising junior doctors. However daunting this may seem, your primary action should be to prevent Mrs Lemont from receiving too much alendronic acid, which can have severe side effects. Therefore you should ask Dr Lisk to clarify his prescription request (**answer A**). There may be a legitimate reason for once-daily dosing and this will give Dr Lisk the opportunity to explain this to you. If, however, it was a mistake, then Dr Lisk will be able to amend his request. As per the escalation ladder, your next point of contact for advice would be another consultant (**answer D**) followed by the ward pharmacist (**answer C**). The second least appropriate option would be to prescribe the alendronic acid once a week as you were taught in medical school (**answer E**). Dr Lisk is ultimately responsible for Mrs Lemont's care and there may be a reason (unbeknown to you) that he has recommended once-daily dosing. However, the least appropriate option is to prescribe the alendronic acid once daily without clarification (**answer B**). You currently believe this to be the incorrect dosing regimen and so prescribing as per Dr Lisk's request could cause avoidable harm to Mrs Lemont, and is therefore negligent.

	Your rank choice				
Ideal order	1st	2nd	3rd	4th	5th
A	4	3	2	1	0
D	3	4	3	2	1
C	2	3	4	3	2
E	1	2	3	4	3
B	0	1	2	3	4

A161. This question involves two themes: firstly recognising that Mr Edwards may have a different background and belief regarding end-of-life care/DNAR, and secondly that you haven't been involved in DNAR decision planning previously and therefore should not be attempting this alone. Remember: see one, do one, teach one. Therefore, despite your own feeling about Mr Edwards being fit and healthy, the most appropriate option is to escalate this matter to the on-call registrar, who will be better prepared for this discussion and able to complete the DNAR form. You should ask to accompany the registrar so that you can start to learn how to discuss DNAR decision planning (**answer E**). The next most appropriate option would be to seek advice from the on-call registrar (**answer B**). Discussing Mr Edwards's views about DNAR is the next most appropriate option (**answer C**). However, it is ranked third because you will still not be able to sign the DNAR form despite discussing his views and therefore escalating this matter to your registrar is ranked higher. Refusing to sign the DNAR form owing to your own beliefs about Mr Edwards's physical health is not acceptable (**answer D**). You will not always agree with the decisions that patients make but your duty as a doctor is to respect them. Finally, the least appropriate option would be to simply attend the ward and sign the DNAR form as you are not experienced in this matter (**answer A**).

Ideal order	Your rank choice				
	1st	2nd	3rd	4th	5th
E	4	3	2	1	0
B	3	4	3	2	1
C	2	3	4	3	2
D	1	2	3	4	3
A	0	1	2	3	4

A162. This question is focusing on your willingness to make yourself available to Mr Williams, who is clearly anxious and distressed, in order to try to provide reassurance during this difficult time for him. In this scenario, the CT scan has suggested a malignancy and the most compassionate option would be to inform Mr Williams. However, this diagnosis should be delivered by a senior member of the team who will be equipped to answer any subsequent questions Mr Williams may have. Therefore, the most appropriate option is to arrange for the consultant to return to the ward to meet with Mr Williams (**answer E**). The next most appropriate option would be to explain openly that you are unable to interpret the scan result but will try to discuss Mr Williams' concerns (**answer C**). The third most appropriate option would be to reassure Mr Williams that the consultant will return to discuss his result (**answer A**). Patients often develop anxiety as a result of feeling ignored or forgotten. A simple reassurance may provide Mr Williams with some relief. Telling Mr Williams the result of the scan yourself is not appropriate (**answer B**). As alluded to with answer E, it is unlikely that you will be experienced enough to answer Mr Williams' subsequent questions regarding further tests and treatment options. However, the least appropriate option is to provide any form of false hope (**answer D**).

Ideal order	Your rank choice				
	1st	2nd	3rd	4th	5th
E	4	3	2	1	0
C	3	4	3	2	1
A	2	3	4	3	2
B	1	2	3	4	3
D	0	1	2	3	4

A163. This question is based on showing respect for patients at all times (i.e. trying to provide Mr Sheik and his family with some privacy). This scenario can be an all-too-common occurrence on hospital wards owing to open bays and curtains which are by no means soundproof. The most appropriate option would be to cease the conversation temporarily by asking to speak with the registrar urgently (**answer D**). This would stop neighbouring patients from overhearing any more of the conversation. The next most appropriate option would be to suggest relocating the conversation to the relatives' room to provide some privacy (**answer B**). Expressing your concerns to the registrar (**answer A**) is the next most appropriate option but is ranked below answer D and answer B as it does not result in any direct action to improve the situation. Delegating your concerns to the nurse in charge is not appropriate (**answer C**). If you have concerns it is important that you raise them personally. Finally, the least appropriate action would be closing the curtains around the listening patients (**answer E**). The curtains are not soundproof and do not provide Mr Sheik with any privacy during this distressing discussion.

Ideal order	Your rank choice				
	1st	2nd	3rd	4th	5th
D	4	3	2	1	0
B	3	4	3	2	1
A	2	3	4	3	2
C	1	2	3	4	3
E	0	1	2	3	4

A164. This question is based on your ability to consider patent safety at all times (e.g. Miss Archer's need for a CT scan). Although it is common practice for the FY1 to arrange investigations on your consultant's behalf, it is foolish not to understand the reasoning behind them – partly because you will only develop your decision-making skills by doing so, but also because you are responsible for a patient's safety if you have requested an investigation for them. In this scenario, the most appropriate option is to familiarise yourself with Miss Archer's admission and arrange the CT scan as requested (**answer B**). The next most appropriate option is to call the consultant directly to understand the indication (**answer C**). The next most appropriate option would be to discuss your request with a different radiologist as they may be more understanding (**answer A**). Confronting the radiologist and demanding he does the scan is unlikely to work and will probably result in further friction (**answer E**). However, the least appropriate option is to leave the scan until tomorrow as this will put Miss Archer at risk (**answer D**).

Ideal order	Your rank choice				
	1st	2nd	3rd	4th	5th
B	4	3	2	1	0
C	3	4	3	2	1
A	2	3	4	3	2
E	1	2	3	4	3
D	0	1	2	3	4

A165. This question is assessing your ability to gain trust from Jessica in order to treat Charlie. Your main aim is to provide medical treatment for Charlie promptly as you suspect meningitis but, owing to hearsay, Jessica has lost faith in the medical team that you represent. Therefore, the most appropriate option is **answer B** as this allows you to begin treating Charlie. The next most appropriate option would be to discuss Jessica's concerns with her (**answer C**). This will give you the opportunity to explain what Charlie needs and to answer Jessica's concerns. This would encourage Jessica to trust you to treat Charlie as you need to. The next most appropriate action is to escalate your concerns about Charlie to your registrar (**answer D**). They would probably need to attend to Jessica/Charlie and attempt to help disarm the current conflict. The final two options are both poor outcomes as Charlie will be removed from medical care. If a patient is going to go against medical advice they are required to sign a disclosure form to that effect (**answer A**). This is complicated if the patient is unable to make this decision for themselves (owing to illness, lack of capacity, age, etc.) and the decision being made by their next of kin is deemed to put the patient at risk. A court order can be sought to remove the next of kin's authority but this takes time and requires a court process. The least appropriate option is to allow Jessica to simply leave with Charlie (**answer E**).

Ideal order	Your rank choice				
	1st	2nd	3rd	4th	5th
B	4	3	2	1	0
C	3	4	3	2	1
D	2	3	4	3	2
A	1	2	3	4	3
E	0	1	2	3	4

A166. This question is based on your understanding and ability to consider the different needs of a patient. On one hand Susan has come to terms with her incurable diagnosis (e.g. discussing DNAR), but on the other hand is worried about the actual process of death (e.g. pain). It is important to be able to distinguish a patient's concerns and to try to provide as much tailored care as each patient needs (**answer E**). The next most appropriate option is to discuss Susan's concerns with your consultant (**answer D**). They will be able to advise on an appropriate pain regime and to recommend referral to a palliative care service, which would be your next most appropriate option (**answer B**). As an FY1, discussing a decision that the patient has already previously reached is not wrong, but it creates a setting for confusion (**answer C**). A more appropriate option would involve offering to ask the consultant to speak with Susan again regarding the DNAR decision. But discussing the pros and cons of resuscitation is generally not a task taken on without additional experience. Finally, sedation should not be used simply because a patient is anxious or worried and is clearly the least appropriate option (**answer A**). Susan is not currently in pain or agitated and so the use of sedation at this stage is inappropriate.

Ideal order	Your rank choice				
	1st	2nd	3rd	4th	5th
E	4	3	2	1	0
D	3	4	3	2	1
B	2	3	4	3	2
C	1	2	3	4	3
A	0	1	2	3	4

A167. This question is based on your ability to instil confidence in Mrs Brown. In today's climate of internet and social media, 'anti-NHS' and 'negligence' stories are common place. Patient confidence is reduced and your duty as a doctor is to try to restore this by whatever means available. This will include your attitude, presentation, bedside manner and clinical acumen. The most appropriate option in this scenario is **answer B**. Explaining your reasoning openly and clearly, whilst involving Mrs Brown in the decision-making process, is the best way to instil confidence in your diagnosis. The next most appropriate option is to politely refuse to discuss your management plan with her brother (**answer A**). If you appear confident in your management, Mrs Brown will too. Of course, as an FY1 some patients will connect your position with inexperience, and to a certain extent they are correct. Explaining that your plan will be reviewed by a consultant also helps with building confidence from the public (**answer C**). The second least appropriate option would be to discuss your management with Mrs Brown's brother (**answer D**). You are responsible for your clinical decisions and, although Mrs Brown's brother may be a GP, he is not responsible for her medical care. However, the least appropriate option is **answer E**

as it is not true. A guaranteed way of damaging public confidence in healthcare is to be perceived as untruthful or deceitful.

Ideal order	Your rank choice				
	1st	2nd	3rd	4th	5th
B	4	3	2	1	0
A	3	4	3	2	1
C	2	3	4	3	2
D	1	2	3	4	3
E	0	1	2	3	4

A168. This question is assessing your ability to balance patient safety (i.e. a deteriorating patient) with the needs of your other patients (i.e. Mr Xavier). Clearly, the deteriorating patient takes priority over Mr Xavier. However, it is essential not to underestimate the importance a patient will assign to your emotional support following a life-changing diagnosis. Therefore, the most appropriate option is **answer C**. The next most appropriate option would be to ask the nurse to bleep your FY1 colleague (**answer E**). This option will still safeguard the deteriorating patient whilst allowing Mr Xavier to remain supported. Immediately attending the patient would be the next best option as you should always be prepared to prioritise patient safety at all times (**answer A**). Asking the nurse to take over your conversation with Mr Xavier while you assess the deteriorating patient is not a highly ranked option in this scenario (**answer D**). Mr Xavier is likely to have concerns about symptom management, likely investigations and outcome. The nurse would not necessarily be able to answer these questions and may leave Mr Xavier feeling poorly supported. However, the least appropriate option would be **answer B**. Your priority should be patient safety and the delay caused by finding another doctor may lead to patient harm.

Ideal order	Your rank choice				
	1st	2nd	3rd	4th	5th
C	4	3	2	1	0
E	3	4	3	2	1
A	2	3	4	3	2
D	1	2	3	4	3
B	0	1	2	3	4

A169. This question is based on your ability to maintain an appropriate distance from your patient's relatives. The most appropriate option in this scenario is **answer E**. This will maintain your professional distance from Julie whilst showing appreciation for the family's gratitude. The next most appropriate option would be **answer D**. Many relatives will want to demonstrate their gratitude with a gift and the GMC has clear guidance. As a rule of thumb, as long as the gift is of low value and can be shared amongst your colleagues it is generally acceptable (i.e. box of biscuits). The next most appropriate option would be **answer C**. This is honest and open, but may not be as well received by Julie as either answer E or answer D. The next most appropriate option is **answer A**. Remember, sometimes you simply have to be frank but if you can avoid a 'political' statement you'll develop a better rapport with your patients and their relatives. However, the least appropriate option would be to accept Julie's offer (**answer B**). You must develop an appropriate distance from your patients and their relatives in order to remain objective and professional.

Ideal order	Your rank choice				
	1st	2nd	3rd	4th	5th
E	4	3	2	1	0
D	3	4	3	2	1
C	2	3	4	3	2
A	1	2	3	4	3
B	0	1	2	3	4

A170. This question is based on your ability to work jointly with Mrs Toulet about her care. She has requested a non-formulary statin that you are unable to prescribe. However, she has informed you that she will not comply with the formulary statin. Therefore, the most appropriate option to begin with is **answer A**. Exploring Mrs Toulet's concerns will encourage a collaborative relationship to develop and may reveal a reason for her request. The next most appropriate option would be to explain that her GP can prescribe non-formulary but she would need to arrange this. However, in the meantime she should start taking atorvastatin (**answer C**). You could attempt to make contact with the GP yourself (**answer D**) but this does not resolve the current issue of non-compliance. A factual statement such as **answer B** is not an incorrect option but does not attempt to work with Mrs Toulet to resolve the complaint. She may simply agree to stop any further confrontation but she is unlikely to take the intended medications. Finally, the least appropriate option would be to dismiss Mrs Toulet's concerns (**answer E**).

Ideal order	Your rank choice				
	1st	2nd	3rd	4th	5th
A	4	3	2	1	0
C	3	4	3	2	1
D	2	3	4	3	2
B	1	2	3	4	3
E	0	1	2	3	4

A171. This question is based on your reaction to compromised patient safety. A delay of several hours in administering antibiotics in a septic patient can mean the difference between life and death. Therefore, the most appropriate option would be to attempt to re-cannulate Ellie immediately so that she can receive antibiotics urgently (**answer E**). Remember: patient safety, patient safety, and patient safety! The next most appropriate option would be to bleep the on-call doctor and ask whether they could cannulate Ellie (**answer B**). Your shift has ended and the on-call team is in place to assist with tasks that are not finished during the day shift. This will ensure that Ellie receives treatment as necessary, but will also safeguard you from fatigue. Asking Jasmine to refer to the on-call doctor would be the next most appropriate option as it would still achieve the desired outcome (**answer D**). However, it is ranked lower than answer B as this will add an extra process to the task and therefore increase the chance of miscommunication. If possible, always hand over information personally. Converting a patient from IV antibiotics onto oral antibiotics should be a decision based on the patient's clinical situation, not simply because it is easier to administer (**answer C**). This is the next most appropriate option in this scenario because the least appropriate response is clearly to delay administering antibiotics until tomorrow morning (**answer A**). Ellie has a known infection and requires regular antibiotics to recover.

Ideal order	Your rank choice				
	1st	2nd	3rd	4th	5th
E	4	3	2	1	0
B	3	4	3	2	1
D	2	3	4	3	2
C	1	2	3	4	3
A	0	1	2	3	4

A172. This question is assessing your capability to provide reassurance to Mrs Bekir, who is clearly very anxious about undergoing her OGD. The most appropriate option would be to explain the situation to your consultant (**answer B**). He will be able to explore her concerns and provide reassurance as needed. The next most appropriate option would be to ask your consultant for more time with Mrs Bekir so you can attempt to reassure her yourself (**answer A**). This is ranked below the consultant personally reassuring Mrs Bekir as there may be concerns that you are unable to answer as you are not performing the OGD yourself. The next most appropriate option is **answer D**. Although telling Mrs Bekir she will be sedated (**answer C**) is factual, patients rarely appreciate platitudes and these should be avoided. However, the least appropriate option would be to leave Mrs Bekir without reassurance (**answer E**).

Ideal order	Your rank choice				
	1st	2nd	3rd	4th	5th
B	4	3	2	1	0
A	3	4	3	2	1
D	2	3	4	3	2
C	1	2	3	4	3
E	0	1	2	3	4

A173. This question is based on the expectation that all doctors are polite, courteous and present an open manner when dealing with patients. There will be many patients that upset or irritate you throughout your career and an important skill to develop is the ability to remain polite and professional. In this scenario, Peter has not been able to manage this and has been rude to a patient. The most appropriate option is **answer A**, followed by **answer C**. Both options will remove Peter from the antagonistic situation and will prevent any additional conflict. However, Peter should apologise to Mrs Beecham and therefore answer A is ranked higher than C. The next most appropriate option would be **answer D**. However, as this option does not immediately attempt to resolve the conflict (unlike A and C) it is ranked lower. The second least appropriate option is to ignore what you have heard (**answer E**). Peter has acted unprofessionally and you should challenge his behaviour. However, the least appropriate option would be to chastise Mrs Beecham (**answer B**).

Ideal order	Your rank choice				
	1st	2nd	3rd	4th	5th
A	4	3	2	1	0
C	3	4	3	2	1
D	2	3	4	3	2
E	1	2	3	4	3
B	0	1	2	3	4

A174. This question focuses on your willingness to spend time with relatives in difficult circumstances. As a busy junior doctor it can be tempting to assign speaking with relatives a low priority. However, it is important to maintain an approachable manner with patients and their relatives, irrespective of your task list. Therefore, the most appropriate option is **answer E**. There may be questions that Janet and Larry would like to ask you specifically. The next most appropriate option is **answer D** as there may be questions that only the consultant can answer. Arranging a time for Janet and Larry to return to speak with you (**answer B**) is sensible as it allows you to manage your tasks. However, in a difficult situation involving a deteriorating patient it is better to speak to relatives as soon as possible. The next most appropriate option in this scenario would be to explain that as their daughter is under a new team you are unable to discuss her care (**answer A**). This answer is ranked fourth because you should always be willing to spend time with relatives. Telling a family that you are unwilling to speak with them as you are no longer looking after their relative will appear uncaring. Finally, the least appropriate option is **answer C**. Dismissing their request for further information is not appropriate.

Ideal order	Your rank choice				
	1st	2nd	3rd	4th	5th
E	4	3	2	1	0
D	3	4	3	2	1
B	2	3	4	3	2
A	1	2	3	4	3
C	0	1	2	3	4

A175. This question is focusing on patient safety (i.e. a possible undiagnosed bowel perforation), your ability to follow the recommended escalation advice and your ability to achieve a work–life balance. In this scenario the most appropriate option is **answer D**; the night FY1 can check the chest x-ray on your behalf and take any necessary action. As per the escalation ladder, the next most appropriate option is to contact the on-call registrar (**answer C**). This would be followed by the ward nursing staff (**answer B**). The next option would be to return to work and review the chest x-ray yourself (**answer E**). This option is a poor choice in reality owing to fatigue, commuting practicalities and evening commitments (e.g. family, friends and hobbies) and you would ordinarily be able to hand over to a member of the on-call team. If you were unable to hand over then you would need to return to the hospital to ensure the patient was not at risk. The least appropriate option in this scenario is to wait until you return to work the following morning (**answer A**). This would result in delayed diagnosis and management of a possible bowel perforation and could lead to Mrs Brown developing peritonitis.

Ideal order	Your rank choice				
	1st	2nd	3rd	4th	5th
D	4	3	2	1	0
C	3	4	3	2	1
B	2	3	4	3	2
E	1	2	3	4	3
A	0	1	2	3	4

A176. This question is focused on your ability to show empathy towards Mrs Bunton and respond appropriately to her concerns. It is common practice for simple procedures to be conducted as a day case and for patients to be discharged on the same day. In this scenario, Mrs Bunton has had an uncomplicated arthroscopy and has been seen by OT, who feels she is safe to be discharged. However, Mrs Bunton feels differently. Therefore, the most appropriate action would be to explore Mrs Bunton's concerns and act empathetically towards her worries (**answer C**). The next most appropriate action would be to discuss your concerns with Julie. There may be support OT can put in place now that Mrs Bunton has voiced her concerns (**answer B**). It is not appropriate to delay a patient's discharge if they are medically fit and able to go home. Nor it is fair to ask Mr Patel, who is expecting a planned admission, to return tomorrow. Therefore, the next most appropriate option is to explain that Mrs Bunton must leave (**answer A**). In this scenario, your next option would be to have Julie re-assess Mrs Bunton (**answer E**). This has a low ranking as you have already been told that Julie has completed her assessment and therefore re-assessment is not an appropriate use of time or resources. However, the least appropriate option would be to ask Mr Patel to return tomorrow (**answer D**).

He is expecting a planned admission and there may be medications that need to be given overnight or investigations that need to be completed (e.g. ECG or blood tests).

Ideal order	Your rank choice				
	1st	2nd	3rd	4th	5th
C	4	3	2	1	0
B	3	4	3	2	1
A	2	3	4	3	2
E	1	2	3	4	3
D	0	1	2	3	4

A177. This question is focusing on your understanding that patients have different backgrounds and beliefs (i.e. religious ceremonies / traditions regarding death). As the FY1 often completing the death documentation, having a brief understanding of this is important. If your clinical commitments allow then you should attempt to accommodate these requests. Therefore, the most appropriate option is **answer C** as your consultant will be able to assess your clinical requirements on the ward round. The next most appropriate option is **answer B**; this is below answer C as your clinical commitments (e.g. ward round) are a higher priority than death certification. There may be another doctor who meets the requirements to complete Mrs Greenberg's death certificate and is currently free and therefore asking the bereavement office is the next most appropriate option (**answer E**). Completing a death certificate may not score highly on your priorities as a junior doctor, but you should be willing to complete them promptly to ease the family's stress at such a difficult time. Therefore, **answer A** is the second least appropriate option. However, equally inappropriate is a disregard for your clinical duties (e.g. ward round) and therefore attending the bereavement office without excusing yourself from the ward round is the least appropriate option (**answer D**).

Ideal order	Your rank choice				
	1st	2nd	3rd	4th	5th
C	4	3	2	1	0
B	3	4	3	2	1
E	2	3	4	3	2
A	1	2	3	4	3
D	0	1	2	3	4

A178. This question is focusing on patient safety and your genuine interest in Siobhan as your patient. You are suspecting she may have been under the influence of an illicit substance which led to her harm. She has now recovered and the temptation could be to discharge her as she is now medically fit. However, the most appropriate action would be to sensitively explore your concerns with Siobhan (**answer A**). The next most appropriate option is **answer D**. Your consultant will have experience with this type of scenario and be able to advise you as necessary. The next most appropriate option would be to refer Siobhan to the drugs and alcohol services (**answer E**); this is ranked below A and D as you should explore your concern first to ensure a referral is appropriate. Asking the nurse to increase the frequency of observation is not necessary as Siobhan is now alert (**answer C**) and therefore it is ranked low. However, the least appropriate option would be **answer B**. Siobhan is now alert and therefore you cannot justify testing her urine for opiate use without discussing your concerns with her first. Of course, if she was still unresponsive then you could test for opiate use with a view to reversing its effect.

Ideal order	Your rank choice				
	1st	2nd	3rd	4th	5th
A	4	3	2	1	0
D	3	4	3	2	1
E	2	3	4	3	2
C	1	2	3	4	3
B	0	1	2	3	4

A179. This question is assessing your willingness to make yourself available to Mrs Lewis in order to provide her with continuity of care. Therefore, the most appropriate option is **answer A**. The next most appropriate option is **answer D**. This attempts to appease Mrs Lewis whilst balancing your clinical commitment to her. If you are unable to assist with Mrs Lewis then you should explain this in person (**answer C**). Discussing Mrs Lewis's request with your registrar is unlikely to add any value to this scenario as you are either willing to oversee Mrs Lewis or you're not (**answer E**). Finally, the least appropriate option would be to refuse Mrs Lewis's request (**answer B**). It is important to attempt to provide continuity of care as it reduces the risk of errors and enhances the patient's experience during admission.

Ideal order	Your rank choice				
	1st	**2nd**	**3rd**	**4th**	**5th**
A	4	3	2	1	0
D	3	4	3	2	1
C	2	3	4	3	2
E	1	2	3	4	3
B	0	1	2	3	4

A180. This question is assessing your ability to work jointly with your patient about their care. In this scenario, Elsie is non-compliant with her anti-epileptic medication and consequently has been admitted with life-threatening status epilepticus. Your aim as her doctor is to attempt to educate and support her to manage her epilepsy. It is important not to act judgementally as this will usually cause your patient to withdraw from healthcare even further. Therefore, the most appropriate option is **answer C**. The next most appropriate option is **answer E**; managing complex and chronic medical conditions can be greatly improved with a supportive network of family and friends. The next most appropriate response would be to refer Elsie to an adolescent support group (**answer B**); this is ranked below C and E as you should attempt to explore your concerns before making a referral. It would also be wise to ensure her GP is involved in her epilepsy management (**answer A**). However, this would not alter the immediate concern of non-compliance and is thus ranked second least. Finally, the least appropriate response in this scenario is to criticise Elsie (**answer D**).

Ideal order	Your rank choice				
	1st	**2nd**	**3rd**	**4th**	**5th**
C	4	3	2	1	0
E	3	4	3	2	1
B	2	3	4	3	2
A	1	2	3	4	3
D	0	1	2	3	4

A181. This question relies on your understanding of the different needs a patient may have (i.e. Mr Higgins's urgent need to be discharged) and your ability to prioritise this. In this scenario Mr Higgins has a non-medical need but as his doctor you should still make an attempt to accommodate this. Another senior member of the team will be able to assess Mr Higgins's suitability for discharge (**answer D**). The next most appropriate option would be to call your registrar and discuss Mr Higgins over the telephone (**answer A**). With sufficient information (e.g. planned discharge date, patient's observations, recent blood tests, outpatient follow-up, etc.) they would be able to make an informed decision. If you are unable to arrange for Mr Higgins to be discharged then you must inform him that there will be a delay. In this scenario it would be advisable for him to contact his mother to discuss her appointment (**answer B**). Ultimately, if you are unable to accommodate a patient's request it is advisable to apologise (**answer E**). The least appropriate option would involve agreeing to discharge Mr Higgins without discussing it first (**answer C**). Remember: FY1s do not discharge patients.

Ideal order	Your rank choice				
	1st	2nd	3rd	4th	5th
D	4	3	2	1	0
A	3	4	3	2	1
B	2	3	4	3	2
E	1	2	3	4	3
C	0	1	2	3	4

A182. This question is assessing your willingness to prioritise meeting Mrs Leeming to discuss her husband's current admission. Although you have mandatory teaching, it is important that Mrs Leeming is given an update when she arrives at hospital as her husband is very unwell and has been admitted to CCU. However, as you are due in a teaching session it would be courteous to explain the situation to the trainer. Therefore, the most appropriate option is **answer C**. The next most appropriate option would be **answer D**. This is ranked below answer C as it shows no consideration to your teaching session. Arranging for another doctor to meet with Mrs Leeming is an option but is not ideal as they wouldn't be able to provide as much information about the patient as you would (**answer A**). However, at least Mrs Leeming would have some information. The next most appropriate option is **answer B**. Asking Mrs Leeming to wait for up to 2 hours to have an update about her critically unwell husband displays a lack of empathy or compassion, and therefore this option is ranked below C, D and A. However, the least appropriate option would be refusing to speak with Mrs Leeming this afternoon and recommending she visits tomorrow when the consultant is available (**answer E**).

Ideal order	Your rank choice				
	1st	2nd	3rd	4th	5th
C	4	3	2	1	0
D	3	4	3	2	1
A	2	3	4	3	2
B	1	2	3	4	3
E	0	1	2	3	4

A183. This question is assessing your ability to gain trust from patients. In this scenario you suspect Miss White is a victim of domestic abuse and therefore your approach needs to be sensitive and tactful in order to convince Miss White that you are trying to help her. The most appropriate option is **answer B**. She may acknowledge your concerns and allow you to offer her help. The next most appropriate option is **answer A**; this is ranked below B because, although reassuring Miss White may increase her trust in you, it doesn't attempt to resolve the issue. In this scenario it would be important to explore Miss White's social network (e.g. mother, sister, friends, colleagues) because in cases of domestic violence the victim often needs many different avenues of support (**answer C**). It would also be important to exclude other potential risks in her social network. Contacting the hospital domestic abuse advisor would be sensible to provide you with assistance, but without Miss White's trust you are unlikely to achieve a positive outcome (**answer E**). However, the least appropriate option in this scenario would be confronting Miss White with a blunt statement (**answer D**). This could cause her to withdraw from any potential help you would try to offer her.

Ideal order	Your rank choice				
	1st	2nd	3rd	4th	5th
B	4	3	2	1	0
A	3	4	3	2	1
C	2	3	4	3	2
E	1	2	3	4	3
D	0	1	2	3	4

A184. This question is assessing your ability to maintain appropriate professional distance from Neil. It is not uncommon to become fond of a patient when you are caring for them for a prolonged period of time. However, there is a fine balance between 'professional fondness' and 'unprofessional attachment', and it is vital that you develop this balance as a junior doctor. In this scenario Neil is clearly fond of you, but it would not be appropriate to develop a friendship with a previous patient. However, you should always be polite and courteous towards patients and so the most appropriate option is **answer D**. The next most appropriate option is **answer B**. This is ranked below answer D as the language used in B is less polite than in D. The next most appropriate option is **answer E**. This is polite, but mentioning guidelines to Neil is likely to seem 'institutional' and impersonal. Discussing a gift from a patient with their consultant is not normally required. However, in this scenario Neil is being treated for a psychiatric disorder and as the gift was a framed photograph of you it would be wise to mention this to his psychiatrist (**answer C**). The least appropriate option would involve visiting Neil socially (**answer A**).

Ideal order	Your rank choice				
	1st	2nd	3rd	4th	5th
D	4	3	2	1	0
B	3	4	3	2	1
E	2	3	4	3	2
C	1	2	3	4	3
A	0	1	2	3	4

A185. This question is based on your ability to prioritise patient safety at all times and take necessary action. In this scenario Mr Patel may be very unwell owing to a cardiac abnormality shown on the ECG and it is important not to ignore what you have recognised. You must review Mr Patel urgently to assess his clinical state (**answer B**) and it would be wise to ask the nursing staff to perform venepuncture simultaneously owing to the potential urgency of this scenario (**answer D**). Finally, you should inform your registrar immediately (as per the escalation ladder) so that he can advise you appropriately (**answer H**).

It is important not to ignore abnormal test results of any nature or assume your senior colleague has noticed and/or acted upon them as this could jeopardise patient safety (**answer A**). However, it is also important not to overreact when a patient is potentially unwell. Arranging urgent angiography based purely on an ECG finding is not appropriate (**answer E**). In this scenario asking your FY1 colleague (**answer C**) is not marked as correct because the SJT assumes all FY1s are equally competent. If you believe the ECG shows ischaemia then your FY1 colleague will too. Therefore this answer is akin to not acting, which is generally not appropriate. This is similar reasoning as to why **answer F** is incorrect. The scenario already states the ECG findings and so a repeated ECG will not provide any additional information that would alter your top three choices. Finally, informing the consultant before discussing the situation with the registrar is inappropriate escalation (**answer G**).

A	B	C	D	E	F	G	H
0	4	0	4	0	0	0	4

A186. This question is based on showing empathy towards Mrs Barrons, who is clearly upset following her diagnosis of cancer. In these situations, the most important action is to provide support for the patient. Therefore it would be appropriate for you to leave the ward round to spend time with Mrs Barrons (**answer G**) and arrange for the specialist nurse to review Mrs Barrons (**answer D**). They will be able to offer a holistic approach to treatment. It would also be appropriate to apologise for the abrupt manner in which the consultant delivered her diagnosis (**answer A**). Often patients can be upset not only by the diagnosis but also by the manner in which it is delivered.

Although the consultant has not acted with the upmost tact, reporting him to the GMC is clearly not necessary (**answer C**). Nor is it appropriate to ignore a patient who is evidently upset to simply continue with your workload (**answer H**). Offering to answer Mrs Barrons's questions may seem correct, but you are not adequately experienced or qualified to lead such a conversation (**answer B**). This should be done by a consultant with the help of a specialist cancer nurse. Finally, offering support by other means, such as a ward nurse (**answer F**) or chaplaincy (**answer E**), is not inappropriate per se, but you should be willing to spend time with a distressed patient yourself.

A	B	C	D	E	F	G	H
4	0	0	4	0	0	4	0

A187. This question is based on your ability to recognise that Mr Robin's needs should be at the centre of this situation and understanding how best to manage his delirium (i.e. his need for bright lighting, family, kindness). This situation does not warrant sedation. As with all scenarios involving a distressed or deteriorating patient, it is important that you review their clinical state (**answer F**). However, you should also familiarise yourself with Mr Robin's case to ensure all that can be done for his delirium is being done (**answer E**). Finally, delirious patients will often respond well to their next of kin and so asking them to visit Mr Robin is appropriate (**answer A**).

Importantly, unless a patient is at actual risk of self-harm and you have tried all non-sedative methods, you should avoid sedating delirious patients (**answer H**). Occasionally soft restraints are required to protect patients from harm, but as you have not yet assessed Mr Robin you would not be in a position to recommend their use (**answer B**). You should never refuse to review an agitated patient (**answer G**). There are many pathologies that may cause agitation on top of delirium (e.g. acute stroke, acute confusional state (ACS)) and this would be missed if you assumed it is simply secondary to delirium. This scenario does not lend itself to requiring security at this stage as no patients or staff members are at risk (**answer C**). Finally, suggesting the staff nurse attempts to calm Mr Robin down is not the correct approach to this situation (**answer D**). They will have already spent much time and effort trying to calm Mr Robin before resorting to calling the on-call doctor.

A	B	C	D	E	F	G	H
4	0	0	0	4	4	0	0

A188. This question is focusing on patient safety (i.e. prescription error) and preventing future recurrences. In this scenario it would be vital to amend the prescription (**answer C**) so that the 'correct' Patricia Brown receives antibiotics as per the indication. However, to prevent future errors occurring whilst both patients remain on the ward it would be wise to ensure that every member of the ward team is conscious of the identical names (**answer G**). This scenario highlights a fault on your ward that needs to be changed. Normally, a ward will have a system to ensure identical patient names are acknowledged (e.g. identical names on admission board written in different colour to other names, or coloured magnets placed next to identical names). To introduce a similar system you would require the cooperation of the nurses and the administrative staff. The simplest way to coordinate this would be to discuss your ideas with the ward manager, who can implement change (**answer E**).

Designing a protocol (**answer B**) would be beneficial only if the ward manager is in agreement with your idea. Therefore, it would be necessary to meet with them first. In this scenario you would complete an incident form owing to the prescription error, but not as an immediate priority (**answer D**). It would be wise to inform the FY1 that a mistake had been made, but this would not be a top three answer (**answer F**). Remember: act now, report later! Calling the night FY1 now is not appropriate either, as they will be post night shift and likely asleep (**answer H**). Finally, discussing this incident with the FY1's educational supervisor is not appropriate (**answer A**). If you are concerned then you should discuss this with your educational supervisor, who can then liaise with the other FY1's educational supervisor if deemed necessary.

A	B	C	D	E	F	G	H
0	0	4	0	4	0	4	0

A189. This question is based on your ability to show a genuine interest in a patient's wellbeing. Although James may be 'medically fit for discharge' with regard to his dislocated shoulder, he may have an unrelated medical problem which should be taken seriously as your approach to patient care should be holistic. In this scenario you would need to gather more information before you can make an assessment. Therefore, it would be sensible to ask the nurse to elaborate on her concerns (**answer C**). You would also need to raise these concerns with James sensitively as any help you can offer James will require his consent (**answer B**). Finally, you should discuss these new concerns with your consultant as it may alter their decision to discharge James (**answer E**).

It is not appropriate to discharge a patient when new concerns have been raised without investigating them (**answer A**). Discussing James's alcohol history with his GP is a sensible approach and would have been the 'fourth' option in this scenario (**answer D**). However, it is possible the GP will have no record of alcohol misuse and so answers B, C and E will address this problem more directly. Referring James to a community alcohol service without discussing your concerns with him first is inappropriate and a waste of your time if James is not willing to interact with services (**answer F**). Delaying James's discharge to review signs of alcohol withdrawal is clinically dangerous. You should not wait for a patient to develop delirium tremens before initiating treatment owing to the risk of seizure (**answer G**). Finally, asking James's GP to monitor his alcohol intake does not address the problem directly and shows a disregard for James's overall health (**answer H**).

A	B	C	D	E	F	G	H
0	4	4	0	4	0	0	0

A190. This question is assessing your understanding that patients have different needs. In this case, Mrs William no longer requires active curative treatment but instead requires compassion and caring to enable a peaceful and painless death – the so-called 'good death'. You would need to have a DNAR form completed urgently so that Mrs William did not have to undergo unnecessary resuscitation (**answer B**). It would also be sensible to prescribe end-of-life medication on the 'as required' side of the drug chart so that Mrs William remains comfortable (**answer G**). Finally, as Mrs William appears to have deteriorated and may pass away shortly it would be appropriate to update her NOK so that they have the option to sit with her when she eventually passes away (**answer D**).

As an FY1 you aren't able to sign the DNAR form yourself (**answer A**). However, you are able to support Mrs William in other ways (answers B and G) and so asking Sarah to liaise directly with the registrar is not appropriate (**answer C**). Escalating Mrs William's care to ITU is completely unacceptable (**answer F**). The consultant responsible for Mrs William has clearly documented the plan and her family is in agreement. There is also no need to call your consultant as an agreed plan is already in place (**answer E**). Finally, you should speak with Mrs William's NOK personally to explain that she has deteriorated. This is not a task that should be delegated to the ward nurses (**answer H**).

A	B	C	D	E	F	G	H
0	4	0	4	0	0	4	0

A191. This question is based on prioritising patient safety at all times. In this scenario, the nurse is concerned that Susy is having an allergic reaction to the antibiotics you prescribed. Your immediate action should be to return to the ward and assess Susy (**answer G**). You should also update her medical notes and drug chart to prevent this happening again (**answer C**). Finally, it is important to be open with patients and their relatives and so you should discuss this incident with Susy and her parents (**answer A**).

Delaying your assessment of Susy is not appropriate (**answer B**). If she is having a true reaction to the penicillin as the nurse suspects she will become very unwell, very quickly. Remember, you should always prioritise patient safety above all else. It is also equally inappropriate to put out a cardiac arrest call when the patient is not in cardiac arrest or peri-arrest (**answer H**). Informing your registrar would be a sensible idea, but not until you have reviewed Susy and corrected her drug chart. Therefore **answer F** is not in the top three choices. It is important that you do not ever destroy medical documentation. Adding Susy's allergy status to her medical notes and drug chart can be done without destroying the current chart and therefore **answer E** is not correct. Finally, the nurse has acted correctly by bleeping you and, although a set of observations may assist you, this can be done as you're making your way to the ward. Do not chastise nurses for calling you about unwell patients (**answer D**).

A	B	C	D	E	F	G	H
4	0	4	0	0	0	4	0

A192. This question is assessing your ability to instil confidence in Mrs Harris regarding her current consultant, Mr Carey. As with any grievance or complaint, there is often an element of miscommunication or misunderstanding. Therefore your initial action would be to explain that Mr Carey is fully informed about her progress (**answer B**). This may alleviate Mrs Harris's anxieties. It would also be sensible to ensure that Mrs Harris has not developed any new clinical concerns (**answer A**) before discussing this issue with Mr Carey himself (**answer D**).

It would not be appropriate to tell Mrs Harris that Mr Carey will review her tomorrow before speaking to him first (**answer C**). Nor would it be advisable to corroborate Mrs Harris's views on your consultant's ward round technique (**answer F**). However, if Mrs Harris did pursue her complaint then you should advise her to liaise with the PALS (**answer G**). This answer is incorrect in this scenario as you haven't yet attempted to address her concerns (e.g. answers B, A and D). It is unlikely that the ward matron would be willing or able to influence the consultant ward round (**answer E**). Finally, you should always avoid dismissing a patient's concerns even if they are unfounded. Remember, a good junior doctor will explore a patient's ideas, concerns and expectations. Therefore **answer H** is not correct.

A	B	C	D	E	F	G	H
4	4	0	4	0	0	0	0

A193. This question is based on your consideration for Ivanov's different needs (e.g. alcohol addiction) compared with his pure medical needs. Your actions should be based around raising your concerns (**answer B**) with Ivanov and reassuring him that you are willing to help him with his addiction (**answer H**). Finally, if you discover a patient has additional problems you must inform your consultant so that they can make appropriate decisions about the patient's care (**answer D**).

Directly asking Ivanov if he is drinking when he leaves the ward (**answer C**) or telling him he will not be treated if his behaviour continues (**answer A**) are both confrontational approaches and may result in his withdrawing from help. It is also not appropriate to change a patient's antibiotic without your consultant's agreement, especially as the reasoning is to allow Ivanov to leave hospital (**answer G**). It is sensible to discuss your concerns with an advisory agency, but at this stage in the scenario you haven't attempted to discuss your concerns with Ivanov, which you should attempt to do first. Therefore **answer F** is not correct. Finally, telling Ivanov that you cannot review him unless he is at his bedside will not prevent him leaving the ward once the ward round has finished. Therefore **answer E** is not a sustainable solution.

A	B	C	D	E	F	G	H
0	4	0	4	0	0	0	4

A194. This question is focused on the different beliefs that patients may have. In this scenario, Mr Xiou does not believe in Western medicine and is unwilling to be treated by you. However, in his attempt to express his non-belief in Western medicine he has now become abusive. Therefore you should clearly explain that this type of behaviour will not be accepted (**answer A**). You should also explore his concerns regarding treatment in an attempt to come to an agreement (**answer G**). Ultimately, if a patient has capacity to make this decision then you cannot force a treatment plan. Therefore, you would need to assess Mr Xiou's capacity (**answer F**).

Currently, Mr Xiou has not committed a crime or been physically aggressive towards staff members and so calling police (**answer C**) and security (**answer B**) are not warranted. Furthermore, you should avoid sedating a patient unless every non-pharmaceutical attempt to calm them down has been tried. Therefore **answer D** is not appropriate at this stage. It is sensible to ensure that the other patients have not been upset by Mr Xiou's behaviour (**answer E**) but as this doesn't attempt to resolve the immediate issue it is not a top three answer. Finally, asking Mr Xiou to leave the hospital is not appropriate (**answer H**). He has been admitted with a serious condition that can be life-threatening and every effort should be made to calm Mr Xiou down and to work with him to find an agreeable treatment plan.

A	B	C	D	E	F	G	H
4	0	0	0	0	4	4	0

A195. This question is assessing your ability to show compassion and empathy towards Mr Archer's family and your willingness to spend time with them following his death. Initially you should offer to spend some time with Mr Archer's NOK as they may have questions that you can assist with (**answer A**). However, if you are going to do this then try to arrange for your bleep to be diverted so that you are not disturbed (**answer D**). Finally, the death of a loved one can be very confusing and obviously upsetting so offering other services (e.g. chaplaincy) can provide additional support (**answer G**).

This scenario is not focusing on Mr Archer's management and there is no indication that he was mismanaged and so confirming whether the furosemide was started is not necessary (**answer E**). Furthermore, asking the registrar whether you could have done anything else is sensible as it helps you learn, but can be done once Mr Archer's NOK have left (**answer B**). Asking the ward nurse to sit with Mr Archer's NOK (**answer C**) and returning to your job immediately (**answer H**) demonstrates a lack of willingness on your behalf to spend time with relatives. Finally, although it is important to try to transfer your bleep, with your registrar's approval, it is not acceptable to simply turn off your bleeper as you are still on call and may be needed urgently (**answer F**).

A	B	C	D	E	F	G	H
4	0	0	4	0	0	4	0

A196. This question is based on maintaining patient safety at all times (i.e. delayed transfusion of urgent blood products). Your concern in this scenario should be the wellbeing of Mrs Sweeny. Therefore it would be appropriate to review her to ensure she hasn't deteriorated as she has not received your treatment plan (**answer B**). You also need to expedite the transfusion so you should liaise with Peter to ensure the transfusion actually starts (**answer H**). However, this is an important lesson regarding handover and so in future you should hand over only in person to minimise errors (**answer F**).

Prescribing iron tablets will not replace Mrs Sweeny's haemoglobin and is not recommended (**answer C**). Nor does Peter require reporting to the ward manager without speaking to him first. There may be a legitimate reason for the delay (**answer A**). Completing an audit (**answer E**) and discussing protocol use (**answer D**) are both sensible actions to take in the future but they do not protect Mrs Sweeny immediately, which is the basis of this question. Finally, informing Mrs Sweeny's consultant about this incident is recommended, but only once you ensure Mrs Sweeny is out of any immediate danger (**answer G**). Therefore answer G would have been a good 'fourth' choice in this scenario.

A	B	C	D	E	F	G	H
0	4	0	0	0	4	0	4

A197. This question is focusing on the different background and beliefs a patient may have, in this case a Jehovah's Witness's belief regarding blood products. This is a common theme in ethical questions, but it is important that doctors have an understanding of different cultures. Put simply, if a patient has capacity to make decisions regarding their health, then they can choose to refuse a blood transfusion – irrespective of the reasons behind their decision. Therefore your role would be to support them as best you can with other means (**answer H**). However, by exploring Noah's belief and explaining the differences between blood products he may realise that there are certain treatments he can accept (**answer G**). Finally, most hospitals will have an advisor for Jehovah's Witnesses and discussing your concerns with them may allow you to help Noah (**answer D**).

There is no indication in this scenario that Noah lacks capacity. Therefore giving him a treatment against his wishes would be a criminal offence. Therefore **answers B** and **C** are inappropriate. Your role as a doctor is to advise your patients accurately and clearly; therefore it is not appropriate to scare your patient (**answer F**) or attempt to change their views (**answer E**). Finally, offering to call Noah's NOK does not attempt to resolve the current issue and therefore it is not a 'top three' option (**answer A**).

A	B	C	D	E	F	G	H
0	0	0	4	0	0	4	4

A198. This question is assessing your ability to work jointly with patients about their care, in this case insulin use in a diabetic patient. Liam's diabetes control is clearly poor and your aim should be to attempt to improve this. You should discuss your concerns with Liam and explore his understating and belief about his diabetes (**answer F**). This may reveal a misunderstanding or a problem, which you can try to solve. In a department that has a nurse specialist they are often best utilised for this type of patient (**answer B**), as they are able to spend longer with the patient than you may be able to and will normally be able to provide community support (e.g. community nursing, support groups). Finally, it would also be wise to arrange a family meeting so that Liam has support to help him manage his diabetes (**answer D**).

Appearing judgemental to Liam will only make him feel ostracised further and this should be avoided (**answer C**). It is also important to remember that, as Liam is 19, you would need to seek his permission before discussing his diabetes with his parents. Therefore **answer G** is not appropriate. Whilst you are discussing your concerns with Liam (e.g. answer F) you would be able to assess his understanding of the risks of poor compliance, and therefore **answer H** is not a correct option. Remember: if two options are similar they are not usually both correct.

There is no evidence that Liam is being abused by his parents and so a safeguarding referral is not required (**answer A**). Finally, although insulin is occasionally stopped in patients at high risk of hypoglycaemia (e.g. the elderly, patients with memory impairment), discussing this option with your consultant is not appropriate as Liam is young and requires insulin (**answer E**).

A	B	C	D	E	F	G	H
0	4	0	4	0	4	0	0

A199. This question is assessing your ability to show compassion towards Mrs Dudley's daughter following her mother's deterioration and palliation. In this situation, you should agree to speak with the daughter and sensitively answer any questions she may have (**answer H**). However, before you do this it would be a sensible idea to arrange for the palliative nurse specialist to join you to provide added support (**answer E**). Finally, this type of conversation should occur in a quiet, peaceful room where you are unlikely to be disturbed, such as the relatives' room (**answer A**).

It is not appropriate to have this conversation at Mrs Dudley's bedside (**answer D**). Nor should you refuse to speak to Mrs Dudley's daughter (**answer B** and **answer F**). Asking the staff nurse to speak with the daughter demonstrates an unwillingness to spend time with relatives during difficult circumstances and is not correct (**answer C**). Finally, there is no indication in the scenario that Mrs Dudley is not comfortable and so your priority would be speaking with her daughter. Therefore **answer G** is not correct.

A	B	C	D	E	F	G	H
4	0	0	0	4	0	0	4

A200. This question is assessing your willingness to spend time with relatives. Although you may be busy, it is still important to spend time with relatives. In this scenario, you would need to gain Mr Couldridge's permission before disclosing his medical information (**answer H**). It would also be sensible to refresh your memory as to why Mr Couldridge was admitted (**answer E**) before you spoke with his relative. Finally, as with any patient-related conversation, it should be done in the relatives' room (**answer D**).

Any discussion you have with a patient or their relatives should be documented clearly in the patient's medical notes and so **answer B** is sensible, but would be the 'fourth' option in this scenario as H, E and D take priority. Disclosing Mr Couldridge's medical information without his consent is not appropriate as it is a breach of patient confidentiality (**answer A**). Asking the staff nurse to speak with Mr Couldridge and his relative (**answer C**), or refusing owing to being too busy (**answer F**), demonstrates an unwillingness to spend time with relatives and so both are incorrect. However, if you genuinely cannot meet with a relative you should attempt to explain the reason, and importantly arrange a time when you are available to meet with them. In this scenario, you are able to discuss Mr Couldridge's admission and therefore **answer G** is not required and so incorrect.

A	B	C	D	E	F	G	H
0	0	0	4	4	0	0	4

8. Domain 5 – working effectively as part of a team

The significance of being able to work effectively as a team is one of the most important attributes as an FY1 and has been demonstrated to improve patient care. There are four key areas of effective teamwork that can be assessed within domain 5 of the SJT:

1. Ability to work effectively as part of a multidisciplinary team (MDT)
2. Demonstrating your ability to encourage an open, collaborative and respectful environment where the views of all members of the team are taken into consideration
3. Delegating tasks appropriately between members of the team and offering assistance or advice, where possible, to other members of the team
4. Understanding team roles and your own position within the team.

Overall, the role of the ward FY1 is rarely medical. Remember, you are in foundation training to develop your clinical understanding of medicine. However, a vital skill that the FY1 should possess is the ability to maintain harmony within their team, and to coordinate the administration of daily tasks. Understanding this role and your responsibilities within the team can seem daunting. However, this is an important self-analysis to undertake as it will allow you to recognise the roles of other team members. This understanding will enable you to identify the most appropriate member of the team for each specific task. This will help you to develop and maintain rapport with members of your team and to work effectively together.

During your time as a foundation doctor it may seem that as the junior member of the team you do not have valid contributions. This is not the case. It is important to be able to demonstrate that you can support other members of your team, both clinically and non-clinically if the need arises. You should be willing to offer assistance to your team, but also to the overall workload in general. If given the opportunity, make sure that you give sound advice and value the advice others give you. There may be occasions where you will be expected to show leadership and effective delegation. These opportunities should not be shied away from. It is important that all members of the team are flexible in their roles, allowing the team to develop an effective and dynamic approach to providing care on the ward.

Finally, no member of the team is too big or too small to take direction from others. Be open and willing to learn from your colleagues, but also to share your knowledge and experience when necessary. Remember, successful teamwork is fundamental to providing good clinical care to patients.

The following practice questions have been developed to provide an opportunity for you to demonstrate how to deal correctly with these topics. Remember, it is what you **should** do, not what you **would** do!

Q201. You are the FY1 on the acute medical assessment unit. You have just seen Mr Stevenson who has been admitted with a chest infection. Your consultant advises oral antibiotics, physiotherapy assessment and discharge home. Chloe, the ward physiotherapist, tells you that Mr Stevenson has passed his functional assessment and is fit to be discharged. However, she is concerned that your consultant has overlooked the patient's mild confusion and wonders if we should be investigating him further for dementia.

Rank in order the following actions in response to this situation (1 = most appropriate; 5 = least appropriate):

A. Explain to Chloe that you will add a request for Mr Stevenson's GP to investigate his confusion.

B. Tell Chloe that she should stick to physiotherapy and leave medicine to doctors.

C. Tell Mr Stevenson that you will delay his discharge and request a confusion screen.

D. Review Mr Stevenson to ascertain whether he has additional medical needs.

E. Discuss Chloe's concerns with the consultant.

> What are the components of a successful MDT?

Q202. You have started your final rotation as an FY1 in care of the elderly medicine. You are surprised to discover a rather old-fashioned firm where Dr Michaels, the consultant, demands that all members of the medical team are present on the ward round for each patient. He also shows little regard for the nurses and therapists when discharge planning. This has made your role very difficult as you find you are having to liaise with other healthcare professionals to ensure the patient is safely discharged. You ask your SHO what they think of Dr Michaels and they tell you it is easier not to try to change the ward as you're here for only 4 months.

Rank in order the following actions in response to this situation (1 = most appropriate; 5 = least appropriate):

A. Ignore what the SHO has told you and make a formal complaint about Dr Michaels.

B. Arrange for a weekly MDT meeting to be started so that all members of the team can discuss patient care.

C. Discuss your concerns with your registrar.

D. Agree with your SHO and try to work with Dr Michaels.

E. Ask the ward manager whether they could arrange for a member of each ward team to be present at the daily board round.

Q203. You have been allocated to urology for your surgical FY1 placement. You have been working for 3 weeks now and realise you have a fairly easy rotation. You generally have less than 10 patients per day to care for and never have to work past 4 pm. You have been able to assist in theatre several times and are happy with your development. Your colleague Ben works on the same ward covering endocrine surgical patients. He is often much busier than you and is frequently still working when you leave at 4 pm. He has mentioned that he really wishes he could occasionally assist in theatre too as he is hoping to apply for core surgical training after his foundation training. Today you have come into work and have even fewer patients than usual as your consultants have been on leave at a conference last week. Ben appears to be busy as usual.

Rank in order the following actions in response to this situation (1 = most appropriate; 5 = least appropriate):

A. Suggest that Ben speaks with his educational supervisor about the disparity in surgical firms.

B. Tell Ben that he can ask for your help on other days too if he is busy.

C. Go to the doctors' mess and have a break as you have completed your immediate tasks.

D. Stay on your ward but offer to assist Ben only if his patients are very unwell.

E. Offer to assist Ben with his workload today.

Q204. You are on call in the adult assessment unit (AAU) today. You have been asked to clerk Mr Peters, a 76-year-old man, who has presented with chest pain and shortness of breath. He has a previous history of ischaemic heart disease and you are worried that this may be acute coronary syndrome (ACS). After you finish clerking Mr Peters you ask one of the nurses to carry out an ECG and to take routine bloods including those for suspected ACS. The nurse asks whether you want to give initial ACS treatment protocol, but you want to wait until the ACS blood tests have been processed. Your SHO overhears your plan and interrupts explaining that this presentation is very likely to be ACS and you shouldn't wait for the blood tests to be processed before giving initial ACS treatment protocol as per trust protocol.

Rank in order the following actions in response to this situation (1 = most appropriate; 5 = least appropriate):

A. Discuss your concerns about being undermined with the on-call registrar.

B. Follow the SHO's advice but explain that you are not happy to be undermined in front of a colleague.

C. Tell the SHO to mind their own business, as this is your patient.

D. Prescribe the initial ACS protocol and read the trust's ACS protocol so that you are familiar with what to do once the initial protocol has been given.

E. Take the SHO's direction and prescribe the initial ACS protocol. The SHO is more experienced and is trying to help.

Q205. You are working as an FY1 on gastroenterology. You are in your first week and have been asked by one of the nurses to review Mrs Suize, a 37-year-old known alcoholic woman. She has been admitted with severe sepsis and despite active management appears to be worsening. You review Mrs Suize and discover that she is bleeding from her mouth. You review her bloods results and can see that she has severely low platelets and her clotting function is severely deranged. You are worried that she is at risk of spontaneous haemorrhage. You search the trust guidelines for alcoholic management but cannot find any information about low platelets. You ask the nurse what the normal protocol is for these patients, but she explains that she is temporary and doesn't normally work on this ward. You are unsure of what to do.

Rank in order the following actions in response to this situation (1 = most appropriate; 5 = least appropriate):

A. Call the on-call haematologist and ask for their advice about alcoholic platelet derangement.

B. Repeat Mrs Suize's blood tests and review her in the afternoon once you have confirmed her results.

C. Ask the nurse to monitor Mrs Suize more closely and bleep you if her observations deteriorate.

D. Call your registrar and ask for advice.

E. Give a platelet transfusion as this should improve her low platelet count.

> What is the correct escalation order?

Q206. You have been working together with your SHO Jessica for 3 months. One month ago Jessica explained that her mother had been diagnosed with breast cancer. She seemed to be coping well over the last few weeks and her mother was doing well from all accounts. This morning Jessica is quieter than normal and seems down. You notice that when she returns from the toilet she looks like she has been crying. She doesn't mention anything at the time and you felt awkward asking whether anything is the matter. Throughout the day you try to engage her in conversation but Jessica is uninterested and distant. You have FY1 teaching at lunchtime so aren't able to speak to Jessica. When you return from teaching Jessica is sitting in the doctor's office crying.

Rank in order the following actions in response to this situation (1 = most appropriate; 5 = least appropriate):

A. Give Jessica some tissues and explain that you'll work from the nurses' station for as long as she needs.

B. Do not enter the doctor's office, as you do not want to disturb Jessica.

C. Suggest to Jessica that she should go home, as she is not able to work while she is upset.

D. Ask Jessica if she'd like to take a break and you'll cover her on the ward.

E. Make Jessica a tea and ask if she'd like to talk about what is upsetting her. You'll cover her on the ward if she'd rather be alone.

Q207. You are working on a very busy medical ward. It is only you and the SHO working today; however, you have been allocated a final-year medical student, Yani, for this week. You finish the ward round at 1 pm and have a long list of jobs to complete. You are worried that you will not finish by 5.30 pm. You need to leave work on time this evening as you have agreed to attend an evening lecture about your career path. Your SHO is also keen to leave on time tonight as she is attending the same lecture. The medical student asks whether they can shadow you this afternoon.

Rank in order the following actions in response to this situation (1 = most appropriate; 5 = least appropriate):

A. Bleep your SHO half way through the afternoon to ensure you are both on schedule with your jobs. Redistribute any jobs between yourself and the SHO to equalise each other's job lists.

B. Divide the jobs fairly between you and the SHO. Suggest that the SHO takes the unwell patient reviews and you will take more of the procedural tasks.

C. Ask Yani whether she would mind going to the library and studying this afternoon as you are too busy to offer her any supervision.

D. Ask Yani what skills she is confident with and allocate tasks that involve those to her. Explain that if she experiences any difficulties to find you immediately and you will help her.

E. Leave at 5.30 pm even if you have not completed the tasks because it is important to show commitment to developing your career.

Q208. You are working as an FY1 on a breast and endocrine firm. The ward clerk Deborah takes you to one side and asks for your advice. She explains that this morning when she was showering she noticed a lump in her breast. It wasn't painful and she tells you that she also noticed that the skin around her nipple looked different to normal. Deborah is clearly very upset and worried. She explains that her mother died of breast cancer when she was around the same age as Deborah and asks you if you think it might be cancer. She asks what your advice would be. You are aware that a painless lump with skin changes is a worrying sign and it might very well be cancer.

Rank in order the following actions in response to this situation (1 = most appropriate; 5 = least appropriate):

A. Tell Deborah she has nothing to worry about, as you do not want to upset her further. You're sure she'll visit her GP if she is worried.

B. Tell Deborah that it is not appropriate for her to ask your professional opinion, as you are colleagues. You are not impressed by being put into this compromising position.

C. Explain to Deborah that you cannot comment on whether it might be cancer but she should arrange an appointment with her GP if she is worried.

D. Offer to examine Deborah's breast and arrange urgent imaging.

E. Tell Deborah that what she has described warrants further investigation and she should visit her GP urgently to have this looked into correctly.

Q209. You are working in a large tertiary referral centre for neurology. There are two FY1s, three SHOs and two registrars, Ben and Martin. You have only been working for a few days but it has become clear that there is a personality clash between Ben and Martin. They often disagree with each other's management plans and sometimes they will quibble over which tasks should be delegated to the other members of the team. One of the SHOs, Michelle, is a core medical trainee wishing to become a neurologist. Today Ben has asked whether you would be interested in coming to clinic with him to develop your examination skills. You agree and are looking forward to this afternoon's clinic. Martin finds out that Ben has arranged for you to attend clinic and tells you that this is unacceptable, as Michelle should take priority as her MRCP exams are soon approaching.

Rank in order the following actions in response to this situation (1 = most appropriate; 5 = least appropriate):

A. Tell Martin that on this occasion you are happy to step aside so that Michelle can prepare for her MRCP examination but that you would also like the chance to develop your clinical acumen.

B. Arrange another clinic to go to so that Michelle can attend this afternoon's clinic.

C. Tell Martin that you want to go to clinic and you do not care that Michelle has MRCP examinations coming up.

D. Call Ben and tell him that Martin is trying to swap you and Michelle and you are unhappy about this.

E. Ask Martin whether perhaps you and Michelle could both go to clinic, as the other FY1 and SHOs are on the ward this afternoon.

> How can you maintain harmony in your team?

Q210. Your team has been caring for Mrs Omu for 3 weeks following her recent stroke. She has made a good recovery and she is reaching the stage where she will be declared medically fit and ready for discharge. Occupational therapy and physiotherapy have been working intensively with Mrs Omu and are also happy that she will be ready for discharge shortly. Your consultant has asked for Mrs Omu to be seen in the stroke clinic in 6 weeks' time for a follow-up.

Rank in order the following actions in response to this situation (1 = most appropriate; 5 = least appropriate):

A. Ask Mrs Omu's GP to arrange an outpatient stroke clinic in her discharge summary.

B. Telephone your consultant's secretary and arrange a follow-up appointment in 6 weeks' time.

C. Ensure you have documented this request in Mrs Omu's current medical admission notes. Medical records will see the entry and arrange for the appropriate follow-up.

D. Speak to your ward clerk and ask them to book Mrs Omu into your consultant's clinic in 6 weeks' time.

E. Add this appointment to the follow-up section of your discharge summary. When you send the patient home your ward clerk will see your note and make the appropriate arrangements.

Q211. Katerina and you are both FY1s. You are working together on the respiratory ward. You notice that Katerina is very quiet and doesn't contribute to conversations very often. When she does contribute you usually disagree with her and she often leaves the conversation. You feel that her views are outdated and can't bear to hear them. She is a very conscientious doctor but you do not see yourself becoming anything more than colleagues. Two weeks into this rotation your registrar, Katerina and you are discussing the local election that took place. You are upset because the borough lost its Labour seat and you are worried a Conservative councillor will change the hospital ethos. Katerina begins to explain her view when you ask the registrar what they think. The registrar tells you to show more respect to Katerina and allow her to give her views.

Rank in order the following actions in response to this situation (1 = most appropriate; 5 = least appropriate):

A. Make a conscious effort to allow Katerina to share her views in the future.

B. Explain that you are sorry for seeming disrespectful but you think that Katerina's views are outdated.

C. Tell the registrar that you have work to do and leave the conversation.

D. Apologise to Katerina and ask her what she thinks of the local election.

E. Apologise to Katerina.

Q212. You are on call when you receive a cardiac arrest bleep. You arrive at the patient and a nurse has started chest compressions. You are the only member of the cardiac arrest team to have arrived so far and the nurse is asking you what to do next. You have recently completed your advanced life support (ALS) course but have not had to lead a genuine cardiac arrest. You ask one of the other nurses to bring the cardiac arrest trolley over, at which point the on-call locum SHO turns up. You are initially relieved to see them, as they will take over as leader. However, the SHO seems unsure of what to do and asks where the registrar is. You know you are wasting precious time and are aware that you should have applied the defibrillator by now.

Rank in order the following actions in response to this situation (1 = most appropriate; 5 = least appropriate):

A. Take the lead in the situation. Ask the nurses to apply the defibrillator and ask the SHO to help the nurses with chest compressions.

B. Tell the SHO they must take charge and ask what you should be doing.

C. Continue helping the nurses with chest compressions and wait for the registrar to attend the call. They can then make the decision.

D. Tell the SHO that you think they should apply the defibrillator but you are not taking responsibility for the decision.

E. Ask a nurse to repeat the cardiac arrest call as the registrar has still not arrived.

Q213. You have just started your first rotation as an FY1. You were a conscientious student and spent most of your clinical teaching on the ward. However, you realise that during your time as a student you weren't given much opportunity to work with other healthcare professionals such as physiotherapists or clerical staff. Today your consultant asks you to arrange a follow-up cardiology outpatient appointment for Mrs Skinner. She is due to be discharged tomorrow. Your registrar is on study leave today and you don't want to seem silly by asking your consultant how to do this.

Rank in order the following actions in response to this situation (1 = most appropriate; 5 = least appropriate):

A. Visit the cardiology outpatient clinic and ask the clinic receptionist how you can arrange an outpatient appointment.

B. Ask Mrs Skinner to arrange an appointment with her GP who can refer her to cardiology as an outpatient.

C. Ask the ward clerk whether they would be able to arrange this appointment on your behalf.

D. Ask the ward sister to arrange Mrs Skinner's outpatient cardiology appointment.

E. Call the on-call cardiologist and explain that Mrs Skinner needs to be reviewed. If the cardiologist feels further investigation is needed they can arrange a clinic appointment directly.

Q214. You are the FY1 on gastroenterology. You have come to the end of your first week and are updating the patient notes before the weekend. You recall being told at the beginning of the week that there is an electronic weekend handover to which patients should be uploaded if they require a weekend review. It is 6.30 pm and you have agreed to meet your friends tonight for a catch-up. You have missed the previous two evenings that your friends have met and are very keen to see them. Your registrar is in clinic but has told you that they will come back to the ward before they go home. You are aware that there are two patients that have weekend reviews documented in their notes.

Rank in order the following actions in response to this situation (1 = most appropriate; 5 = least appropriate):

A. Leave now so that you can meet your friends. The nurses will bleep the on-call doctor to review the patients tomorrow.

B. Text your registrar explaining that you have to leave and two patients need to be uploaded to the electronic handover.

C. Leave a note asking your registrar to upload the patients, as they will be returning to the ward anyway.

D. Upload the patient details to the electronic handover.

E. Upload the patient details to the electronic handover and text your friends to explain that you will be late.

Q215. You are working as the FY1 in haematology. You are very interested in haematology and would like to pursue this as your chosen career. You have just returned from a conference where you were given a very interesting talk on new oral anticoagulants (NOAC) guidelines. You are keen for your team to know the new information but when you speak to your SHO about this they tell you that you shouldn't bother as they are really expensive and unlikely to be useful. They prefer warfarin and don't see the benefit of changing.

Rank in order the following actions in response to this situation (1 = most appropriate; 5 = least appropriate):

A. Speak to your consultant and ask whether you can give a short presentation to the team to explain what you have learned from the conference.

B. Photocopy the information you were given about NOAC and leave it in the haematology MDT room for people to read.

C. Update your e-portfolio with your attendance at the conference.

D. Agree with the SHO and ignore what you learned at the conference.

E. Tell the SHO that you think they are being short-sighted as NOAC will replace warfarin in the future and they should work harder to keep up to date with prescribing advice.

Q216. You have been working as an FY1 for 4 months and are enjoying your rotation so far. You have been getting on well with your team and feel that you are developing well as a junior doctor. Your ward is very busy and you often have to work late to complete all your tasks. The SHO on the ward is in a similar position and you have both noticed that your registrar often asks you to complete additional tasks, explaining that it is good development for you both. You are keen to learn and want to develop but you are concerned that your workload is becoming too large. Your SHO does not want to say anything as they feel that it will make the registrar lose respect for you both. This afternoon the registrar has asked whether you would be willing to lead the MDT meeting. You still have four discharge letters to write and are worried that you will not be able to complete all of your tasks on time.

Rank in order the following actions in response to this situation (1 = most appropriate; 5 = least appropriate):

A. Agree to lead the MDT and stay late to complete your other tasks.

B. Ask the SHO whether they would be able to help with your tasks this afternoon so that you can lead the MDT meeting.

C. Tell the registrar that you are too busy to take on any more tasks.

D. Ask the registrar whether they would be able to relieve you of some tasks this afternoon so that you can lead the MDT meeting.

E. Explain to your registrar that you appreciate the effort they are making to develop you, but your workload is too large to cope with.

Q217. You are on call in A&E seeing medical patients. Your colleague Emma is also on call with you. It is very busy and there are seven patients waiting to be seen. Your registrar is allocating patients to you and Emma. You have seen your patient and when you report back to the registrar to find out who needs to be seen next you see them telling Emma that she needs to speed up. Later on that day you see Emma and ask how things are going. She says 'ok' and rushes off to see another patient. The waiting room is filling up and there are more patients to be seen than earlier. You haven't seen Emma for several hours but when you next see her she is arguing with a nurse, which is out of character for Emma.

Rank in order the following actions in response to this situation (1 = most appropriate; 5 = least appropriate):

A. Take Emma to one side and advise her to take a break before seeing another patient.

B. Ignore what you saw as it has nothing to do with you.

C. Offer to help Emma with her tasks.

D. Discuss what you have seen with the on-call registrar.

E. Take Emma aside and ask whether everything is ok. Explain that you are concerned because she normally gets on so well with nurses.

> What are the signs of stress?

Q218. Today is your first day in your new role as an FY1 in cardiology. You have joined the ward round this morning and are working on your tasks. You have been introduced to Grace, your SHO, and David, your registrar. The doctor's office is very small so you have decided to work at the main reception desk computer. You can hear Grace and David laughing and joking with each other. You have finished your urgent tasks and plan to go to lunch.

Rank in order the following actions in response to this situation (1 = most appropriate; 5 = least appropriate):

A. Go to the canteen and meet your FY1 colleagues for lunch.

B. Ask Grace and David whether they would like to join you for lunch.

C. Ask Grace and David whether they would like to join you for lunch. Suggest inviting any nurses and therapists that are free to join you too.

D. Tell Grace and David that you are going for lunch and will be back on the ward soon.

E. Suggest to Grace and David that it would be nice to go for an after-work drink.

Q219. You are the FY1 working on orthogeriatrics. You have two registrars, Michelle and Sarah, on your ward. You have been caring for Mr Issac, who was admitted with a fractured neck of femur, over the past week. He has responded well to treatment and is keen to be discharged. Sarah tells you she wants to do further investigations on Mr Issac before he can be discharged. She is worried that we haven't fully investigated the reason Mr Issac fell in the first place. However, Michelle tells you that Mr Issac is medically fit for discharge and should be allowed to go home. You are unsure whether you should listen to Sarah or Michelle.

Rank in order the following actions in response to this situation (1 = most appropriate; 5 = least appropriate):

A. Ask your consultant whether they would be able to offer advice as the registrars cannot agree.

B. Tell Sarah and Michelle that as they cannot decide what is best for Mr Issac you will not become involved.

C. Discuss with both Sarah and Michelle together their differing opinions.

D. Discharge Mr Issac as per Michelle's wishes.

E. Ask Sarah why Mr Issac needs further investigation and ask Michelle why Mr Issac is fit for discharge.

Q220. You are one of the FY1s working in the adult assessment unit (AAU). Sophie, a staff nurse, and James, another FY1, have an argument over the care of one of the patients. They now refuse to work together or communicate with each other when they are on the same shift. This has made working on AAU very awkward. More importantly, you are worried that this will compromise patient safety.

Rank in order the following actions in response to this situation (1 = most appropriate; 5 = least appropriate):

A. Arrange a work night out and invite them both so that they can make up.

B. Act as a communication aid between Sophie and James to ensure patient safety.

C. Arrange a meeting with your educational supervisor so that you can discuss your concerns and ask for advice.

D. Report Sophie and James to human resources.

E. Take Sophie and James aside separately and discuss why they have fallen out. Explain that you are concerned that this may impact on patient care and they should put their differences aside.

Q221. You are working on the gastroenterology ward. Yesterday one of your patients, Mr Cumming, was diagnosed with bowel cancer. Your consultant explained the diagnosis and immediate plan with him and his wife. Today, Mr Cumming has asked whether you could answer a few questions he has since speaking with the consultant yesterday. You are discussing these questions with him and his family when Tom, an inexperienced nurse, comes to you worrying that a different patient, Mrs Wood, has 'had a funny turn' even though her observations have continued to remain stable. Tom is known for being anxious.

Rank in order the following actions in response to this situation (1 = most appropriate; 5 = least appropriate):

A. Ask one of the senior nurses to review Mrs Wood.

B. Ask Tom to repeat Mrs Wood's observations in 30 minutes and you will review her then.

C. Ignore Tom and continue your discussion with Mr Cumming.

D. Ask Peter, your FY1 colleague, to continue your discussion with Mr Cumming while you review Mrs Wood.

E. Ask Tom to continue your discussion with Mr Cumming while you review Mrs Wood.

> Are you prioritising patient safety?

Q222. You and Jason are both FY1s on the clinical decision unit (CDU). You went to medical school together and are good friends. Jason is normally very outgoing and happy. You have noticed that Jason seems 'low' and is constantly busy. He often finishes late and you have overheard your SHO telling him that he is no good at his job. You are discussing this with Jason over lunch and he tells you that he would prefer to ignore it and not take things further. After all, you have only 2 weeks left on this rotation.

Rank in order the following actions in response to this situation (1 = most appropriate; 5 = least appropriate):

A. Discuss how Jason is managing his workload and offer advice where appropriate.

B. Suggest he should speak to his educational supervisor.

C. Accept his choice and leave things as they are.

D. Tell your SHO that their behaviour could come across as bullying.

E. Tell your SHO's educational supervisor what they said to Jason.

Q223. Julie, a senior nurse on your ward, doesn't get on well with you and refuses to do the jobs that you ask of her. You are not sure what you have done wrong as Julie seems to get on well with your other FY1 colleagues. You are upset by this situation as you always felt that you were polite and professional to Julie. You are worried about raising your concerns as Julie is married to your educational supervisor.

Rank in order the following actions in response to this situation (1 = most appropriate; 5 = least appropriate):

A. Ask Julie to join you in the meeting room and discuss your concerns.

B. Speak to your educational supervisor and tell them you are having difficulties with the nursing team but don't mention any names.

C. Explain the situation to your clinical supervisor and ask what they think you should do.

D. Discuss this matter with your work colleague, Susan, who is also an FY1.

E. Ignore Julie, as it is obviously an issue that she has.

Q224. You and your FY1 colleague Michael are currently on call in A&E. There are several managers in the department and you are being put under pressure to see patients quickly as the hospital is very busy. Last month several patients breached the 4-hour target and the managers are trying to prevent this happening again. You and Michael have been working for over 8 hours without a break. Michael faints in the reception area but regains consciousness after 2 minutes. He isn't injured but is clearly very embarrassed.

Rank in order the following actions in response to this situation (1 = most appropriate; 5 = least appropriate):

A. Ask one of the nurses to help you transfer Michael onto a bed.

B. Give Michael a blanket and a glass of water. Continue to see patients while Michael recovers.

C. Inform the on-call registrar that Michael has fainted and ask if you may both take a break.

D. Ask Michael whether he will be able to continue working.

E. Reassure the patients in the waiting room that they will be seen shortly but you are very busy at the moment.

Q225. You have been working on the cardiology ward for 3 months. Your hospital is the regional heart attack centre and is very busy. You routinely have between 50 and 60 patients under your consultant's care and four junior doctors to complete the daily tasks. It has been snowing heavily overnight and there is widespread disruption to travel. You arrive at work and are told by the ward manager Stephen that two of your colleagues have called to explain that they are unable to make it to work owing to the snow. There have been four new admissions overnight requiring urgent coronary catheterisation by your consultant. He asks you and your FY1 colleague to start the ward round in his absence.

Rank in order the following actions in response to this situation (1 = most appropriate; 5 = least appropriate):

A. Ask the other FY1 to start at the bottom of the list and you'll start at the top of the list. You will eventually meet and discuss tasks that need to be completed.

B. Politely tell your consultant that you do not feel this is appropriate as you and the other FY1 are very inexperienced.

C. Arrange a quick meeting with the other FY1 and Stephen to identify patients who need to be seen first.

D. Tell the consultant you are unwilling to see patients without senior cover.

E. Inform the medical staffing department that you need senior assistance on the ward.

Q226. You and Nick, another FY1, have been working together on the respiratory ward for 3 weeks. Nick is very quiet and seems shy. He is often unwilling to offer any suggestions on the ward round and seems uninterested. When you and Nick are alone he is very knowledgeable and when Nick interacts with patients he has a very caring approach. This morning the consultant tells Nick that he should show more enthusiasm on the ward round. You speak to Nick after the ward round and he is upset by what the consultant has said.

Rank in order the following actions in response to this situation (1 = most appropriate; 5 = least appropriate):

A. Suggest that Nick speaks to his educational supervisor about what happened.

B. Tell Nick that he should be more enthusiastic on the ward round as the consultant is forming the wrong opinion of him so far.

C. Tell Nick that he shouldn't let little things like this bother him. He needs to work with this consultant for only 4 months.

D. Explain to Nick that you think he is very knowledgeable and has a very caring approach towards patients. He should feel confident that he is a good doctor.

E. Ask Nick whether he would like to go for a coffee break so that you can discuss what happened this morning.

Q227. It is August and you have started working as an FY1 for the first time. You were a conscientious student and spent most of your clinical time at medical school shadowing junior doctors. You have been sent your working agreement and can see that your contractual hours are 8.30 am to 5.30 pm. You have been arriving at 8.30 am each morning since you started working but your consultant hasn't been turning up until 9 am. Your ward is very short-staffed and you are the only junior doctor. You were told by the previous FY1 that in this time your responsibility is to update the patient list and prepare the patient notes for the ward round. You live over 60 minutes from the hospital and could benefit from an extra 30 minutes of sleep by turning up at 9 am instead of 8.30 am.

Rank in order the following actions in response to this situation (1 = most appropriate; 5 = least appropriate):

A. Continue to arrive at 8.30 am and use this time to complete your compulsory e-learning modules.

B. Update the patient lists at the end of each day so that you do not need to do this the following morning.

C. Ask your consultant whether they would have any objection to you also coming in at 9 am.

D. Start arriving at 8.55 am so that your consultant doesn't realise any difference.

E. Continue to arrive at 8.30 am and use this time to prepare the daily patient lists and update their medical notes as necessary.

Q228. You are the FY1 on the orthopaedic ward. It is very busy and you are under pressure from the discharge coordinator to maintain high patient turnover. You have been caring for Cheryl who was recently involved in a skiing accident. She has damaged the cruciate ligaments in her knee and is being seen daily by Sharon, the senior physiotherapist on the ward. Cheryl is still unable to weight-bear fully but the discharge coordinator is asking you whether she can be discharged. You tell the discharge coordinator that you will double-check with your consultant and get back to them. You are unable to reach your consultant but their plan in the notes is 'discharge when mobilising'.

Rank in order the following actions in response to this situation (1 = most appropriate; 5 = least appropriate):

A. Call the discharge coordinator and tell them that your consultant has said Cheryl is not fit for discharge.

B. Explain to Sharon that you are being asked to discharge Cheryl and what community services are available.

C. Tell the discharge coordinator that you were unable to contact your consultant.

D. Discharge Cheryl and ask her GP to refer her to community physiotherapy.

E. Ask Sharon how Cheryl is coping and whether she is fit to be discharged.

> Is this patient safe to be discharged?

Q229. You are working on an endocrine ward as an FY1. There are two other junior doctors on your ward, Henry and Sham, who are both FY2s. All three of you were on surgery together in your previous rotation. You had a few minor disagreements with Henry previously and do not get on well with him. Today you are looking after Marie, a 66-year-old woman, who has been admitted to hospital with diabetic ketoacidosis. She is very unwell and you are unsure of how much insulin to give her. You have searched the trust intranet but you cannot find a protocol. You are aware that Henry had a similar case last week and Sham is on call today.

Rank in order the following actions in response to this situation (1 = most appropriate; 5 = least appropriate):

A. Research DKA protocols online and prescribe as per their recommendation.

B. Ask Henry how he treated his patient last week and explain that you would appreciate support with Marie.

C. Give 10 units of insulin and re-assess Marie in 30 minutes.

D. Ask the ward nurse what they are used to seeing prescribed in patients with DKA.

E. Bleep the on-call registrar and ask for their advice.

Q230. You are on call in the CDU. You overhear Mitch, a locum SHO, talking to another SHO about a patient he has clerked. He is unsure of exactly which antibiotic he should be prescribing as he has been working in this hospital for only 3 weeks. The other SHO is unsure too. You are confident that you know which antibiotic should be used as you had FY1 teaching yesterday lunchtime from the chief pharmacist in your hospital. The topic of the teaching session was antibiotic prescribing.

Rank in order the following actions in response to this situation (1 = most appropriate; 5 = least appropriate):

A. Give Mitch the pharmacy extension and suggest that he phone for advice.

B. Politely tell Mitch which antibiotic he should be prescribing.

C. Wait until the SHOs have stopped discussing this case before offering any assistance.

D. Do not say anything because the SHOs will think you are being arrogant.

E. Explain to Mitch that you had teaching on antibiotic prescribing yesterday and ask whether he would like your suggestion.

Q231. You are working on the stroke rehabilitation ward. One of your patients, Judith, has been admitted following a minor stroke. She asks to speak with you and confides that she was not coping at home before the stroke. Now she is worried that she will be even less likely to cope. On this morning's ward round your consultant told Judith she was doing much better and would be able to go home soon. Judith asks you whether there is anything you can do to help.

Rank in order the following actions in response to this situation (1 = most appropriate; 5 = least appropriate):

A. Ask your ward physiotherapist to assess Judith and consider her suitability for being at home.

B. Ask your ward occupational therapist (OT) to assess Judith and consider her suitability for being at home.

C. Ask your registrar to assess Judith and consider her suitability for being at home.

D. Ask your consultant whether Judith's discharge can be delayed until she is feeling more able to cope at home.

E. Ask social services to assess Judith and consider her suitability for being at home.

Q232. You have started working on the intensive therapy unit (ITU) as an FY1 in a supernumerary position. Your working hours are comfortable and you are gaining good practical experience. You have noticed that the ITU nurses seem to have additional skills compared with ward nurses and often suggest decisions to the SHOs looking after the patients. You are sitting in the staffroom when James, one of the SHOs, asks you what you think about the nurses telling doctors what to do. He asks you about one nurse in particular who routinely tells the other nurses that they are really 'in charge' of the patients, not the doctors.

Rank in order the following actions in response to this situation (1 = most appropriate; 5 = least appropriate):

A. Tell James that you can see how it might be frustrating, but it is workplace banter and he shouldn't take it personally.

B. Explain to James that you think it is important for every staff member to have an opinion and feel valued.

C. Discuss James's concerns and suggest he listens to the nurses' opinions. They spend more time with each patient and may notice something he doesn't.

D. Tell James that you are surprised when nurses make suggestions.

E. Tell James that you normally ignore what the nurses tell you because they don't have responsibility for the patient.

Q233. Sarah and you are both FY1s. You are on call today in A&E seeing medical patients who need to be admitted to hospital. The department is very busy and you are both struggling to see patients quickly enough. The on-call registrar has already told you both that you need to be quicker as otherwise the hospital will be fined for having ambulances waiting outside A&E unable to hand over patients. You manage to see patients faster, but Sarah seems to be struggling. She has two patients who have returned from x-ray and she has been asked by the registrar to see another patient who has just arrived. It is several hours into your shift and neither of you has had a break.

Rank in order the following actions in response to this situation (1 = most appropriate; 5 = least appropriate):

A. Speak with Sarah and ask whether there is anything you can help with in between seeing your own patients.

B. Inform the registrar that you and Sarah have not had a break.

C. Bring Sarah a cup of tea and suggest she takes 5 minutes to refocus her thoughts.

D. Ask Sarah whether she would like to work together seeing patients for the rest of the shift.

E. Tell the registrar that you and Sarah are both working as hard as you can and you do not find it helpful being constantly berated.

> Are you at risk of fatigue? Could this lead to a patient error?

Q234. You have been working on the respiratory ward for 6 weeks. The ward is very busy and has its own high-dependency unit for patients on CPAP / BiPAP (continuous positive airway pressure / bilevel positive airway pressure). You often feel the ward is very chaotic and that you are not clear what the plans are for each patient. You feel that this problem is arising because you are not receiving sufficient information from your colleagues in handover. You haven't said anything yet because you were hoping it would improve, but you are worried that you may make a mistake or miss something with a patient because you were not given the correct information. The handover is very haphazard in terms of structure and attendance.

Rank in order the following actions in response to this situation (1 = most appropriate; 5 = least appropriate):

A. Discuss your concerns with the rest of the respiratory team and ask whether anybody has any ideas to improve handover.

B. Ask your educational supervisor for advice on how to resolve your concern.

C. Create a formal handover protocol.

D. Ask more questions during handover to ensure you have sufficient information.

E. At the beginning of your shift ask the senior nurse about your patients and double-check the plan in their notes.

Q235. You are working on the adult assessment unit. You and your consultant see Mrs Bloomsbury. She is a 97-year-old woman who has been admitted because her son is worried that she has been experiencing visual hallucinations. Your consultant diagnoses Charles–Bonnet syndrome and explains to Mrs Bloomsbury that treatment is not required and she can be discharged home. You complete the discharge summary and tell the nurse in charge that she can go. Later that day the ward OT James tells you that he doesn't think Mrs Bloomsbury can go home because she was very 'wobbly' on her feet. She seemed fine when you saw her earlier in the day.

Choose the most suitable **three** options from the following list:

A. Discuss James's concerns and ask whether Mrs Bloomsbury has any further need for therapy input.

B. Acknowledge James's concerns and ask the GP to monitor blood pressure.

C. Inform your consultant about James's concerns.

D. Ask the on-call SHO to assess Mrs Bloomsbury.

E. Ask the staff nurse to assess Mrs Bloomsbury and to let you know whether she has any concerns.

F. Acknowledge James's concerns but discharge Mrs Bloomsbury as your consultant has already made his decision.

G. Re-assess Mrs Bloomsbury.

H. Ask James to re-assess Mrs Bloomsbury later to see whether she is steadier.

Q236. You have been asked to review Mr Isaac on Ward 4A. He was admitted for observation following a fall at home. Mr Isaac is clinically stable and keen to be discharged. You explain that he will be admitted overnight and the consultant will see him in the morning to discuss discharge planning. As you are making your entry into his medical notes you notice that Mr Isaac has had three falls in the past 6 months. When you review the current plan you can see that the medical registrar has written that Mr Isaac is 'independent of all ADLs' as he has been 'witnessed mobilising on the ward'.

Choose the most suitable **three** options from the following list:

A. Complete your entry for this evening noting that Mr Isaac is stable.

B. Speak to the ward nurses and remind them that Mr Isaac has had a fall. He should not be mobilising independently until cleared by occupational therapy/physical therapy (OT/PT).

C. Remind Mr Isaac that if he feels unsteady when mobilising to ask the nurses for assistance.

D. Bleep OT/PT and ask them to add Mr Isaac to their review list.

E. Speak to the ward nurses and ask them whether they have any concerns about Mr Isaac mobilising independently.

F. Tell Mr Isaac not to leave his bed until he has been seen by OT/PT.

G. Make an entry that OT/PT need to assess Mr Isaac owing to his falls history.

H. Bleep OT/PT and ask them whether Mr Isaac is safe to mobilise independently.

Q237. You are the FY1 working on medical care for the elderly. Your team has been caring for Mrs Daley, who was admitted earlier this week with severe sepsis. She has been treated with fluid resuscitation and antibiotics. Your registrar referred Mrs Daley to ITU but they decided that, owing to her co-morbidities, ITU would not be suitable escalation. Today Mrs Daley is doing much worse and appears distressed with her illness. The decision is taken to withdraw active treatment and treat Mrs Daley symptomatically only. Her daughter asks to speak to one of her mother's doctors and your registrar asks you to speak with her.

Choose the most suitable **three** options from the following list:

A. Offer to help your registrar with their tasks so they are free to speak with Mrs Daley's daughter.

B. Remind your registrar that you are only an FY1 and you feel it is unfair to ask you to have this conversation.

C. Tell your registrar that you do not feel this conversation is appropriate for an FY1.

D. Explain to Mrs Daley's daughter that you have been asked to speak to her. Answer her questions as openly as possible.

E. Tell Mrs Daley's daughter that her mother is very unwell and despite treatment she is unlikely to survive.

F. Explain to your registrar that you do not feel this conversation is appropriate for an FY1, but you would like to be involved so that you can learn how to approach this subject.

G. Decline your registrar's request.

H. Ask Mrs Daley's daughter to wait in the relatives' room.

Q238. You have started working on general surgery. The department is very large and also very busy. You frequently work with different doctors and nurses on a daily basis. You do not feel that the ward has a particularly close team spirit as everybody seems to focus on their own work.

You have noticed that you do not know your colleagues' names and everybody just calls you 'doctor' despite introducing yourself on a first-name basis.

Choose the most suitable **three** options from the following list:

A. Organise a social event for your department.

B. Speak to the ward manager and suggest introducing a short meeting at the beginning of each shift to introduce everyone.

C. Make a conscious effort to introduce yourself to other members of the ward staff.

D. Create a social media page so that you can get to know the staff in the department.

E. Speak to the ward manager and suggest introducing a staff picture wall.

F. Arrange to meet with your FY1 colleagues for lunch each day.

G. Make a conscious effort to complete your work quickly so that you can go home.

H. Discuss your concerns and ideas with your educational supervisor.

Q239. You and Alex are both FY1s working on cardiology. Last week Alex was on call on the adult assessment unit. When you see Alex this morning he seems very distant and uninterested in the ward round. You ask him what is the matter and he explains that last week he clerked a patient with hyperkalaemia who was moved to a ward before he was seen by the consultant. Alex was very busy and forgot to have him reviewed. He found out the next day that this patient had a cardiac arrest and did not survive. He has been told that the case will have to go to the Coroner's Court and he is likely to be called to give his statement.

Choose the most suitable **three** options from the following list:

A. Tell Alex that you're sure everything will be fine and he should concentrate on work as a distraction.

B. Ask Alex whether he thinks it is a good idea being at work after such a serious mistake.

C. Tell Alex that everyone ends up in the Coroner's Court at some point and he shouldn't let it worry him.

D. Tell Alex that you're sure everything will be fine but maybe he should avoid seeing ill patients for the time being.

E. Test Alex on the treatment for hyperkalaemia.

F. Take Alex to the doctor's office and offer to make him a hot drink. Tell him you will finish the ward round.

G. Advise Alex to speak to his clinical supervisor.

H. Ask Alex whether he would like to talk more about what happened after work.

Q240. You are on call on the acute medical intake in A&E. You are not busy and there are currently no patients waiting to be seen. You and your registrar go to the canteen for a coffee and when you return to A&E there are still no patients waiting to be seen. You have been on call for the past 5 days and are appreciative of the quiet morning. You bump into Jasmine in the corridor. She is the on-call SHO covering the medical wards. You ask her how things are on the wards and she tells you she is very busy with three ill patients requiring medical review.

Choose the most suitable **three** options from the following list:

A. Tell Jasmine it is busy in A&E and wish her luck with the rest of her shift.

B. Tell Jasmine to bleep the on-call registrar to discuss extra support.

C. Ask Jasmine whether she would like your help.

D. Tell Jasmine that she can give the ward nurses your bleep for the next hour so that she can make progress with her job list.

E. Empathise with Jasmine agreeing that ward cover is always busy.

F. Speak to your registrar. Explain the situation on the wards and ask whether they would mind you helping.

G. Offer to buy Jasmine a coffee so that she can have a quick break.

H. Ask Jasmine if she would like your help to review one of the sick patients. If she still needs help later you can reconvene to divide jobs.

Q241. You are the FY1 on the respiratory ward. Dan, a final year medical student, is being mentored by your SHO. Dan has been asked to take blood from a patient and you overhear him asking the nurses to help. They tell him they are too busy and he should ask the SHO supervising him for help. Dan asks you whether you have seen the SHO and you tell him he has gone to the mortuary to complete a death certificate and may be some time.

Choose the most suitable **three** options from the following list:

A. Ask the ward sister to take the patient's blood as Dan has been unsuccessful.

B. Offer to go with Dan and help him take blood from the patient.

C. Share your experience with Dan and give him some tips for taking blood. Tell him to get you if he is still unable to perform the blood test.

D. Tell Dan to bleep the SHO and ask whether the bloods are definitely needed.

E. Offer to teach Dan about important blood results that he will need to be confident with as an FY1.

F. Carry on with your tasks as you are not responsible for Dan.

G. Tell Dan to wait until the SHO has returned and ask him to help him.

H. Tell Dan that he should keep trying because as an FY1 you will be expected to be competent at taking blood.

> What are your duties towards medical students in accordance with *Good Medical Practice*?

Q242. You are an academic FY1 in a tertiary referral centre. You are working in virology with an esteemed team and are very happy to have this post. You have been asked by your academic supervisor to prepare an introductory piece of work discussing the benefits of a new method of viral polymerase chain reaction (PCR) technology. You are keen to impress your supervisor but are struggling to find the time to do this work as you are still on your clinical rotation and aren't due to start your academic post for 8 months. Your recent meeting with your clinical supervisor did not go well as you have missed several important clinical tasks owing to focusing on your academic project. You are worried that you may have taken on too much.

Choose the most suitable **three** options from the following list:

A. Tell your clinical supervisor that you will make an effort to improve but your academic post is very important to you.

B. Postpone your initial piece of work until you start your academic rotation.

C. Ask your clinical supervisor if you could be excused from clinical tasks so that you can develop your academic work.

D. Discuss your concerns with your academic supervisor. Explain that you have other commitments currently with your clinical post.

E. Ask your housemate Michael, another FY1, if he can help with your clinical commitments for the time being.

F. Ignore your last clinical meeting as your next one will be better.

G. Discuss your concerns with your clinical supervisor.

H. Carry on balancing your workload as it will benefit your career.

Q243. You are working in a busy district general hospital. You normally have a daily consultant ward round. Dr Andrews, your consultant, told you yesterday that, owing to a hospital management meeting, he would be unable to attend the ward until the afternoon. He has asked you to do a ward round in his absence but he will be available to discuss any concerns you have. Your registrar is at a conference today and unable to help on the ward. You have just seen Mr Patel who seems very confused today. You are unsure of what the cause might be.

Choose the most suitable **three** options from the following list:

A. Ask the nurses to increase the frequency of Mr Patel's observations and inform you if anything changes.

B. Wait for Dr Andrews to return to the ward in the afternoon and discuss your concerns about Mr Patel.

C. Ask the nurse to put out a cardiac arrest call.

D. Complete the remainder of the ward round.

E. Send Mr Patel for an urgent MRI scan in case.

F. Attempt to call Dr Andrews on his mobile telephone and update him about Mr Patel.

G. Ask the senior nurse what they think you should do.

H. Call the on-call registrar and ask for assistance with Mr Patel.

Q244. You are on call in A&E. You have been seeing Mr Franklin, a 78-year-old man, who is complaining of abdominal pain. You believe he is suffering from acute diverticulitis and are aware that an urgent abdominal CT scan and erect CXR should be ordered. You order these investigations and report to the on-call registrar to discuss your plan. They tell you that the history sounds more likely to be irritable bowel syndrome (IBS) and that you should cancel the abdominal CT scan.

Choose the most suitable **three** options from the following list:

A. Ask the on-call consultant to review the patient because you and the registrar have had a difference of opinion.

B. Document your conversation with the registrar in Mr Franklin's medical notes.

C. Continue with your plan as Mr Franklin is your patient.

D. Revise the investigation and management of IBS.

E. Cancel the abdominal CT scan.

F. Ask Mr Franklin to come back tomorrow, when a different registrar will be on call.

G. Cancel the abdominal CT scan documenting that you do not agree with the decision.

H. Cancel the abdominal CT scan and tell Mr Franklin that you didn't agree with the registrar's opinion.

Q245. You have been asked to help with a teaching session for the medical students attached to your hospital. The session has been organised by two SHOs and involves clinical scenarios in small groups of medical students. You arrive at the teaching venue and neither SHO is there. The medical students have turned up and are asking you what they should do.

Choose the most suitable **three** options from the following list:

A. Attempt to call the SHOs.

B. Ask the medical students to make tea or coffee whilst you arrange the session.

C. Explain that you will only be able to supervise one group of students so the rest will have to leave.

D. Separate the medical students into small groups and ask them to discuss the scenarios as planned.

E. Send a text message to the SHOs.

F. Apologise to the medical students and explain that you will have to cancel the session as the SHOs aren't here.

G. Ask the medical students to wait 30 minutes and see whether the SHOs turn up.

H. Tell the medical students that as the SHOs haven't arrived you aren't able to run the session.

Q246. You are currently working on general surgery with Miriam, another FY1. You have been working together for 6 weeks when she asks if you would be willing to swap your on-call shift with her. She explains that there is a religious holiday approaching that she would like to celebrate. You do not support religion and were hoping to take leave the week Miriam is asking you to swap. However, you are yet to submit your leave request.

Choose the most suitable **three** options from the following list:

A. Tell Miriam that you will not swap your shift as you were planning on taking leave.

B. Show interest by enquiring as to what the celebration involves.

C. Agree to swap with Miriam.

D. Suggest Miriam asks another FY1.

E. Explain that you do not support religion and are unwilling to swap on call because of religious holidays.

F. Ask Miriam how she can believe in religion as a doctor.

G. Confirm a future swap date with Miriam so that you can take your planned leave.

H. Apologise to Miriam but explain that you do not think it is fair that you should have to re-arrange your leave so that she can take religious leave.

Q247. You are working on the gastroenterology ward with Charles, another FY1. You have known him since medical school and are aware that his mother recently passed away from complications of alcoholic liver disease. This morning Miss Lerbort has been admitted with decompensated liver cirrhosis. Your consultant explains that there is nothing that the team can do and she is informed that she is likely to pass away in the near future. Over the next 2 days she deteriorates rapidly and passes away. Charles is clearly upset but tells you that he will be fine. You notice this morning that Charles is quieter than normal and has made several mistakes during the ward round.

Choose the most suitable **three** options from the following list:

A. Take Charles into the doctor's office and discuss your concerns with him. Tell him you will cover his patients on the ward today and he should go home.

B. Discuss your concerns with your consultant explaining the relevance of Miss Lerbort passing away.

C. Suggest Charles speaks to his educational supervisor.

D. Tell Charles to snap out of it. Miss Lerbort was an alcoholic and probably expected to die early.

E. Tell your consultant that Charles should be sent home. He is only likely to delay your work today anyway.

F. Report Charles to the GMC as you don't think he is fit to practice.

G. Tell your SHO that Charles should be moved to another ward owing to his mother dying of a gastroenterology disease.

H. Ask Charles if he would like to go to the pub after work to discuss what has happened.

Q248. You are the FY1 working in the endocrine and diabetes team. The ward is very busy and the team is quite large. There are three other FY1s, two FY2s, four core medical trainees and two registrars. There are also two nurse consultants who specialise in diabetes management. You have been seeing Henry, a 17-year-old patient with insulin-controlled diabetes. This is his third admission this year owing to poor compliance with his insulin. One of SHOs is cross that the consultant has asked a nurse specialist to review Henry instead of a doctor. The SHO doesn't think the nurse specialist is sufficiently trained to deal with complicated patients.

Choose the most suitable **three** options from the following list:

A. Discuss the pros and cons of working with the nurse specialists.

B. Tell the SHO that they are being childish and their only focus should be patient care.

C. Advise the SHO to complain to the consultant.

D. Suggest the SHO tells the nurse specialists what they think about their role.

E. Listen to the SHO's concerns.

F. Review Henry once the nurse specialist has finished.

G. Suggest the SHO spends some time with the nurse specialists to see the benefit of their time with each patient.

H. Ignore the SHO.

> Is the SHO demonstrating an understanding of the role of nurse specialists?

Q249. You are the FY1 working in trauma and orthopaedics. The ward is very busy and the team is quite small. There are no other FY1s and only one core surgical trainee and one registrar. Alex, a final-year medical student, has been allocated to your firm for 4 weeks. He seems very competent and is very enthusiastic. He is hoping to become an orthopaedic surgeon in the future. Today your consultant has a complicated procedure to complete and needs both the registrar and core trainee to assist. You are very busy as several patients are due to go home today.

Choose the most suitable **three** options from the following list:

A. Ask Alex to help with blood taking and preparing discharge summaries.

B. Call the consultant and ask whether the core trainee could be released to help with the ward tasks.

C. Arrange a quick meeting with the senior nurse and explain that you are very busy. Politely ask her what tasks the nurses would be able to help with.

D. Work through the list, but accept that jobs may be left over until tomorrow.

E. Ask Alex to use today as a study day because you are too busy to supervise him safely.

F. Compile a clear list of today's tasks.

G. Ask Alex to briefly summarise the medical notes of any patients that need to be seen today while you work through the job list.

H. Cancel patient discharges to ease your workload.

Q250. You are on call and have been bleeped by James, a staff nurse on Cedar Ward. He has asked you to assess the DNAR status of Mr Peters, an 88-year-old man with palliative metastatic lung cancer. James tells you that the consultant ward round confirmed that Mr Peters is not for resuscitation but there was no DNAR form available at the time. You can see in the medical notes that the ward round entry from the consultant this morning mentions Mr Peters is 'not for escalation of care', but does not specifically mention DNAR. When you briefly assess Mr Peters he is unresponsive but appears comfortable. You acknowledge that he is likely to pass away shortly.

Choose the most suitable **three** options from the following list:

A. Sign a DNAR form.

B. Call the on-call registrar and explain the situation. Ask them to assess Mr Peters and to sign a DNAR form if they agree.

C. Ask James to speak to the ward clerk tomorrow ensuring there are DNAR forms available in the future.

D. Call the patient's NOK and inform them of his current medical state.

E. Call the consultant and ask whether they meant DNAR instead of 'not for escalation'.

F. Call the ITU registrar and ask them to assess Mr Peters as he is unresponsive and currently for resuscitation.

G. Tell James that you will not sign the DNAR form, as the consultant has not made it clear in the medical notes.

H. Ask James to bleep the on-call SHO.

ANSWERS

A201. This question is focusing on your ability to work effectively within a multidisciplinary team. In this scenario, a colleague has raised a concern about a patient's wellbeing. Other members of the MDT will often spend longer with the patient each day during therapy sessions than you will as a doctor. Therefore, it is highly likely that they may notice a subtle problem (e.g. cognitive impairment) that may not have been detected within your short ward round exposure. In this case it would be wise to re-assess the patient yourself to confirm whether there is any cognitive impairment (**answer D**). The next most appropriate action would be to discuss Chloe's concerns with the consultant (**answer E**), who may already be aware of the patient's cognitive impairment or may suggest additional investigations once made aware of this new concern. As this concern does not relate to an immediate risk to the patient, a sensible approach at this point would be to acknowledge Chloe's opinion and ask the patient's GP to investigate any cognitive impairment in the community (**answer A**). Delaying Mr Stevenson's discharge to carry out a confusion screen in a non-acute onset is inappropriate (**answer C**); the patient's GP is more than qualified and experienced to investigate this concern. **Answer B** is clearly the least appropriate answer; this attitude is completely unacceptable and will lead to patient harm if you discourage an open and multidisciplinary working environment.

Ideal order	Your rank choice				
	1st	2nd	3rd	4th	5th
D	4	3	2	1	0
E	3	4	3	2	1
A	2	3	4	3	2
C	1	2	3	4	3
B	0	1	2	3	4

A202. This question is assessing your ability to demonstrate your willingness to encourage an open, collaborative and respectful environment where the views of all members of the team are taken into consideration. The most effective method of maintaining an MDT approach to patient care is to have a structured forum for MDT members to meet and discuss their concerns, usually as a weekly MDT meeting. To implement this change as an FY1 you would benefit from the support of your seniors. Therefore, the most appropriate action would be to discuss this with your registrar (**answer C**). The next most appropriate choice would be to arrange a weekly MDT meeting (**answer B**). If you do not have the support for a weekly MDT meeting then the next most appropriate option would be to encourage MDT attendance at the daily board meeting (**answer E**). This will allow for a brief discussion of each patient and will include the medical, therapist and social needs of the patient. Agreeing with your SHO is a poor choice (**answer D**). This would be seen as ignoring the problem and highlights your inability to have conviction about your concerns.

However, the least appropriate action would be to complain formally. Dr Michaels has not acted in such a way as to warrant a formal grievance (**answer A**).

Ideal order	Your rank choice				
	1st	2nd	3rd	4th	5th
C	4	3	2	1	0
B	3	4	3	2	1
E	2	3	4	3	2
D	1	2	3	4	3
A	0	1	2	3	4

A203. This question is focusing on your ability to offer assistance with a colleague's workload. In this scenario it is clear that Ben is overworked whilst you are underworked. This is not uncommon if a ward is shared, as your workload will depend greatly on which type of patients are admitted to your ward. The most appropriate choice in this scenario would be to offer to help Ben with his immediate workload (**answer E**). However, you should also tell Ben that he can ask for your help whenever he is busy (**answer B**). It is important to recognise that your colleague is struggling and offer assistance when necessary. In this situation it may be advisable for Ben to discuss his concerns with his educational supervisor. This may lead to additional support being arranged for future placements or even additional support currently. Therefore, the next most appropriate choice would be to advise Ben speaks with his educational supervisor (**answer A**). Staying on the ward and offering to help Ben only if one of his patients becomes ill is a poor attempt at offering assistance. Perhaps his patient wouldn't become unwell if he had more time to monitor them because you are helping with other routine tasks. However, **answer D** is more appropriate than **answer C**, which shows no regard for your colleague and is therefore the least appropriate option in this scenario. You should always endeavour to support your colleagues as you yourself would like to be supported.

Ideal order	Your rank choice				
	1st	2nd	3rd	4th	5th
E	4	3	2	1	0
B	3	4	3	2	1
A	2	3	4	3	2
D	1	2	3	4	3
C	0	1	2	3	4

A204. This question is focusing on your ability to take direction from other team members, a vital skill in effective teamwork. In this scenario, the SHO has recommended a different plan to your own. Remember, although you are a valued member of the team as an FY1, the SHO does have more experience in medicine and you should be open to their direction. Therefore, the most appropriate choice would be **answer D** as this demonstrates you are open to direction but also enables you to learn from this situation by familiarising yourself fully with the ACS protocol. The next most appropriate choice would be **answer E**. However, this does not indicate an attempt to better your practice, unlike D. **Answer B** is the next most appropriate choice as this still follows the SHO's direction. However, chastising the SHO for attempting to help is not an advisable approach. Discussing this situation with the registrar (**answer A**) or being rude to the SHO (**answer C**) are both inappropriate choices. The SHO has correctly altered your management plan and didn't undermine you and so discussing this with the registrar is unlikely to make any difference. The nurse is likely to be in agreement with the SHO as she was already querying your management plan.

Ideal order	Your rank choice				
	1st	2nd	3rd	4th	5th
D	4	3	2	1	0
E	3	4	3	2	1
B	2	3	4	3	2
A	1	2	3	4	3
C	0	1	2	3	4

A205. This question is focusing on your ability to seek advice appropriately. You are clearly out of your depth and are unsure how to proceed. This is not uncommon in FY1 and you should seek advice immediately. Therefore the most appropriate choice is **answer D**. Your registrar will be experienced in gastroenterology and will be able to give you the most appropriate advice initially (always remember the escalation ladder). Your next point of call should be the on-call haematologist (**answer A**), who will be able to give you generic advice about the deranged blood results and importantly what may be wrong with Mrs Suize. The next most appropriate choice would be to closely monitor the patient (**answer C**). Repeating Mrs Suize's blood tests and arranging to review her in the afternoon (**answer B**) is not a safe approach. You already know her blood tests are deranged and the nurse has told you that she is getting clinically worse. This answer is similar to 'watching and waiting' – an approach that is rarely correct in SJT questions. If a patient is unwell you need to take immediate action and blood tests are rarely wrong; therefore in this situation there would be little benefit in repeating them.

However, the least appropriate choice (and most dangerous action) would be to transfuse a patient when you are unsure how to do so (**answer E**).

Ideal order	Your rank choice				
	1st	2nd	3rd	4th	5th
D	4	3	2	1	0
A	3	4	3	2	1
C	2	3	4	3	2
B	1	2	3	4	3
E	0	1	2	3	4

A206. This question is focusing on your ability to provide non-medical support to your colleagues. In this scenario, Jessica is clearly upset by something and the decent approach to take would be to allow Jessica to talk about it if she wishes (**answer E**). The next most appropriate choice would be to explain that you will cover the ward, allowing Jessica to leave and take a break (**answer D**). Jessica may just need a short break to compose herself and this would enable her to do so. However, something is clearly wrong and Jessica has been upset all day. She may not be fit to work as she may not be in the right frame of mind. Therefore, the next most appropriate choice would be to suggest she goes home sick (**answer C**). Sick leave does not refer simply to a physical illness. Offering Jessica a box of tissues and explaining that you will give her as long as she needs is not very compassionate (**answer A**); she should be given the opportunity to talk about what has upset her. If she'd rather be alone that is fine too, but it should not be on the ward where she may be disturbed. Finally, the least appropriate choice is to shy away from Jessica and offer no assistance (**answer B**). Doctors should feel comfortable talking to other people, be it patients or colleagues, when they are upset. You can provide an open and non-judgemental shoulder for that person to cry on, whether figuratively or literally. This is a vital element of any successful team and should be encouraged.

Ideal order	Your rank choice				
	1st	2nd	3rd	4th	5th
E	4	3	2	1	0
D	3	4	3	2	1
C	2	3	4	3	2
A	1	2	3	4	3
B	0	1	2	3	4

A207. This question is assessing your ability to delegate and share tasks effectively. In this scenario, you and the SHO will have to work closely to ensure effective teamwork and, more importantly, effective task delegation. The most appropriate action here is to divide your jobs fairly between you and the SHO, taking into consideration the SHO's greater experience (**answer B**). The next most appropriate option would be **answer D**; medical students do have skills that you can maximise whilst providing an opportunity for them to develop confidence and a feeling of autonomy. As a final-year student, Yani is likely to be competent in simple skills such as venepuncture, cannulation and writing discharge summaries. Therefore you should view a medical student as an added member of the team with a certain skill set – not a burden that requires your constant supervision. However, an important caveat is to explain you are freely contactable to help if the student has any difficulties. The next most appropriate choice is **answer A**. Do not be afraid to reconvene, re-evaluate jobs and redistribute outstanding jobs as necessary. Asking Yani to revise for the afternoon is a poor choice (**answer C**). She has been allocated to your firm to learn clinical medicine and should be given that opportunity. If you feel burdened by your medical students then you are viewing them incorrectly. However, the least appropriate choice is **answer E**. Patient safety must always be your priority.

Ideal order	Your rank choice				
	1st	2nd	3rd	4th	5th
B	4	3	2	1	0
D	3	4	3	2	1
A	2	3	4	3	2
C	1	2	3	4	3
E	0	1	2	3	4

A208. This question is focusing on your willingness to provide advice to your colleague. You are clearly worried about breast cancer and you are obliged to give appropriate medical advice even though Deborah is not one of your patients. The most appropriate action would be for Deborah to visit her GP for referral to an urgent one-stop breast lump clinic (**answer E**). You are clearly suspicious that this lump may be malignant, but you may not wish to comment either way (**answer C**); advising Deborah to visit her GP if she is worried is a suitable approach, although it may not impose the appropriate urgency, unlike E. Examining Deborah's breast may not seem like the next most appropriate choice. However, you are a doctor on a breast firm and she is requesting your medical advice (**answer D**). If Deborah consents and you have a chaperone as per any other patient this is the next most appropriate action in this scenario as answers B and A below are both inappropriate. Chastising Deborah for seeking your advice (**answer B**) is not appropriate; you should aim to encourage an open and supportive working environment and your colleagues may wish to seek your advice from time to time. However, clearly the least appropriate choice would be to give Deborah unsafe advice / false hope (**answer A**).

Ideal order	Your rank choice				
	1st	2nd	3rd	4th	5th
E	4	3	2	1	0
C	3	4	3	2	1
D	2	3	4	3	2
B	1	2	3	4	3
A	0	1	2	3	4

A209. This question is focusing on your ability to maintain harmony within your team. In this scenario, Ben and Martin would probably take this as another opportunity to disagree with each other. Michelle does have an important examination coming up, but at the same time you do deserve the opportunity to develop. An enviable skill to develop when part of a large team is the ability to diffuse situations and allay developing conflicts. **Answer A** diffuses the immediate situation as Ben and Martin would have no need to argue. You've kindly stepped aside showing that you are a keen team player but subtly telling Martin that you will be seeking these opportunities too. This is a mature attempt to maintain team harmony. The next most appropriate action would be to simply re-arrange your clinic attendance (**answer B**). This would solve the conflict but does lend itself towards you being overlooked by Martin again in the future. Asking if you and Michelle can attend clinic together is a suitable approach at this point, but it may put you back at square one if Martin says no (**answer E**); therefore this choice is less appropriate than A and B. Calling Ben is likely to cause further conflict between him and Martin and would be an undesirable choice (**answer D**). Remember, if you can select an answer that resolves conflict locally that is better than an answer that may lead to escalation. However, the least appropriate choice is **answer C**, as this would cause conflict between yourself and Martin, which is not currently where the problem centres.

Ideal order	Your rank choice				
	1st	2nd	3rd	4th	5th
A	4	3	2	1	0
B	3	4	3	2	1
E	2	3	4	3	2
D	1	2	3	4	3
C	0	1	2	3	4

A210. This question assesses your ability to identify the most appropriate member of the team to complete the task at hand. In this scenario, you are attempting to book a follow-up outpatient appointment, which is the role of the ward clerk. In most circumstances the ward clerk will process patient discharge summaries and would see follow-up requests made. However, to ensure that you have a good working relationship with your ward clerk, it would be best to speak with them in person to make this arrangement (**answer D**). You should still include this information on your discharge summary so that the ward clerk will also see a written request (**answer E**); this will prevent any miscommunication from occurring. If you do not have a ward clerk, or they are unable to make the appointment, you should call the consultant's secretary directly (**answer B**). Asking the GP to make a follow-up appointment is not the usual process (**answer A**). You are relying on the GP receiving the discharge summary in a timely fashion and also on the GP having access to specific outpatient clinics. However, the least appropriate option is to simply document in the current medical notes (**answer C**). Medical notes are not routinely screened by secretarial staff and this type of request would be easily omitted.

Ideal order	Your rank choice				
	1st	2nd	3rd	4th	5th
D	4	3	2	1	0
E	3	4	3	2	1
B	2	3	4	3	2
A	1	2	3	4	3
C	0	1	2	3	4

A211. This question focuses on showing respect for your colleagues. In this scenario you are clearly not showing the due respect that Katerina deserves by constantly dismissing her views and, on this occasion, speaking over her. The most appropriate action is clearly to apologise. However, you should also encourage Katerina to share her views (**answer D**). You may feel that her views are outdated but she has just as much right as you do to share her thoughts. The next most appropriate choice is to simply apologise (**answer E**). In order to maintain effective teamwork and a harmonious relationship you should also make a conscious effort to encourage Katerina in future conversations (**answer A**). It is unlikely that you will always see eye-to-eye with every single colleague and so you must develop a professional demeanour whilst at work and show your colleagues due respect. In this scenario, the next most appropriate choice would be to leave the conversation (**answer C**) because the least appropriate choice would be to criticise a colleague's opinion openly (**answer B**). At this point there is nothing to indicate that Katerina's views are inappropriate and warrant challenging (unlike the bigoted views covered in domain 1).

You simply do not agree with them and therefore Katerina has an equal right to her views as you do to yours.

Ideal order	Your rank choice				
	1st	2nd	3rd	4th	5th
D	4	3	2	1	0
E	3	4	3	2	1
A	2	3	4	3	2
C	1	2	3	4	3
B	0	1	2	3	4

A212. This question is focusing on your ability to adapt your role within the team and become the leader. You have recently passed your ALS course and are now certified to run this exact scenario. It may seem daunting, especially if a more senior colleague is in attendance, but an important skill is identifying that, whilst you are not the senior member of the team, you may be the most suitable for that role (e.g. the locum SHO may not have a current ALS certificate). The most appropriate choice is to take charge and begin necessary management (**answer A**). The next most appropriate action would be to repeat the cardiac arrest call, as you still need more support and will not be able to do much more without it (**answer E**). This is one of the rare occasions where repeating an action in the SJT is ranked highly – attempting ALS without the appropriate team is futile; therefore you must try to assemble the rest of the cardiac arrest team. Continuing chest compressions while you wait for the registrar (**answer C**) is the next most appropriate choice, as it will do less harm than the SHO potentially acting incorrectly (**answer B**). However, giving advice to the SHO is the least appropriate choice in this scenario as they are clearly not competent (**answer D**). You must take the lead if the patient has any chance of surviving in this scenario, and understanding your role within a team is a vital skill to develop.

Ideal order	Your rank choice				
	1st	2nd	3rd	4th	5th
A	4	3	2	1	0
E	3	4	3	2	1
C	2	3	4	3	2
B	1	2	3	4	3
D	0	1	2	3	4

A213. This question is assessing your understanding of the responsibilities of other members of the MDT. In this scenario, the ward clerk would be the most appropriate member of the team with whom to liaise (**answer C**). Their responsibilities include arranging follow-up appointments, maintaining patient medical notes, arranging transport for patient discharges and coordinating the administration of the ward. The next most appropriate action would be for you to visit cardiology yourself (**answer A**). However, remember as an FY1 you will be very busy and needlessly visiting other departments will soon take a toll on your workload. If this can be avoided by asking other members of your team then it is best to do so. The next most appropriate decision would be to ask the ward sister (**answer D**). Although they will not arrange the appointment directly, they will be aware of overall tasks that are outstanding on the ward. Therefore they will be able to liaise with the appropriate member of the team (i.e. the ward clerk) to ensure all tasks are completed. Asking the patient to visit their GP to arrange an outpatient appointment is a suitable choice if the outpatient appointment is unrelated to their admission. However, in this scenario your consultant has requested a follow-up appointment be arranged for Mrs Skinner and therefore this should be done before she is discharged (**answer B**). However, the least appropriate choice is **answer E**. Asking an on-call doctor to review your patient in the hope that they will alter your consultant's decision and therefore rid you of a task is not appropriate – especially as the main reason for doing so is because you are unsure of how to carry out said task.

Ideal order	Your rank choice				
	1st	2nd	3rd	4th	5th
C	4	3	2	1	0
A	3	4	3	2	1
D	2	3	4	3	2
B	1	2	3	4	3
E	0	1	2	3	4

A214. This question is focusing on your understanding of your responsibilities in the team as an FY1. The FY1 is responsible for administering clinical tasks. This will include updating the ward list daily, ordering blood tests, ordering scans and handing over patient reviews (this may be in person or electronically). Therefore, in this scenario it is your responsibility to ensure that the two patients requiring weekend review are uploaded to the electronic handover. If you have another event to attend, your priority must be completing your clinical responsibilities first; however, a text message to inform your friends is sensible (**answer E**). This is more appropriate than simply completing the electronic handover without informing your friends (**answer D**). Your registrar will not take kindly to having to complete your tasks. However, if you are going to leave then you must ensure your registrar is aware. A text message (**answer B**) is far more reliable than a note (**answer C**). The least appropriate choice is **answer A,** as you cannot rely on another member of the team noticing your request from the day before.

Ideal order	Your rank choice				
	1st	2nd	3rd	4th	5th
E	4	3	2	1	0
D	3	4	3	2	1
B	2	3	4	3	2
C	1	2	3	4	3
A	0	1	2	3	4

A215. This question is focusing on your ability to share your knowledge with all members of the team, including senior members. In this scenario, you have been given new information about a drug class that may benefit patient care. A successful team will be willing and able to learn from all of its members. Therefore you should persist and arrange to give a small talk on what you have learned from the conference (**answer A**). The next most appropriate choice would be to leave copies of the conference literature in the MDT room, allowing team members to read it in their own time (**answer B**); however, the risk with this strategy is that nobody will read the information. In this scenario, the next most appropriate option would be to update your e-portfolio (**answer C**); this is an important aspect of your career development and evidence is important when applying for roles later in your career. The next option is unnecessarily confrontational (**answer E**) and so less appropriate than updating your e-portfolio. The SHO may be short-sighted but telling him to work harder is likely to lead to friction. Finally, the least appropriate option is to agree with the SHO (**answer D**) as you have a responsibility to share new knowledge with the team.

Ideal order	Your rank choice				
	1st	2nd	3rd	4th	5th
A	4	3	2	1	0
B	3	4	3	2	1
C	2	3	4	3	2
E	1	2	3	4	3
D	0	1	2	3	4

A216. This question is focusing on your willingness to make others aware of your workload whilst also balancing your career development. The most appropriate choice would be first to see whether your registrar can help with your workload (**answer D**). This would allow you to attend the MDT meeting for your development whilst also demonstrating that your workload is too large without assistance. Failing this, the next most appropriate choice would be **answer E**. You (and the SHO) are clearly very busy and have large workloads. It is not practical for the SHO to take on any of your tasks and so explaining to the registrar that you appreciate their effort but simply do not have time is the correct action. **Answer C** is the next most appropriate choice. Your workload is too large to take on any additional tasks. The final two choices are both poor options as neither you nor the SHO can handle any more tasks. However, asking the SHO to take on your workload so that you may attend a meeting is not acceptable in this situation. Therefore the next most appropriate choice is to stay late yourself in order to develop your own career (**answer A**). The least appropriate option is **answer B** as the SHO is clearly not in a position either to take on additional tasks.

Ideal order	Your rank choice				
	1st	2nd	3rd	4th	5th
D	4	3	2	1	0
E	3	4	3	2	1
C	2	3	4	3	2
A	1	2	3	4	3
B	0	1	2	3	4

A217. This question focuses on recognising that your colleague, Emma, is struggling to cope with the pressure of a busy on-call shift. Feeling overwhelmed or under pressure will often result in behaviour out of character for an individual. In this case you see Emma arguing with a fellow colleague. The most appropriate action is to take Emma to one side and explain your concerns (**answer E**). This will give Emma an opportunity to talk to somebody and may relieve some of her stress. You may also be able to offer her advice on how you cope with busy shifts. Following this, offering to assist with Emma's workload (**answer C**) is the next best option. Clearly Emma could benefit from some help during this busy shift and a key skill for foundation doctors is willingness to offer advice and / or assistance when necessary. Advising Emma to take a break (**answer A**) is only a temporary solution, but may be all it takes for her to regain composure and continue with the remainder of her shift. Informing the on-call registrar (**answer D**) may be necessary if the above three options are not viable, as Emma does need support; however, discussing your concerns with the registrar would not be your priority. Finally, the least appropriate choice would be **answer B**. It is completely inappropriate to ignore your concerns over Emma. Both the patients and Emma are likely to be adversely affected by this situation.

Ideal order	Your rank choice				
	1st	2nd	3rd	4th	5th
E	4	3	2	1	0
C	3	4	3	2	1
A	2	3	4	3	2
D	1	2	3	4	3
B	0	1	2	3	4

A218. This question is assessing your willingness to attempt to build rapport and establish relationships. You are new to cardiology and it is clear that Grace and David get on well. It can seem overwhelming to join a new team, but it is important that you are able to build rapport with colleagues and develop your professional relationships. In this scenario, the most appropriate choice would be to encourage a team lunch (**answer C**). This would allow you to get to know the team and vice versa. Remember: the better a team knows each other the better they will work together. Inviting Grace and David for lunch will still develop rapport between the three of you, but is a suboptimal choice in this scenario, as this would not allow you to get to know the other members of your MDT (**answer B**). Although an after-work social event may seem like a good idea, many people will have evening commitments or differing shift patterns that prevent them from attending (**answer E**). Therefore this option is less appropriate than getting to know your colleagues over lunch. Going for lunch without your colleagues is not advisable when you start a new rotation, as it may seem unfriendly (**answer D**). Although it can seem reassuring to have lunch with the other FY1s, this will not encourage you to develop a good working relationship with your colleagues (**answer A**). Try to avoid this comfort blanket when you join a new team.

Ideal order	Your rank choice				
	1st	2nd	3rd	4th	5th
C	4	3	2	1	0
B	3	4	3	2	1
E	2	3	4	3	2
D	1	2	3	4	3
A	0	1	2	3	4

A219. This question identifies conflict resolution between healthcare professionals (Sarah and Michelle) and focuses on your ability to maintain harmony. The best course of action in these situations is to discuss the conflict openly without being seen to take sides. Therefore the most appropriate option is **answer C**. If this is not possible you could attempt to diffuse the situation by individually seeking each side of the argument so that you fully understand each request (**answer E**). If Sarah and Michelle are unable to agree with a management plan you would have no choice but to escalate this conflict to your consultant as they will be able to make the final decision (**answer A**). Refusing to become involved in patient care (**answer B**) is neither practical nor acceptable as a doctor; you have a responsibility for Mr Issac and your aim should be to resolve the conflict between Sarah and Michelle in order to ensure the best outcome for the patient. However, the least appropriate action would be to discharge Mr Issac (**answer D**) – a conflict has been discovered and so it would be inappropriate to act according to the wishes of either party involved as there may be a problem with this plan. You would require a non-biased intermediary to help (e.g. consultant).

Ideal order	Your rank choice				
	1st	2nd	3rd	4th	5th
C	4	3	2	1	0
E	3	4	3	2	1
A	2	3	4	3	2
B	1	2	3	4	3
D	0	1	2	3	4

A220. This question focuses on your ability to resolve professional conflict between Sophie and James. As this is likely to be an inflamed situation, the best approach would be to discuss your concerns separately with both Sophie and James (**answer E**). Seeking advice in these situations is often wise. In this scenario, discussing your concerns with your educational supervisor is the next most appropriate choice. Your educational supervisor is normally free from possible bias and will be able to give you advice confidentially (**answer C**). The next most appropriate action would be to report your concerns to human resources (**answer D**). Although this may seem like a drastic step to take, you are concerned that patients are at risk and are left with no option. Acting as a communication aide between Sophie and James (**answer B**) is not professional or sustainable, and is ranked fourth for these reasons. Finally, the least appropriate answer is to attempt to arrange a social event in the hope that James and Sophie will 'make up' (**answer A**). Sophie and James are both professionals and should be able to put their differences aside to ensure good patient care. If this is not the case then a social event is unlikely to resolve the issue.

Ideal order	Your rank choice				
	1st	2nd	3rd	4th	5th
E	4	3	2	1	0
C	3	4	3	2	1
D	2	3	4	3	2
B	1	2	3	4	3
A	0	1	2	3	4

A221. This question is focusing on your ability to value the opinions of your colleagues and listen to their concerns. Tom is clearly concerned about his patient and, although he may be known for being anxious, it is still important that you value his opinion and act accordingly. In this scenario, the most appropriate action would be to listen to Tom's concerns and assess his patient promptly. However, you still have to consider Mr Cumming and so asking your colleague to continue your discussion is acceptable (**answer D**). The next most appropriate choice would be **answer A**. A senior nurse will have ample experience to assess an unwell patient and advise you as necessary. This will allow you to continue your discussion with Mr Cumming while showing Tom that you value his opinion. **Answer B** would be the next most appropriate option, as it attempts to prioritise Mr Cumming without dismissing Tom's concerns. Asking Tom to continue your discussion with Mr Cumming is not appropriate (**answer E**); as he is inexperienced it is unlikely that he will be able to answer Mr Cumming's questions and provide sufficient information about his cancer diagnosis. Finally, the least appropriate choice would be ignoring Tom and dismissing his concerns (**answer C**). This is unprofessional and unlikely to develop a safe, welcoming and collaborative working environment.

Ideal order	Your rank choice				
	1st	2nd	3rd	4th	5th
D	4	3	2	1	0
A	3	4	3	2	1
B	2	3	4	3	2
E	1	2	3	4	3
C	0	1	2	3	4

A222. This question is assessing your ability to identify that Jason is struggling with his current rotation. Your initial action should involve discussing your concerns with Jason directly and offering support (**answer A**). This will allow Jason to confide in you whilst providing practical advice to improve Jason's experience on this rotation. Following this, your next most appropriate option would be to advise Jason to seek advice from his educational supervisor (**answer B**). Remember, whenever you face a confrontational situation it is better to advise the individual as if you are involved, rather than to actually become involved. Therefore, at this point the next most appropriate option is **answer C** as the final two options require you to become involved in the conflict. Confronting the SHO directly (**answer D**) or reporting the SHO to their educational supervisor (**answer E**) is not appropriate. However, D is slightly more appropriate than E as confronting the SHO directly at least attempts to resolve the conflict at a local level.

Ideal order	Your rank choice				
	1st	2nd	3rd	4th	5th
A	4	3	2	1	0
B	3	4	3	2	1
C	2	3	4	3	2
D	1	2	3	4	3
E	0	1	2	3	4

A223. This question is focusing on working effectively with others, in this case Julie. It is clear that, for reasons unbeknown to you, Julie and you do not get on. In these situations the most appropriate action is to discuss your concerns directly with the individual concerned (**answer A**). This scenario does not involve confrontation and therefore attempting to resolve this issue is a good idea. Both parties can express their concerns to each other and work through any difficulties that are discovered. The next most appropriate option would be to discuss this problem with your educational supervisor (**answer C**) who is there to support you and, although it may seem daunting owing to his relationship with Julie, he will be professional and advise you correctly. **Answer B** is your next choice but is less appropriate than C as you should always be open and honest as a doctor. Discussing your concerns with Susan, a fellow FY1, is not appropriate in this scenario as it is likely to be seen as gossiping (**answer D**). There is a clear chain of escalation during your foundation training and if you are having problems with other members of the team you should discuss these with the correct people. However, the least appropriate option is ignoring Julie (**answer E**); even if the problem between you two is completely one-sided you should demonstrate the ability to work together effectively in an MDT.

Ideal order	Your rank choice				
	1st	2nd	3rd	4th	5th
A	4	3	2	1	0
C	3	4	3	2	1
B	2	3	4	3	2
D	1	2	3	4	3
E	0	1	2	3	4

A224. This question is dealing with your management of a colleague in difficulty. In this scenario, Michael has probably fainted as a result of overworking. However, as with any patient, you should ensure that Michael has not suffered any harm and the most appropriate initial treatment would be to move him onto a bed so that he can recover (**answer A**). Following this, you should inform the on-call registrar immediately as you and Michael will be unable to see patients currently whilst you review Michael (**answer C**). However, as Michael has fainted it is likely that you are also overworked and could also benefit from a break. The next most appropriate course of action would be to update the patients in the waiting room (**answer E**). They may have been shocked to see a doctor faint and there will now be a delay as you and Michael take a break. The final two options are both poor choices. Leaving Michael to recover alone demonstrates a lack of compassion and comradery (**answer B**); Michael is likely to welcome a friendly face while he recovers. Finally, ignoring the fact that Michael has fainted and asking whether he can continue working demonstrates no insight (**answer D**). He has fainted as he is overworked and is more likely than not going to feel unable to continue working.

Ideal order	Your rank choice				
	1st	2nd	3rd	4th	5th
A	4	3	2	1	0
C	3	4	3	2	1
E	2	3	4	3	2
B	1	2	3	4	3
D	0	1	2	3	4

A225. This question is based on your ability to adapt your role within the team. In this scenario, owing to the adverse weather you and your FY1 colleague are now the 'senior' doctors on the ward. Your consultant is needed elsewhere and so you need to adapt your role and become the reviewing doctor. The most appropriate option is **answer C** as this prioritises patient safety. The next most appropriate option is **answer A**. This will still result in all the patients being seen and tasks being prioritised based on clinical need. However, this option is ranked second as this may put at risk patients in the middle of the list if they are unwell, as they will be seen last. Requesting senior assistance is definitely advisable (**answer E**) as the next most appropriate option. However, if your ward is short-staffed the chances are other wards will be as well. The next two options are both inappropriate. Although you may be inexperienced as an FY1 you must be adaptable to succeed in medicine. Your consultant will not be expecting you to make difficult decisions, but by seeing the patients you will identify any who are unwell whilst also ensuring that outstanding plans are being completed. In this scenario, **answer B** is ranked fourth as there is an attempt at justifying your reason for not adapting. The least appropriate option is **answer D**; it leaves patients at risk and inflexibility is not helpful in adverse situations.

Ideal order	Your rank choice				
	1st	2nd	3rd	4th	5th
C	4	3	2	1	0
A	3	4	3	2	1
E	2	3	4	3	2
B	1	2	3	4	3
D	0	1	2	3	4

A226. This question is focusing on your ability to support Nick in a non-task-related problem. It may seem that this is not a problem with which you should concern yourself. However, team dynamics are crucial to providing safe patient care. Every team member has a responsibility to support each other emotionally as well as professionally. In this scenario, Nick clearly lacks confidence and this is being reflected in his performance with your consultant. The most appropriate option would be trying to give Nick a confidence boost (**answer D**). The next most appropriate option would be offering to discuss this morning's incident with Nick as he is upset (**answer E**). Nick could benefit from discussing this problem with his educational supervisor (**answer A**). This is ranked third as it wouldn't deal with the immediate incident, unlike D and E. **Answer B** is the next most appropriate option, although it is clearly not helpful, as Nick is likely to be aware that the consultant is forming the wrong opinion following this morning's ward round incident. Finally, the least appropriate option is **answer C**; ignoring problems that arise is never the correct approach.

Ideal order	Your rank choice				
	1st	2nd	3rd	4th	5th
D	4	3	2	1	0
E	3	4	3	2	1
A	2	3	4	3	2
B	1	2	3	4	3
C	0	1	2	3	4

A227. This question is based on your responsibilities as an FY1. Updating the patient list is not an uncommon task for an FY1 and the expectation would be for you to arrive with plenty of time to update it before the consultant starts the ward round. You shouldn't be expected to arrive earlier than your shift, but in this scenario your working day starts at 8.30 am. Therefore the most appropriate option is to continue arriving on time and updating the list daily (**answer E**). The next most appropriate option would be updating the list the previous evening (**answer B**). Unfortunately, this would mean any patient admitted after you have gone home would not appear on the list. Following this, **answer A** is the next most appropriate option. You are contractually (and morally) obliged to attend your place of work from 8.30 am as a minimum. Choosing to work on your e-learning is a noble endeavour, but your time would clearly be better spent on clinical work at this time of the morning. The final two choices are both poor, as you should be willing and able to meet the requirements of your position. However, discussing your working hours with your consultant (**answer C**) shows more integrity than **answer D**, which is clearly the least appropriate option.

Ideal order	Your rank choice				
	1st	2nd	3rd	4th	5th
E	4	3	2	1	0
B	3	4	3	2	1
A	2	3	4	3	2
C	1	2	3	4	3
D	0	1	2	3	4

A228. This question is assessing your understanding of a physiotherapist's role in discharge planning. In this scenario, Cheryl has been declared ready for discharge once she is safely mobilising. The best staff member to assess Cheryl's mobility is the physiotherapist, not the doctor. Therefore, the most appropriate option is **answer E**. The next most appropriate option would be to discuss with Sharon your need to discharge Cheryl (**answer B**). There are many community services available that could be suitable for Cheryl, thus allowing her safe discharge. The third most appropriate action is **answer C**. This is not ranked higher because it does not show any regard for hospital pressures. Although pressure to discharge is irritating it is usually owing to high demand from new admissions, and answers E and B both take Cheryl's safety into consideration and should therefore be attempted first. **Answer A** is the next option. This will remove the pressure from the discharge coordinator whilst Sharon is completing her assessment. However, it is ranked low as lying is not acceptable. Integrity is a key attribute that all doctors must have. However, the least appropriate option would be to discharge Cheryl without physiotherapy agreement (**answer D**) as this may impair Cheryl's recovery.

Ideal order	Your rank choice				
	1st	2nd	3rd	4th	5th
E	4	3	2	1	0
B	3	4	3	2	1
C	2	3	4	3	2
A	1	2	3	4	3
D	0	1	2	3	4

A229. This question is focusing on your willingness to seek help from others to benefit your patient's outcome. This is complicated in this scenario by a personal grievance you have with another member of the team. The most appropriate option is to ask Henry for advice (**answer B**). You must be able to put grievances to one side if you require help with your patients. Henry will be able to advise you on the management of DKA as he had a similar patient last week – or, at a minimum, to advise you on where to find appropriate help if he isn't confident. If in doubt, ask! The next most appropriate answer is to ask the on-call registrar (**answer E**) in accordance with the escalation ladder. The ward nurses are often very experienced in protocols and will have managed many patients requiring insulin therapy, so asking for their advice is the next most appropriate option (**answer D**). If you are unable to seek help from your colleagues you can consult approved internet sources such as BMJ Best Practice (http://us.bestpractice.bmj.com/best-practice/welcome.html) for guidance (**answer A**). However, this should be used with caution owing to the risk of error online. Finally, the least appropriate option is to prescribe a regimen of which you are unsure (**answer C**); it is dangerous and may put patients at risk.

Ideal order	Your rank choice				
	1st	2nd	3rd	4th	5th
B	4	3	2	1	0
E	3	4	3	2	1
D	2	3	4	3	2
A	1	2	3	4	3
C	0	1	2	3	4

A230. This question is based on willingness to offer advice. Willingness to seek advice goes hand in hand with willingness to offer advice. In this scenario, you are confident that you are able to advise Mitch appropriately and benefit the patient's outcome. Although you may be an FY1 you should feel confident that you are a valued member of the team and can offer advice when necessary. The most appropriate option is therefore **answer E**, followed by **answer B**. It is very unlikely that an SHO will have any objection to taking advice from an FY1, but on the rare occasion that this may be a problem explaining the reason behind your advice is likely to lessen any problem. That is why answer E is ranked higher than answer B. The next most appropriate option would be to suggest the SHO calls pharmacy (**answer A**) as the pharmacy staff will be fully aware of the antibiotic prescribing guideline and be able to recommend as required. Waiting until the SHOs have stopped their discussion (**answer C**) is the next most appropriate option. It still indicates you are willing to offer advice but not necessarily at the right time. Finally, the least appropriate option would be to say nothing (**answer D**). You should feel confident to offer a suggestion to any colleague, regardless of their grade. Your willingness to offer help should be equally met by their willingness to seek help.

Ideal order	Your rank choice				
	1st	2nd	3rd	4th	5th
E	4	3	2	1	0
B	3	4	3	2	1
A	2	3	4	3	2
C	1	2	3	4	3
D	0	1	2	3	4

A231. This question is assessing your ability to identify and utilise the most relevant individual for this situation. In this scenario, Judith has been declared medically fit for discharge but she is worried that she will not be able to cope socially. The most appropriate option is **answer B**. A patient's ability to cope at home is best assessed by OT and they will be able to recommend any social care needed before the patient is discharged. However, this assessment can sometimes be shared with physiotherapy and so the next most appropriate option would be **answer A.** Social services are also involved in arranging care at home. However, they are unable to instigate a care package without recommendation from OT or physiotherapy. Therefore **answer E** would be the third most appropriate option. If you are unable to refer to OT or physiotherapy then it would be wise to discuss Judith's concerns with your registrar. They have more experience with patient care and may be able to carry out a very basic assessment if the patient has no social needs (**answer C**). Finally, the least appropriate option would be to delay Judith's discharge (**answer D**). If she is not coping at home then delaying her discharge will not help – she requires a package of care.

Ideal order	Your rank choice				
	1st	2nd	3rd	4th	5th
B	4	3	2	1	0
A	3	4	3	2	1
E	2	3	4	3	2
C	1	2	3	4	3
D	0	1	2	3	4

A232. This question is based on the importance of valuing people's opinions and listening to their concerns. In this scenario, the most appropriate option is **answer C**. James is clearly irritated by this problem and, although you may or may not agree with him, it is important to try to listen to his concerns. However, nurses do spend more time with patients and routinely notice complications. You should listen to their concerns seriously and value their input; hence the next most appropriate option is **answer B**. You are not agreeing or disagreeing with James, but equally you are not exploring his complaint. In this specific scenario, the nurse's comment is more probably work banter than anything else. However, telling James this (**answer A**) may frustrate him further as he'll feel dismissed and not listened to. The final two options are both inappropriate. They show no respect for the nurses' opinions and that attitude will be detrimental to patient care. **Answer D** is marginally more appropriate than answer E. Although it is clearly short-sighted to expect nurses not to make suggestions, D does not show open disregard for nursing staff; therefore **answer E** is the least appropriate.

Ideal order	Your rank choice				
	1st	2nd	3rd	4th	5th
C	4	3	2	1	0
B	3	4	3	2	1
A	2	3	4	3	2
D	1	2	3	4	3
E	0	1	2	3	4

A233. This question is based on identifying others when they are struggling. You and Sarah are both tired and have been working for several hours without a break. It would be unwise to continue in this manner; either you will feel unwell, or a patient will be put at risk. However, Sarah is struggling more with the demands of this on-call shift. Therefore, the most appropriate option would be to suggest she takes a short break and has a rest before she makes a mistake (**answer C**). The next most appropriate option is to offer to help Sarah (**answer A**). You are busy with your own workload, but if a colleague is struggling you should attempt to help. You will appreciate the favour returned if you are having an off day. At this point, it would be wise to inform the registrar that you and Sarah have not had a break (**answer B**). On a busy on-call shift unwell patients do need to be seen urgently, but at least the registrar is aware and can attempt to plan a break when appropriate. Working together (**answer D**) is not a realistic approach to take, as this will probably result in fewer patients being seen. However, it is more appropriate than confronting your registrar (**answer E**), which is the least appropriate option. The shift is busy and unpleasant, but turning on each other is never beneficial.

Ideal order	Your rank choice				
	1st	2nd	3rd	4th	5th
C	4	3	2	1	0
A	3	4	3	2	1
B	2	3	4	3	2
D	1	2	3	4	3
E	0	1	2	3	4

A234. This question is based on maintaining harmony amongst a busy team. In this scenario, you are finding yourself frustrated at the lack of information sharing. The chances are that if you are annoyed then others will be too. In these situations the best action is to try to alleviate the cause of the frustration, allowing the team to work better together. The most appropriate option is to raise your concerns with your team (**answer A**). This will allow you all to vent your frustrations and come up with ideas. The next most appropriate action is to create a formal handover to improve information exchange (**answer C**). The third most appropriate option would be **answer D**; this may help reduce your frustration but is unsustainable as it will depend on your presence at handover. A formal handover protocol would be a better system. You should always feel comfortable to approach your educational supervisor to discuss any concerns that you have (**answer B**); however, in this scenario you should discuss these within your team first. The least appropriate option is to ask the nurses for a medical handover each morning (**answer E**); the nurses will be busy with their daily tasks and may have only met the patient that morning (due to their shift pattern).

Ideal order	Your rank choice				
	1st	2nd	3rd	4th	5th
A	4	3	2	1	0
C	3	4	3	2	1
D	2	3	4	3	2
B	1	2	3	4	3
E	0	1	2	3	4

A235. This question is assessing your understanding of a colleague's role in the MDT, in this case that of an occupational therapist. Mrs Jones has been declared medically fit for discharge, but James's assessment has suggested she is not safe to be mobilising at home. You should assess this new development with James to confirm what impact it will have on her discharge (**answer A**). Social services may be able to start a package of care this afternoon thus allowing Mrs Bloomsbury still to be discharged. It would be advisable to re-assess Mrs Bloomsbury, as there has been a change in her condition since you saw her this morning (**answer G**). Her 'wobbly' legs may be the result of hypotension or hypoglycaemia. Finally, any potential change to a patient's management plan must be discussed with your consultant, as they are ultimately responsible for that patient's care (**answer C**).

Asking the on-call SHO (**answer D**) or staff nurse (**answer E**) to assess Mrs Bloomsbury is not necessary. You should be assessing her for any change, as she is your patient. Acknowledging James's concerns but discharging Mrs Bloomsbury anyway is not appropriate (**answer B** and **answer F**). A patient's discharge relies on a multidisciplinary approach and each element of their care is equally important. Although she may be medically fit for discharge, if she is not safe to be at home she should not be discharged. Asking James to re-assess Mrs Bloomsbury in the afternoon (**answer H**) is not completely unreasonable. There may have been a simple reason for her earlier 'wobble' that has since resolved. However, it is not one of the three most appropriate options as it does not address the immediate issue. Doing nothing, or waiting and watching, is rarely the correct approach to SJT.

A	B	C	D	E	F	G	H
4	0	4	0	0	0	4	0

A236. This question is based on appreciating that allied healthcare colleagues (e.g. occupational therapy, physiotherapy, speech and language, dietitian) have a salient role in the safe management of patients. Importantly, the doctor (i.e. medical registrar in this situation) is not the best-trained person to make an assessment of a patient's mobility. Your concern in this scenario should be the need for occupational therapy (i.e. fall history) being overlooked by the medical registrar. Therefore you should inform OT/PT about Mr Isaac (**answer D**). They will be able to perform their own assessment. You should also liaise with the nursing staff to ensure that Mr Isaac is appropriately supervised whilst on the ward (**answer B**). Finally, you should always document any referral or addition to a patient's management plan (**answer G**).

It is not appropriate to ignore what you have read (**answer A**) or to rely on Mr Isaac to ask for assistance (**answer C**) as this will leave him at risk of falling. Asking the ward nurses whether they have any concerns is always a good idea, as they will have a reasonable idea about a patient's mobility. However, nurses are not the appropriate members of the team to conduct this assessment (**answer E**). OT will not be able to assess a patient's safe mobilising without seeing them in person (**answer H**); therefore this is not a correct answer. Finally, telling Mr Isaac to stay in bed until he is assessed is unfair and will make him more likely to develop pressure sore areas (**answer F**). There are many different levels of safety; Mr Isaac may be safe to sit in his chair once he is helped to it.

A	B	C	D	E	F	G	H
0	4	0	4	0	0	4	0

A237. This question is focusing on your awareness of your own role within a team and, as a general rule of thumb, FY1s do not deliver bad news. They should be actively involved in the discussion around delivering bad news and, if practical, observe the senior doctor's interaction with the patient and relatives. In this scenario, it would be advisable to tell your registrar that you do not think it is appropriate for you to discuss Mrs Daley's poor prognosis with her daughter alone. However, it is important to learn and so you should ask to be involved (**answer F**). Offering to assist with the registrar's tasks would enable more time for the registrar to talk with Mrs Daley's daughter (**answer A**). In the meantime, you should ask

Mrs Daley's daughter to wait in the relatives' room, as this news should be discussed somewhere quiet and private (**answer H**).

In this situation it would be inappropriate for you to discuss Mrs Daley's poor prognosis yourself (**answer D** and **answer E**). These conversations are very upsetting and best managed by experienced members of the team. It is important to explain that you are uncomfortable with the request made by the registrar, and why, but you should always demonstrate your eagerness to learn. Therefore, although **answer B** and **answer C** are appropriate actions to take, they are poorer versions of F, and therefore incorrect. Finally, declining a request made by your registrar with no justification is simply impertinent (**answer G**).

A	B	C	D	E	F	G	H
4	0	0	0	0	4	0	4

A238. This question is based on establishing relationships and building rapport when joining a new team. You will often find yourself amongst a new team during your training and it is beneficial to learn to establish relationships quickly. In this scenario, you can easily start with simple improvements, such as learning your colleagues' names (**answer C**). It would be a good idea to arrange a daily meeting each morning (**answer B**). This is common practice in high-state roles (such as operating theatres and on-call shifts) and would provide an opportunity to get to know the team. Finally, organising a social event is an appropriate way of building rapport amongst new colleagues (**answer A**). This gives everybody the chance to talk to each other in a relaxing environment without the stresses of their workload interfering.

The other options in this question are not 'wrong' but they are less ideal than answers A, B and C. Creating a social media page (**answer D**) will exclude any colleagues who do not have a social media account. A staff picture is a good idea but would rely on members of the team spending time looking at the picture board – which is unlikely on a busy ward (**answer E**). Arranging to meet with your FY1 colleagues for lunch (**answer F**) would be an appropriate method for getting to know the other FY1s on the team but would not solve the problem with senior colleagues and other members of the MDT. Trying to work quickly so that you can leave as soon as possible (**answer G**) is an approach that is not recommended. You will need your colleagues for more than just social interaction and building a good rapport will make it easier to achieve your tasks. It is important to try to develop professional relationships whilst working – even if it is just for a rotation. Finally, if you find that you are not able to build a working relationship then discussing it with your educational supervisor is a good idea (**answer H**). However, it is worth attempting to resolve this issue yourself in the first instance.

A	B	C	D	E	F	G	H
4	4	4	0	0	0	0	0

A239. This question is assessing your ability to provide non-task-related support to Alex in a stressful, difficult situation. The most important support you can provide in these situations is listening (**answer H**). Alex is clearly not in the right frame of mind to be on the ward round this morning, so it would be wise to suggest he takes a break (**answer F**). It would also be advisable for Alex to speak with his clinical supervisor sooner rather than later as there will be due process in an unexpected death (**answer G**).

In this situation it is important not to disregard Alex's concerns with non-empathetic platitudes such as false reassurances (**answer A** and **answer D**), nonchalant dismissal (**answer C**) or insensitive probing (**answer B**). Once Alex has been through the appropriate process following a patient death, it may be deemed that additional education is required. However, now is not the time as Alex would be unlikely to appreciate your 'teaching' (**answer E**).

A	B	C	D	E	F	G	H
0	0	0	0	0	4	4	4

A240. This question is based on your willingness to offer Jasmine assistance with her workload. Although it is important to ensure that you are available to carry out your assigned role (i.e. A&E clerking), it is usual to offer to help your colleagues when the workload is so disproportionate. However, if you are going to leave your work area it is important your registrar is aware of this (**answer F**). The most appropriate way of helping Jasmine is to offer to assess one of the ill patients, as they are likely to require time (**answer H**). You can also provide Jasmine with your bleep so that she can ask the ward nurses to contact you for a short period to relieve her of new jobs (**answer D**). This will allow her to complete some of her immediate tasks.

It is important to show willingness to support your colleagues, as some will not feel comfortable asking for help; therefore **answer B** and **answer C** are not appropriate. Do not wait to be asked for help if you know a colleague would benefit from your assistance. Offering to buy Jasmine a coffee is very kind, but with three ill patients she is unable to take a break (**answer G**). In a stressful, busy situation any empathy may be well received, but it will not alter the situation (**answer E**). Finally, **answer A** is completely inappropriate as it is not true.

A	B	C	D	E	F	G	H
0	0	0	4	0	4	0	4

A241. This question is assessing your willingness to offer assistance to your colleagues, in this case Dan, the medical student. In this scenario, it is clear that Dan is struggling to carry out his venepuncture and is looking for help. The ward nurses are unable to help and you know that your SHO is likely to be delayed in the bereavement office. This is something that you are able to help with and Dan would appreciate your time to develop his skills. Therefore it would be appropriate to help Dan with this procedure (**answer B**). Another approach you could take would be to give Dan some advice, but with the caveat that he can find you if he is still unable to take blood (**answer C**). This allows Dan to attempt to take blood and develop confidence, but still considers the safety of the patient, as the blood test will not be delayed. Finally, Dan will be approaching his final examinations and so teaching him about blood results will be well received (**answer E**).

Although you have not been asked directly by Dan for help, you are aware that he would appreciate assistance. It is not acceptable to ignore this (**answer F**). Nor is it advisable for Dan to keep trying without any adjustment (**answer H**). This is his final year of medical school and he should be encouraged to seek help now whilst he does have an FY1 to assist him in gaining confidence. There is no reason to believe that the blood test can be delayed (**answer G**) or cancelled (**answer D**) and so those approaches are not appropriate. Finally, as the ward nurses have already told Dan they are unable to help, it is very unlikely they would suddenly be able to help when you ask (**answer A**). Remember, doing nothing (or an action that results in no change) is usually a poor choice in the SJT.

A	B	C	D	E	F	G	H
0	4	4	0	4	0	0	0

A242. This question is based on your ability to make your clinical team aware of your academic workload, and vice versa. In these situations the best approach is to be completely open and honest. Meeting with your academic supervisor (**answer D**) and your clinical supervisor (**answer G**) will give you an opportunity to discuss your heavy workload and how best to manage your commitments. However, ultimately you have taken a clinical post as a Foundation Programme trainee and your priority must be to your clinical workload. Therefore postponing your project until you start your academic rotation is appropriate (**answer B**).

As mentioned, your post is predominantly clinical and you have allocated time to work on your academic project; therefore allowing it to affect your clinical work is inappropriate. Simply telling your clinical supervisor you will try harder but caveating this is not professional (**answer A**). Asking your clinical supervisor for dispensation is not appropriate (**answer C**); it puts unfair demands on the remainder of the team. Nor is it fair to expect another FY1 to increase their workload to allow you time away from clinical work (**answer E**). You are clearly not balancing your workload and so continuing with this is not an option (**answer H**). Finally, ignoring your last clinical meeting is not advisable (**answer F**). Although your ambition may be academic medicine, you still need to complete your annual review of clinical progression (ARCP) and negative comments from your clinical team may jeopardise this.

A	B	C	D	E	F	G	H
0	4	0	4	0	0	4	0

A243. This question is focusing on your willingness to consult with others to seek advice. In this scenario, you are unsure of how to proceed with a patient and do not have an immediate senior to turn to. As per the escalation ladder in Chapter 3 'Top tips', your first point of call should be your team, in order of seniority, followed by the on-call team. Unfortunately, your team is not available and so the first point of escalation is the on-call team (**answer H**). You should attempt to update Dr Andrews, as Mr Patel is his patient (**answer F**). It is also important to remember that, although Mr Patel may not be well, once you have sought advice you should continue to see the other patients on the ward (**answer D**).

It is not appropriate to adopt the 'wait and watch' approach when you have an unwell patient, as this may put them at unnecessary risk (**answer A** and **answer B**). Nor is it appropriate to activate the cardiac arrest team (**answer C**). Mr Patel may be unwell, but there is no indication he is in approaching cardiac arrest. Sending Mr Patel for an urgent MRI is not appropriate (**answer E**). It is clear in the question that you are unsure how to proceed and your aim should be to seek advice appropriately, not to blindly investigate. Finally, asking a senior nurse what they think you should do is often a wise decision, but would not be ranked in the top three in this question (**answer G**). Remember the escalation ladder: the on-call team should be contacted before nursing staff.

A	B	C	D	E	F	G	H
0	0	0	4	0	4	0	4

A244. This question is assessing your ability to take direction from others, in this case the on-call registrar. You should always be willing to take direction from your colleagues as you are in foundation training to develop your clinical acumen. The on-call registrar is experienced and has a different opinion to you. This should not discourage you from attempting to form clinical diagnoses because this is a crucial skill you are developing. However, the registrar's opinion does take priority in this scenario and you should alter your plan as per their recommendation (**answer E**). It is also important to document your discussion in the patient's notes (**answer B**). It would be wise to revise IBS, as you didn't make the most appropriate interpretation of the history and examination (**answer D**).

In this situation it would be unreasonable to escalate this to the consultant. The registrar has made a sensible suggestion and you should be willing to take this on board (**answer A**). It is also inappropriate to disregard the advice of the registrar (**answer C**). They have experience that you should learn from, and technically the patient is not 'yours' but is actually the responsibility of the on-call consultant. Asking Mr Franklin to return tomorrow is absolutely unacceptable (**answer F**); it is a waste of resources and exposing a patient to unnecessary radiation should be avoided. You should also avoid discussing your difference in opinion with the patient as this risks damaging their trust in your hospital and the care it provides (**answer H**). Finally, documenting your disagreement with the registrar in a manner such as **answer G** is not appropriate. Your registrar has reviewed your plan and made an alteration – you should be willing to accept this and learn from their advice.

A	B	C	D	E	F	G	H
0	4	0	4	4	0	0	0

A245. This question is based on your ability to adapt within your role. In this instance you are required to become the leader and salvage this teaching session. A sensible approach to this problem would be to delay the medical students (**answer B**) and try to call the SHOs to clarify whether they are simply running late or are now unable to attend (**answer A**). You should then be willing to run the teaching session as best you can (**answer D**), as otherwise you and the medical students will have wasted your time. Being able to adapt in adverse conditions is a vital skill to succeed in your Foundation Programme.

In these types of scenarios you are ultimately making the best of a bad situation, and you should be honest with the students. However, they will understand that the session may be less smooth than planned. Generally, advising certain students to stay and others to leave is not a good idea (**answer C**); it will seem unfair and will be very hard to arrange. Sending a text message to the SHOs is also a poor choice (**answer E**). You may not receive an immediate response (unlike a phone call) and the session will be delayed indefinitely while you wait. Remember: watching and waiting is rarely correct in the SJT. **Answer G** is not correct for that same reason. Although waiting for the SHOs is an option, it would be far better for you to take on the role of session leader. Your last resort should be cancelling the session (**answer F** and **answer H**).

A	B	C	D	E	F	G	H
4	4	0	4	0	0	0	0

A246. This question is based on accepting different perspectives; in this case religion. Although you may not follow religious practice, you should be willing to accept that somebody else may and attempt to support them where necessary. As you have yet to submit your holiday request, the kindest action to take would be to swap with Miriam so that she can celebrate her religious festival (**answer C**). However, it would be a good idea to arrange your swap at the same time so that there isn't any future problem (**answer G**). Finally, building rapport and developing relationships is also important during your foundation training and so you should show interest in Miriam's religion by asking her about the celebration (**answer B**).

Surviving your foundation training will involve negotiations and shift swaps, not only for others but also for you. As you did not have any leave set in contract, it is generally a good idea to try to accommodate, as you may need a similar favour in the future. Therefore denying Miriam's request is not a good option (**answer A**). Furthermore, it is not appropriate to express an opinion about Miriam's religious belief (**answer E** and **answer H**). Suggesting that Miriam ask another FY1 is an appropriate response but will not earn you any favours and in this scenario isn't in the top three choices (**answer D**). Finally, **answer F** is confrontational and not relevant to her request.

A	B	C	D	E	F	G	H
0	4	4	0	0	0	4	0

A247. This question is focusing on your ability to recognise that your colleague, Charles, is struggling to deal with the emotive nature of Mrs Lerbort's presentation. It is not uncommon to come across a situation that reminds you of an upsetting personal experience. In this scenario, Mrs Lerbort is reminding Charles of his mother's recent death. The most appropriate action is to ensure that Charles has support in this difficult time, but that he also realises he may not be fit to work so close to his mother's death (**answer A**). You should also advise Charles to arrange a meeting with his educational supervisor (**answer C**). Their role is to provide support and continuity throughout your foundation training. Finally, it would be wise to discuss your concerns sensitively with your consultant, as they are responsible for their team (**answer B**).

In these situations it is not helpful to tell somebody to 'snap out of it' (**answer D**); everybody will be affected differently by patients with whom they interact and you should be supportive towards your colleagues. It is not appropriate for you to suggest that Charles be sent home (**answer E**) or moved to another ward (**answer G**); there is a structured protocol to ensure that employees are adequately supported and your consultant will ensure that this is followed correctly. Offering to take Charles to the pub is not an inappropriate response (**answer H**), as this will give him an opportunity to discuss this situation with you in a relaxed format. However, it does not alter the situation at the present time. Finally, it is not acceptable to report Charles to the GMC for a fitness to practice hearing as there is no evidence that Charles has been negligent (**answer F**).

A	B	C	D	E	F	G	H
4	4	4	0	0	0	0	0

A248. This question is based on appreciating the roles within your team. In this scenario, a member of your team is not happy with a decision that has been made. In the first instance it is advisable to explore the concerns of the individual involved – that is, the SHO (**answer E**). You can discuss the advantages and disadvantages of nurse consultants/practitioners/specialists (**answer A**) as the SHO may not have worked with them previously. Finally, suggesting the SHO spends some time with the nurse consultants would enable them to appreciate their purpose and understand their role with difficult patients (**answer G**).

Admonishing the SHO for their views is unlikely to improve this situation and will create further friction within the team (**answer B**). Nor would it be appropriate for the SHO to share their views with the nurse consultants (**answer D**) or complain to the consultant (**answer C**). The SHO's views are not appropriate as the nurse consultants are more than experienced to see these types of patients. In fact, as they can spend more time with the patient than the SHO could, complicated patients like Henry really benefit from seeing a nurse consultant. Ignoring the SHO may make you feel better, but it would not attempt to solve the problem and is not the correct approach to teamwork (**answer H**). Finally, the consultant has not asked you to review Henry and you will simply be doubling your team's workload if you review every patient seen by a nurse specialist (**answer F**).

A	B	C	D	E	F	G	H
4	0	0	0	4	0	4	0

A249. This question is assessing your ability to delegate and share tasks effectively, in this case using Alex appropriately as a member of the team to complete the tasks required. A final-year medical student should be seen as an asset and not a nuisance. It is likely that Alex will be competent with simple skills such as venepuncture, drafting discharge summaries and summarising admission notes. Delegate these tasks to him and involve him in the team as much as possible (**answer A** and **answer G**). Of course, you need to ensure that Alex is comfortable with what you ask him to do and that he knows he can ask you for help if he needs to. However, when delegating tasks do not forget to involve the ward nurses where practical (**answer C**).

In these situations it can seem burdensome to have to supervise medical students, but you should see them as junior members of the team and work with them to achieve your goal. Avoid sending your medical students off the ward when you are busy (**answer E**) – they are there to learn. It is not acceptable to leave jobs until the next day (**answer D**). You may be busy tomorrow as well and the jobs from yesterday will not be done. Nor is it advisable to delay patient discharges (**answer H**), as a hospital would grind to a halt if all teams stopped discharging patients when it became busy. **Answer F** will not change the actual amount of work you have; appropriate delegation and teamwork are the keys to success. Finally, you have already been told that the consultant needs the other members of the team, so calling the consultant will not alter the situation (**answer B**); this is deemed to be on the same par as not acting.

A	B	C	D	E	F	G	H
4	0	4	0	0	0	4	0

A250. This question is assessing your ability to identify the most appropriate person within your team for a given task, in this case completing a DNAR status. This is very challenging because, on the one hand, you do not know the patient's wishes, those of his family or those of his consultant. However, on the other hand, without a DNAR form the nursing staff are obliged to start resuscitation. In this situation, the on-call registrar is the most appropriate member of the team to sign the DNAR form, and not the FY1 (**answer B**). You should also call the NOK and inform them that he is likely to pass away shortly as they may wish to be present (**answer D**). Finally, ensuring that the ward clerk orders DNAR forms may prevent a similar situation happening again (**answer C**).

Answer A is not an appropriate choice as this is not a decision that should be made by an FY1. Escalating care is not appropriate (**answer F**); although the patient's notes may not make his resuscitation status clear, it is certainly noted that he is 'not for escalation'. Calling his consultant would not solve the problem of having the form signed (**answer E**); you would still require the registrar to sign the DNAR form and so discussing the situation with them first is more appropriate. (**Note**: this is a rare caveat to the escalation ladder because you are not escalating a concern but instead seeking an appropriate person to complete a task.) The on-call SHO is in a similar position to you and would be equally unprepared to sign the DNAR form (**answer H**). Finally, refusing to sign the DNAR form without offering to sort out the problem is not in the patient's best interest (**answer G**). The most important issue is that Mr Peters has a peaceful and non-traumatic death, which is not achieved with 'last ditch' CPR attempts.

A	B	C	D	E	F	G	H
0	4	4	4	0	0	0	0

Recommended reading

Department of Health. (2008). *A High Quality Workforce: NHS next stage review*. London, UK: Department of Health. Online. Available: http://webarchive.nationalarchives.gov.uk/ 20130107105354/http://www.dh.gov.uk/prod_consum_dh/groups/dh_digitalassets/@dh/ @en/documents/digitalasset/dh_085841.pdf (accessed 30 April 2015).

Donaldson, Sir L. (2002). *Unfinished Business: Proposals for reform of the Senior House Officer grade*. London, UK: Department of Health. Online. Available: http://webarchive. nationalarchives.gov.uk/20130107105354/http://www.dh.gov.uk/prod_consum_dh/groups/ dh_digitalassets/@dh/@en/documents/digitalasset/dh_4018808.pdf (accessed 30 April 2015).

Driver and Vehicle Licencing Agency (DVLA). (2013). *At a Glance Guide to the Current Medical Standards of Fitness to Drive*. Swansea, UK: DVLA. Online. Available: https://www.gov.uk/ government/publications/at-a-glance (accessed 1 May 2015).

General Medical Council (GMC). (n.d.). *GMC Policy on Whistleblowing*. London, UK: GMC. Online. Available: http://www.gmc-uk.org/DC5900_Whistleblowing_guidance___for_ publication.pdf_57107304.pdf (accessed 1 May 2015).

General Medical Council (GMC). (2008). Consent: patients and doctors making decisions together. Read the explanatory guidance. In *Good Medical Practice*. London, UK: GMC. Online. Available: http://www.gmc-uk.org/guidance/ethical_guidance/consent_guidance_ index.asp (accessed 1 May 2015).

General Medical Council (GMC). (2009a). *Tomorrow's Doctors*. London, UK: GMC. Online. Available: http://www.gmc-uk.org/education/undergraduate/tomorrows_doctors.asp (accessed 1 May 2015).

General Medical Council (GMC). (2009b). *Confidentiality*. London, UK: GMC. Online. Available: http://www.gmc-uk.org/guidance/ethical_guidance/confidentiality.asp (accessed 1 May 2015).

General Medical Council (GMC). (2009c). *Confidentiality: Reporting concerns about patients to the DVLA or the DVA*. London, UK: GMC. Online. Available: http://www.gmc-uk.org/ Confidentiality_reporting_concerns.pdf_55976735.pdf (accessed 1 May 2015).

General Medical Council (GMC). (2012). Raising and acting on concerns about patient safety. Read the explanatory guidance. In *Good Medical Practice*. London, UK: GMC. Online Available: http://www.gmc-uk.org/guidance/ethical_guidance/raising_concerns.asp (accessed 1 May 2015).

General Medical Council (GMC). (2013a). *Good Medical Practice*. London, UK: GMC. Online. Available: http://www.gmc-uk.org/guidance/good_medical_practice.asp (accessed 1 May 2015).

General Medical Council (GMC). (2013b). Honesty in financial dealings. Paragraph 77. In *Good Medical Practice*. London, UK: GMC. Online. Available: http://www.gmc-uk.org/guidance/ good_medical_practice/20466.asp (accessed 1 May 2015).

General Medical Council (GMC). (2013c). Gifts, bequests and donations. Paragraphs 6–7. In *Good Medical Practice*. London, UK: GMC. Online. Available: http://www.gmc-uk.org/guidance/ethical_guidance/21161.asp (accessed 1 May 2015).

General Medical Council (GMC). (2013d). The meaning of fitness to practise. Paragraphs 1–7. In *Good Medical Practice: Learning materials*. London, UK: GMC. Online. Available: http://www.gmc-uk.org/guidance/21721.asp (accessed 1 May 2015).

General Medical Council (GMC). (2013e). Respond to risks to safety. Paragraphs 24–5. In *Good Medical Practice: Learning materials*. London, UK: GMC. Online. Available: http://www.gmc-uk.org/guidance/good_medical_practice/respond_to_risks.asp (accessed 1 May 2015).

General Medical Council (GMC). (2013f). Social media. Explanatory guidance paragraph 5. In *Good Medical Practice: Doctors' use of social media*. London, UK: GMC. Online. Available: http://www.gmc-uk.org/guidance/ethical_guidance/21186 (accessed 1 May 2015).

General Medical Council (GMC). (2013g). Maintaining boundaries. Explanatory guidance paragraph 11. In *Good Medical Practice*. London, UK: GMC. Online. Available: http://www.gmc-uk.org/guidance/ethical_guidance/21186 (accessed 1 May 2015).

General Medical Council (GMC). (2013h). The benefits and risks of using social media. Explanatory guidance paragraph 9c. In *Good Medical Practice: Doctors' use of social media*. London, UK: GMC. Online. Available: http://www.gmc-uk.org/guidance/ethical_guidance/21186.asp (accessed 1 May 2015).

Humphreys, R. A., Lepper, R., & Nicholson, T. R. J. (2014). When and how to treat patients who refuse treatment. *BMJ, 348*, 33–37.

Kruger, J., Wirtz, D., & Miller, D. T. (2005). Counterfactual thinking and the first instinct fallacy. *J Pers Soc Psychol, 99*, 725–735.

Lievens, F., & Sackett, P. R. (2007). Situational judgement tests in high-stakes settings: Issues and strategies with generating alternate forms. *J App Psych, 92*, 1043–1055.

McDaniel, M. A., Morgeson, F. P., Finnegan, E. B., et al. (2001). Use of situational judgment tests to predict job performance: A clarification of the literature. *J App Psych, 86*, 730–740.

Mid Staffordshire NHS Foundation Trust. (2013). *Public Enquiry (chaired by Robert Francis QC). Final Report*. Online. Available: http://www.midstaffspublicinquiry.com/report (accessed 1 May 2015).

Paice, E., Rutter, H., Wetherell, M., et al. (2002). Stressful incidents, stress and coping strategies in the pre-registration house officer year. *Med Educ, 36*, 56–65.

Patterson F, Archer V, Kerrin M, et al. (2010). *FY1 Job Analysis Report: Improving selection to the Foundation Programme final report*, pp 149–58. Online. Available: http://www.isfp.org.uk/AboutISFP/Documents/Appendix_D_-_FY1_Job_Analysis.pdf (accessed 1 May 2015).

Patterson, F., Ashworth, V., & Good, D. (2013). *Situational Judgement Tests: A guide for applicants to the UK Foundation Programme*. London, UK: Medical Schools Council. Online. Available: Situational_Judgement_Tests_Monograph_FINAL_August_2013-1-3.pdf (accessed 1 May 2015).

UK Foundation Programme Office (UKFPO). (2015). *FP 2015 Eligibility Information*. In Online. Available: www.foundationprogramme.nhs.uk/pages/home/how-to-apply/FP2015-Eligibility-Information (accessed 1 May 2015).

Weekley, J. A., & Ployhart, R. E. (2005). Situational judgment: Antecedents and relationships with performance. *Hum Perform, 18*, 81–104.

Acts of Parliament

Act, Mental Capacity. (2005). *Norwich.* UK: The Stationery Office. Online. Available: http://www.legislation.gov.uk/ukpga/2005/9/contents (accessed 1 May 2015).

Act, Mental Health. (1983). *Norwich.* UK: The Stationery Office. Online. Available: http://www.legislation.gov.uk/ukpga/1983/20/contents (accessed 1 May 2015).

Act, Mental Health. (2007). *Norwich.* UK: The Stationery Office. Online. Available: http://www.legislation.gov.uk/ukpga/2007/12/contents (accessed 1 May 2015).

Index

Note: Page numbers followed by *b* indicate boxes, *f* indicate figures and *t* indicate tables.